1994
YEAR BOOK OF
CHIROPRACTIC

Statement of Purpose

The YEAR BOOK Service

The YEAR BOOK series was devised in 1901 by practicing health professionals who observed that the literature of medicine and related disciplines had become so voluminous that no one individual could read and place in perspective every potential advance in a major specialty. In the final decade of the 20th century, this recognition is more acutely true than it was in 1901.

More than merely a series of books, YEAR BOOK volumes are the tangible results of a unique service designed to accomplish the following:

- to *survey* a wide range of journals of proven value
- to *select* from those journals papers representing significant advances and statements of important clinical principles
- to provide *abstracts* of those articles that are readable, convenient summaries of their key points
- to provide *commentary* about those articles to place them in perspective.

These publications grow out of a unique process that calls on the talents of outstanding authorities in clinical and fundamental disciplines, trained literature specialists, and professional writers, all supported by the resources of Mosby, the world's preeminent publisher for the health professions.

The Literature Base

Mosby subscribes to nearly 1,000 journals published worldwide, covering the full range of the health professions. On an annual basis, the publisher examines usage patterns and polls its expert authorities to add new journals to the literature base and to delete journals that are no longer useful as potential YEAR BOOK sources.

The Literature Survey

The publisher's team of literature specialists, all of whom are trained and experienced health professionals, examines every original, peer-reviewed article in each journal issue. More than 250,000 articles per year are scanned systematically, including title, text, illustrations, tables, and references. Each scan is compared, article by article, to the search strategies that the publisher has developed in consultation with the 270 outside experts who form the pool of YEAR BOOK editors. A given article may be reviewed by any number of editors, from one to a dozen or more, regardless of the discipline for which the paper was originally published. In turn, each editor who receives the article reviews it to determine whether or not the article should be included in the YEAR BOOK. This decision is based on the article's inherent quality, its probable usefulness to readers of that YEAR BOOK, and the editor's goal to represent a balanced picture of a given field in each volume of the YEAR BOOK. In addition, the editor indicates when to include figures and tables from the article to help the YEAR BOOK reader better understand the information.

Of the quarter million articles scanned each year, only 5% are selected for detailed analysis within the YEAR BOOK series, thereby assuring readers of the high value of every selection.

The Abstract

The publisher's abstracting staff is headed by a physician-writer and includes individuals with training in the life sciences, medicine, and other areas, plus extensive experience in writing for the health professions and related industries. Each selected article is assigned to a specific writer on this abstracting staff. The abstracter, guided in many cases by notations supplied by the expert editor, writes a structured, condensed summary designed so that the reader can rapidly acquire the essential information contained in the article.

The Commentary

The YEAR BOOK editorial boards, sometimes assisted by guest commentators, write comments that place each article in perspective for the reader. This provides the reader with the equivalent of a personal consultation with a leading international authority—an opportunity to better understand the value of the article and to benefit from the authority's thought processes in assessing the article.

Additional Editorial Features

The editorial boards of each YEAR BOOK organize the abstracts and comments to provide a logical and satisfying sequence of information. To enhance the organization, editors also provide introductions to sections or individual chapters, comments linking a number of abstracts, citations to additional literature, and other features.

The published YEAR BOOK contains enhanced bibliographic citations for each selected article, including extended listings of multiple authors and identification of author affiliations. Each YEAR BOOK contains a Table of Contents specific to that year's volume. From year to year, the Table of Contents for a given YEAR BOOK will vary depending on developments within the field.

Every YEAR BOOK contains a list of the journals from which papers have been selected. This list represents a subset of the nearly 1,000 journals surveyed by the publisher and occasionally reflects a particularly pertinent article from a journal that is not surveyed on a routine basis.

Finally, each volume contains a comprehensive subject index and an index to authors of each selected paper.

The 1994 Year Book Series

Year Book of Allergy and Clinical Immunology: Drs. Rosenwasser, Borish, Gelfand, Leung, Nelson, and Szefler

Year Book of Anesthesia and Pain Management: Drs. Tinker, Abram, Kirby, Ostheimer, Roizen, and Stoelting

Year Book of Cardiology®: Drs. Schlant, Collins, Engle, Gersh, Kaplan, and Waldo

Year Book of Chiropractic: Dr. Lawrence

Year Book of Critical Care Medicine®: Drs. Rogers and Parrillo

Year Book of Dentistry®: Drs. Meskin, Currier, Kennedy, Leinfelder, Berry, Roser

Year Book of Dermatologic Surgery: Drs. Swanson, Glogau, and Salasche

Year Book of Dermatology®: Drs. Sober and Fitzpatrick

Year Book of Diagnostic Radiology®: Drs. Federle, Clark, Gross, Madewell, Maynard, Sackett, and Young

Year Book of Digestive Diseases®: Drs. Greenberger and Moody

Year Book of Drug Therapy®: Drs. Lasagna and Weintraub

Year Book of Emergency Medicine®: Drs. Wagner, Burdick, Davidson, McNamara, and Roberts

Year Book of Endocrinology®: Drs. Bagdade, Braverman, Poehlman, Kannan, Landsberg, Molitch, Morley, Odell, Rogol, Ryan, and Nathan

Year Book of Family Practice®: Drs. Berg, Bowman, Davidson, Dietrich, and Scherger

Year Book of Geriatrics and Gerontology®: Drs. Beck, Reuben, Burton, Small, Whitehouse, and Goldstein

Year Book of Hand Surgery®: Drs. Amadio and Hentz

Year Book of Hematology®: Drs. Spivak, Bell, Ness, Quesenberry, and Wiernik

Year Book of Infectious Diseases®: Drs. Keusch, Wolff, Barza, Bennish, Gelfand, Klempner, and Snydman

Year Book of Infertility®: Drs. Mishell, Lobo, and Sokol

Year Book of Medicine®: Drs. Rogers, Bone, Cline, O'Rourke, Greenberger, Utiger, Epstein, and Malawista

Year Book of Neonatal and Perinatal Medicine®: Drs. Klaus and Fanaroff

Year Book of Nephrology: Drs. Coe, Favus, Henderson, Kashgarian, Luke, Myers, and Curtis

Year Book of Neurology and Neurosurgery®: Drs. Bradley and Crowell

Year Book of Neuroradiology: Drs. Osborn, Eskridge, Grossman, and Harnsberger

Year Book of Nuclear Medicine®: Drs. Hoffer, Gore, Gottschalk, Rattner, Zaret, and Zubal

Year Book of Obstetrics and Gynecology®: Drs. Mishell, Kirschbaum, and Morrow

Year Book of Occupational and Environmental Medicine: Drs. Emmett, Frank, Gochfeld, and Hessl

Year Book of Oncology®: Drs. Simone, Longo, Ozols, Steele, Glatstein, and Bosl

Year Book of Ophthalmology®: Drs. Laibson, Adams, Augsburger, Benson, Cohen, Eagle, Flanagan, Nelson, Rapuano, Reinecke, Sergott, and Wilson

Year Book of Orthopedics®: Drs. Sledge, Poss, Cofield, Frymoyer, Griffin, Hansen, Johnson, Simmons, and Springfield

Year Book of Otolaryngology–Head and Neck Surgery®: Drs. Paparella and Holt

Year Book of Pain: Drs. Gebhart, Haddox, Jacox, Payne, Rudy, and Shapiro

Year Book of Pathology and Clinical Pathology®: Drs. Gardner, Bennett, Cousar, Garvin, and Worsham

Year Book of Pediatrics®: Dr. Stockman

Year Book of Plastic, Reconstructive, and Aesthetic Surgery: Drs. Miller, Cohen, McKinney, Robson, Ruberg, and Whitaker

Year Book of Podiatric Medicine and Surgery®: Dr. Kominsky

Year Book of Psychiatry and Applied Mental Health®: Drs. Talbott, Frances, Breier, Meltzer, Perry, Schowalter, and Yudofsky

Year Book of Pulmonary Disease®: Drs. Bone and Petty

Year Book of Rheumatology: Drs. Sergent, LeRoy, Meenan, Panush, and Reichlin

Year Book of Sports Medicine®: Drs. Shephard, Drinkwater, Eichner, Sutton, Torg, Col. Anderson, and Mr. George

Year Book of Surgery®: Drs. Copeland, Deitch, Eberlein, Howard, Luce, Ritchie, Seeger, Souba, and Sugarbaker

Year Book of Thoracic and Cardiovascular Surgery: Drs. Ginsberg, Lofland, and Wechsler

Year Book of Transplantation®: Drs. Ascher, Hansen, and Strom

Year Book of Ultrasound: Drs. Merritt, Babcock, Carroll, Goldstein, and Mittelstaedt

Year Book of Urology®: Drs. Gillenwater and Howards

Year Book of Vascular Surgery®: Dr. Porter

1994

The Year Book of CHIROPRACTIC

Editor

Dana J. Lawrence, D.C.

Professor, Department of Chiropractic Practice, and Director, Department of Editorial Review and Publication, National College of Chiropractic, Lombard, Illinois

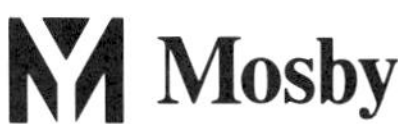

St. Louis Baltimore Boston Chicago London Madrid Philadelphia Sydney Toronto

Vice President and Publisher, Continuity Publishing: Kenneth H. Killion
Sponsoring Editor: Linda Steiner
Illustrations and Permissions Coordinator: Maureen A. Livengood
Manager, Literature Services: Edith M. Podrazik, R.N.
Senior Information Specialist: Terri Santo, R.N.
Information Specialist: Nancy Dunne, R.N.
Senior Medical Writer: David A. Cramer, M.D.
Senior Project Manager: Max F. Perez
Project Supervisor: Tamara L. Smith
Production Editor: Wendi Schnaufer
Senior Production Assistant: Sandra Rogers
Production Assistant: Rebecca Nordbrock
Proofroom Manager: Barbara M. Kelly

1993 EDITION

Printed in the United States of America
Composition by International Computaprint Corporation
Printing/binding by Maple-Vail

Mosby, Inc.
11830 Westline Industrial Drive
St. Louis, MO 63146

Editorial Office:
Mosby, Inc.
200 North LaSalle St.
Chicago, IL 60601

International Standard Serial Number: 1066-484X
International Standard Book Number: 0-8151-6733-4

Contributing Editors

Alan H. Adams, D.C., M.S., D.A.C.B.N.
Vice President for Professional Affairs, and Professor, Clinical Sciences, Los Angeles College of Chiropractic, Los Angeles, California

Jeffrey Ameen, D.C.
Clinical Associate Professor, Los Angeles College of Chiropractic, Los Angeles, California

Vaughn M. Given, D.C., B.A., B.S., M.A.
Clinical Associate Professor, Los Angeles College of Chiropractic, Los Angeles, California

Reed B. Phillips, D.C., D.A.C.B.R., Ph.D.
President, Los Angeles College of Chiropractic, Professor, Research Methodology, Los Angeles College of Chiropractic, Los Angeles, California

Nehmat G. Saab, M.A., M.L.S.
Director, Library Services, Los Angeles College of Chiropractic, Los Angeles, California

Shoreh Saljooghi, M.L.S.
Assistant Librarian, Los Angeles College of Chiropractic, Los Angeles, California

Gary Schultz, D.C., D.A.C.B.R.
Associate Professor, and Chairman, Department of Radiology, Los Angeles College of Chiropractic, Los Angeles, California

Table of Contents

Journals Represented

Mosby subscribes to and surveys nearly 1,000 U.S. and foreign medical and allied health journals. From these journals, the Editors select the articles to be abstracted. Journals represented in this YEAR BOOK are listed below.

Acta Neurologica Scandinavica
Acta Orthopaedica Scandinavica
American Family Physician
American Journal of Clinical Nutrition
American Journal of Emergency Medicine
American Journal of Health Promotion
American Journal of Obstetrics and Gynecology
American Journal of Roentgenology
American Journal of Sports Medicine
Angiology
Annals of Emergency Medicine
Annals of Internal Medicine
Annals of Nutrition and Metabolism
Annals of Rheumatic Diseases
Archives of Internal Medicine
Archives of Neurology
Archives of Physical Medicine and Rehabilitation
Arthritis and Rheumatism
Australasian Radiology
Behaviour Research and Therapy
British Journal of General Practice
British Journal of Radiology
British Medical Journal
Canadian Journal of Public Health
Canadian Medical Association Journal
Cephalalgia
Chiropractic Journal of Australia
Chiropractic Sports Medicine
Chiropractic Technique
Clinical Biomechanics
Clinical Imaging
Clinical Journal of Pain
Clinical Orthopaedics and Related Research
Clinical Science
Drug and Alcohol Dependence
Ergonomics
European Journal of Applied Physiology and Occupational Physiology
European Journal of Chiropractic
Family Practice
Gynecological Endocrinology
ICA International Review of Chiropractic
Italian Journal of Orthopaedics and Traumatology
Journal of Biomechanics
Journal of Biomedical Engineering
Journal of Bone and Joint Surgery (American Volume)
Journal of Bone and Joint Surgery (British Volume)
Journal of Chiropractic
Journal of Clinical Epidemiology
Journal of Computer Assisted Tomography
Journal of Family Practice

Journal of Gerontology
Journal of Hand Surgery (British)
Journal of Manipulative and Physiological Therapeutics
Journal of Neurosurgery
Journal of Occupational Medicine
Journal of Orthopaedic Research
Journal of Orthopaedic Trauma
Journal of Orthopaedic and Sports Physical Therapy
Journal of Pediatric Orthopedics
Journal of Pediatrics
Journal of Rheumatology
Journal of Shoulder and Elbow Surgery
Journal of the American Academy of Child Adolescent Psychiatry
Journal of the American Dietetic Association
Journal of the American Medical Association
Journal of the American Osteopathic Association
Journal of the Canadian Chiropractic Association
Journal of the National Cancer Institute
La Presse Medicale
Lancet
Life Sciences
Medical Care
Medical Journal of Australia
Medical Problems of Performing Artists
Medicine and Science in Sports and Exercise
Neurology
Neurosurgery
New England Journal of Medicine
Orthopaedic Review
Pain
Pediatrics
Physical Therapy
Physician and Sportsmedicine
Physiotherapy Canada
Postgraduate Medicine
ROFO. Fortschritte Auf Dem Gebiete Der Rontgenstrahlen Und Der Neuen Bildgebenden Verfahren
Radiology
Scandinavian Journal of Rehabilitation Medicine
Scandinavian Journal of Rheumatology
Scandinavian Journal of Work, Environment and Health
Southern Medical Journal
Spine
Sports Medicine

Standard Abbreviations

The following terms are abbreviated in this edition: acquired immunodeficiency syndrome (AIDS), the central nervous system (CNS), cerebrospinal fluid (CSF), computed tomography (CT), electrocardiography (ECG), human immunodeficiency virus (HIV), and magnetic resonance (MR) imaging (MRI).

Publisher's Preface

We are pleased to introduce the YEAR BOOK OF CHIROPRACTIC and to welcome Dana J. Lawrence, D.C., as its Editor, commencing with this 1994 edition.

Understanding the chiropractic profession and keeping current with the literature in this rapidly growing area present enormous challenges. Dr. Lawrence has reviewed an exhaustive scope of literature and chosen the most important and relevant articles to your practice. Each selection is accompanied by expert commentary and professional interpretation.

The YEAR BOOK OF CHIROPRACTIC was conceived as a means of providing insight into the best of the world's literature as it relates to the specialty. We believe Dr. Lawrence has succeeded admirably in reaching this goal. We hope this YEAR BOOK and its subsequent editions prove to be a valuable resource and a useful addition to your library.

Introduction

The amount of literature published from within the chiropractic profession has been growing exponentially over the course of the past 5 years. This information is, in many ways, changing the face of chiropractic practice. It was not so many years ago that much of this information was difficult to locate and parochial in nature; chiropractors published by themselves for themselves. Today, one can find chiropractic textbooks and journals published by some of the nation's largest and most influential medical publishing companies; a decade ago this would have been unthinkable.

Before the start of this information explosion, chiropractors found themselves in a real Catch-22. We were criticized for not publishing any science (although, of course, we did), but no reputable publisher wanted to publish our science. That left us only "in-house" publication as an avenue for documenting our science. With a rampantly developing research enterprise, we have done so admirably.

This has created its own set of problems. It is now virtually impossible to keep up with all the developments being documented in our literature. Focus groups have demonstrated that the average practitioner is too busy to devote more than one half hour per day (if that) to reading literature. However, the practitioner is obligated to know the material; it may be brought up in court, it may change how he or she practices, and it may contain information that will answer a question arising in clinical practice. Beyond the chiropractic literature, there is a wealth of biomedical and basic science literature that impacts upon the profession. It is a daunting task to stay conversant regarding this material.

This first volume of the YEAR BOOK OF CHIROPRACTIC presents an overview of the pertinent chiropractic literature of 1993. Material such as this plays several important roles in the development of standards of care; indeed, such documents as the proceedings of the Mercy Conference or other consensus panels could not occur in the absence of rigorous scientific information available for examination. It shows what our areas of interest and expertise are. It shows how rigorous our work is. It also shows how well we are integrating with other practitioners and scientists. We have much of which to be proud.

The material in this volume is drawn from chiropractic sources as well as biomedical ones. The papers topics cover management, diagnosis, specific anatomical regions, and politicolegal issues. Many articles demonstrate our interest in assessment, such as those that examine various outcomes tools (visual analogue scale, neck disability index, etc.). There are those that examine reliability, the ability of an examiner to repeat his or her findings or for several examiners to locate the same finding (i.e., differences in intra- and interexaminer reliability). A good deal of material comes from sources not specifically chiropractic in nature, because there is much we can learn from the orthopedists and anatomists, among others.

The political arena is not left untouched. A paper by Eisenberg et al. has garnered a great deal of positive coverage within the chiropractic field for its finding that nearly 30% of Americans have seen some sort of alternative health-care practitioners; these same people regularly do not share this information with their medical practitioner. The authors' conclusions and recommendations are surprising.

The full breadth of material discussed shows once and for all that chiropractors are not simply back specialists. The case reports cover a wide range of conditions and management approaches. Our research covers many areas, from anatomy to immunocompetence, from controlled trials for back pain and headache to those studying electromyography and H-reflex responses.

We are happy to bring to you information you will find helpful, stimulating, and provocative. These are the best and most exciting of times for the chiropractic profession. We have won several major battles and face new ones every day. With information such as this, we will continue to grow and serve our patients to the best of our abilities, to answer questions our skeptics may have, and to serve as an effective force for conservative health care.

Dana J. Lawrence, D.C.

1 Clinical Management

Manual Procedures

MANIPULATION

Paraspinal Autonomic Ganglion Distortion Due to Vertebral Body Osteophytosis: A Case of Vertebrogenic Autonomic Syndromes?

Giles LGF (Griffith Univ, Nathan, Brisbane, Queensland, Australia)

J Manipulative Physiol Ther 15:551–555, 1992 1–1

Introduction.—Motion segment dysfunction via the autonomic nervous system may affect the circulation of blood and CSF near the spinal nerve roots, or it may affect the recurrent meningeal nerve or structures associated with the intervertebral disk. The medical community has neglected functional disturbances that cannot be supported by morphologic findings. The recent finding of a possible relationship between ab-

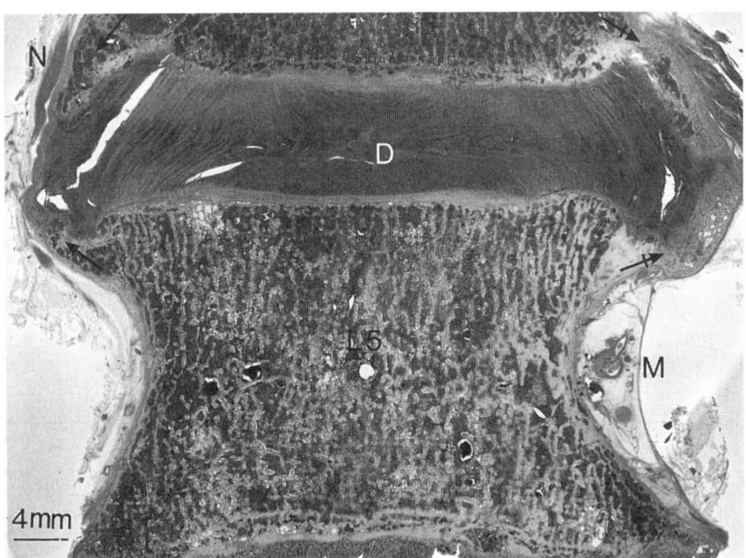

Fig 1–1.—Histologic preparation showing a 200 μm thick section cut in the coronal plane through the fifth lumbar vertebral body (*L5*) with adjacent L4–L5 intervertebral disk (*D*). Note the large osteophytes (*arrows*) that have developed adjacent to the lateral margins of the L4–L5 intervertebral disk bilaterally. A membrane (*M*) encloses parts of the neurovascular structures that are closely related to the spine. On the left side, the osteophytes are distorting the nerve (*N*). (Courtesy of Giles LGF: *J Manipulative Physiol Ther* 15:551–555, 1992.)

normal vascular changes and neural tissue degenerative changes in the intervertebral foramen may explain the clinical impression that spinal manipulation for pain of mechanical origin may offer relief from visceral dysfunction. In a preliminary histologic study, it was ascertained whether vertebral body osteophytosis can compromise the adjacent paraspinal autonomic structures.

Methods.—Histologic sections of the L4 to S1 vertebrae were prepared for morphologic examination using light microscopy. The specimens, taken from elderly subjects in their seventies, were cut in the coronal plane at a thickness of 200 μm.

Findings.—Paraspinal autonomic nerves and ganglia were considerably distorted by the presence of osteophytes. In 1 case, a membrane enclosed parts of neurovascular structures that were usually in close proximity to the spine (Fig 1–1). The nerves were seen to be distorted in their courses as they passed through the osteophytes. In other sections, the paraspinal autonomic ganglion was deformed by claw osteophytes.

Conclusion.—Histologic evidence indicates that the viscera may be affected by osteophytosis of motion segments. Autonomic reflex dysfunction may result from abnormal microvascular circulation in the paraspinal autonomic neural structures or abnormal axoplasmic flow in the neural structures affected by osteophytes. More research into the possible consequences and mechanisms of vertebrogenic autonomic syndrome is needed.

▶ Autonomic reflex phenomena are long-studied theoretical mechanisms offered by chiropractors and osteopaths in their explanations of why manipulative procedures may affect visceral function. In general, these studies have centered around joint fixation as the trigger for the abnormal or nociceptive dorsal horn cell bombardment that leads to altered autonomic function. However, such changes may well be caused by the presence of osteophytic changes. Such potential changes are demonstrated in the histologic changes in the spines of 3 cadavers of elderly individuals. The presence of such osteophytes, which is a regular radiographic finding (particularly in the elderly), carries serious ramifications for chiropractors in understanding the mechanisms that affect and alter autonomic and, therefore, visceral function.—D.J. Lawrence, D.C.

A Meta-Analysis of Clinical Trials of Spinal Manipulation

Anderson R, Meeker WC, Wirick BE, Mootz RD, Kirk DH, Adams A (Mills College, Oakland, Calif; Palmer College of Chiropractic–West, Sunnyvale, Calif; Los Angeles College of Chiropractic, Whittier, Calif)

J Manipulative Physiol Ther 15:181–194, 1992 1–2

TABLE 1.—A Meta-Analysis of Clinical Trials of Spinal Manipulation

Author(s)	n, Sampling	Presenting Condition	Type of Treatment	Reassessed	Conclusions/ Comments
Arkuszewski, 1986 (20)	100, consecutive patients admitted to neurology clinic	LBP ± sciatica with root irritation or compromise	1. Bed rest, Bernard's current, medications, massage 2. Above + traction, mobilization and manipulation described by Lewit*	Variable; post-discharge, 6 months post-discharge	Highly significant differences in average treatment period. Post-treatment: highly significant differences in posture, gait, active spinal movements, pain, "manual examination of the spine" and neurological evaluation. 6 months post-treatment: highly significant differences in all categories above except pain.
Berquist-Ullman and Larsson, 1977 (21)	197, selected light industry and clerical patients reporting to industrial medical department	Acute or subacute LBP localized to lumbosacral region	1. Back school education program 2. Combined physiotherapy including SMT* 3. Shortwave low intensity placebo	10 days, 3 and 6 wk, 3 and 6 months, l year	70% of all subjects recovered within 2 months of initial episode and 86% within 3 months, regardless of treatment type. Back school and physiotherapy patients reported shorter duration of symptoms than the placebo group. Back school patients had shorter duration of sick leave during initial episode than other two groups.
Chrisman et al., 1964 (22)	61, private orthopedic patients	Intervertebral disc syndrome (low back pain with sciatic radiation)	1. Rotational manipulation under anesthesia † 2. Conservative therapy alone (bed rest, medication, heat, traction, corset, exercises)	2-4 days, 6-8 wk, 5-12 months, after 3 yr	51% had good or excellent results at 3-yr follow-up; myelograms showed no changes after manipulation, but those without a defect did better.

(Continued.)

Author(s)	n, Sampling	Presenting Condition	Type of Treatment	Reassessed	Conclusions/ Comments
Coxhead, et al., 1981 (23)	322, multicenter: patients referred to outpatient physiotherapy department of eight hospitals	Sciatic symptoms with or without LBP	1. Traction 2. Exercises 3. Manipulation* 4. Corset	4 wk, 4 and 16 months	In the short term, active physiotherapy with several treatments appears of value in the management of patients with sciatic symptoms, but did not seem to confer any long-term benefit. No conclusive evidence that any of the four individual treatments were effective, but possible that each conferred some benefit, particularly manipulation.
Coyer and Curwen, 1955 (24)	136, unselected orthopedic hospital patients	Acute low back pain	1. Rotational manipulation of the lumbar spine* 2. Bed rest, lumbar pillow and analgesics	Weekly or shorter intervals	Of the patients manipulated, 50% were free of signs and symptoms at the end of one week as compared with 27% in the control group. At the end of 6 wk, only 12% of group 1 were suffering from signs and symptoms, while 28% of group 2 were still affected.
Doran and Newell, 1975 (25)	395, multicenter: patients referred to department of rheumatology of 7 hospitals	LBP localized to the lumbar region	1. Manipulation* 2. "Definitive" physiotherapy 3. Corset 4. Analgesia	3, 6 wk, 3 months, 1 yr	None of the methods showed any great superiority. Analgesics alone fared marginally worse than those on other treatments. Corsets, on long-term basis, were as effective as the others. No clear reason for recommending manipulation over physiotherapy or corset.

Author(s)	n, Sampling	Presenting Condition	Type of Treatment	Reassessed	Conclusions/ Comments
Edwards, 1969 (26)	184, patients referrd to out-patient physical therapy department of 2 hospitals and 2 private practices	1. Central LBP only 2. LBP + radiation to buttock 3. LBP + radiation to knee 4. LBP + radiation past knee	A. Mobilization and manipulation as described by Maitland* B. Heat, massage and exercise	Each treatment (variable)	1A. 82.5% success in 9.7 treatments. 1B. 82.5% success in 4.8 treatments. 2A. 69.5% success in 10.2 treatments. 2B. 78.1% success in 4.3 treatments. 3A. 65.2% success in 8.5 treatments. 3B. 95.7% success in 6.2 treatments. 4A. 51.7% success in 13.3 treatments. 4B. 78.5% success in 6.4 treatments. Success here means the result was acceptable (either good or satisfactory).
Farrell and Twomey, 1982 (27)	48, selected patients presenting to physiotherapy clinics	Acute low back pain of less that 3 week duration	1. Passive mobilization and manipulation ‡ 2. Physical therapy: microwave diathermy, isometric abdominal exercises, ergonomic instructions	1st, 3rd and last treatment, 3 wk	The duration of low back pain symptoms was significantly less for patients who received passive mobilization and manipulation than those who received an alternative conservative treatment.
Gibson et al., 1985 (28)	109, selected hospital out-patients	LBP from 2-12 months duration	1. SMT* 2. Short wave diathermy 3. Placebo (detuned diathermy)	2,4, and 12 wk	Number of patients who reported an immediate benefit of treatment and complete pain relief was very similar across all groups. Reduction of daytime pain and the improvement of spinal flexion were also similar in 3 groups. Neither osteopathic manipulation nor SWD was superior to placebo treatment. Results attest to the magnitude of the placebo response which may be achieved when harmless treatments are applied with conviction.

(Continued.)

Author(s)	n, Sampling	Presenting Condition	Type of Treatment	Reassessed	Conclusions/ Comments
Glover et al., 1974 (29)	84, industrial patients reporting to works medical center	Back pain between inferior angle of the scapula and the lower end of the sacrum	1. Rotational manipulation* 2. Placebo (detuned SWD)	15 min, 3 and 7 days, 1 month	Each of the two treatment groups showed progressive progress and marked improvement in percentage of relief from pain during 7-day period. But there were no demonstrable differences at the end of 7 days, except at the 15-min point immediately after treatment. The relief from pain in the manipulated group was always greater than controls.
Godfrey, et al., 1984 (30)	81, patients recruited from area physicians	Acute low back pain	1. Rotational manipulation, massage † 2. Minimal massage and low level electro-stimulation	Variable	Both treated and control patients improved rapidly in the 2-3 wk observation period. On retest, there was no statistically significant difference between the improvement scores of the treated or control groups on any of the scales.
Hadler et al., 1987 (31)	54, recruited via general practitioners and local advertising	LBP < 1 month duration	1. Placebo mobilization 2. Rotational manipulation (nonspecific)	Day 1 post-treatment, every 3 days for 2 wk	Manipulation group showed significantly greater and faster improvement in stratat with pain beginning 2-4 wk prior to presentation. No significant differences in strata with pain in 2 wk.

Author(s)	n, Sampling	Presenting Condition	Type of Treatment	Reassessed	Conclusions/ Comments
Hoehler et al., 1981 (32)	95, selected patients referred to university back clinic	Low back pain	1. Manipulation therapy † 2. Soft tissue massage	Variable, discharge, and 3 week postdischarge	Patients who received manipulative treatment were much more likely to report immediate relief after the first treatment. At discharge, there were no siginificant differences between the two groups. Because both showed substantial facilitate recovery there is no evidence demonstrating that it affects the long-term prognosis.
Lewith and Turner, 1982 (33)	66, retrospectively selected patients presenting to private medical clinic	Acute low back pain less than 1 wk duration requiring certified sick leave	1. Analgesics, rest, postural advice alone or in any combination 2. Above + manipulation described by Bordillion	N/A	Significantly less mean time for certified sick leave for manipulated group vs. nonmanipulated.
Maitland, 1957 (34)	220, selected patients from private practice and hospital physiotherapy department; 95 patients involved in controlled portion	LBP only, in status quo or deteriorating at time of treatment	1. Heat and back and postural exercises 2. Nonstandardized manual manipulation described by Maitland*	Variable, after resumption of "normal functions"	50% success in group 1 after an average of 23 days of treatment, 96% success in group 2 after an average of 4.5 treatments. Success = a return to "normal function."

(Continued.)

Author(s)	n, Sampling	Presenting Condition	Type of Treatment	Reassessed	Conclusions/ Comments
Mathews et al., 1987 (35)	291, patients presenting to outpatient clinic	a. LBP with asymmetrical restriction of lumbar spine movements b. Above + restriction in straight leg raising and/or positive femoral nerve stretch test	1. Infrared heat 2. Rotational mobilization/manipulation described by Cyriax*	Minimum 4 times with first 2 weeks, 1,3,6 and 12 months	Group a: 10% (nonsignificant) faster recovery rate for manipulated patients. Group b: significantly more patients in manipulation group recovered after 2 wk treatment in addition to significantly quicker recovery after 6 days. When subdivided by sex/age, only females under 48 yr showed significantly greater improvement.
Postacchini et al., 1988 (36)	398, randomly selected among patients presenting to 2 low back clinics	Group IA, LBP < 4 wk duration; group IB, LBP > 2 months duration; group IC, chronic LBP with acute episode; group IIA, acute LBP + radiation, no neurological; group IIB, chronic LBP + radiation, no neurological	1. Chiropractic manipulation 2. (Diclofenac) NSAID 3. Physiotherapy (massage, analgesic currents, diathermy) 4. Placebo, antiedema gel 5. Bed rest 6. Low back school	3 weeks, 2 and 6 months	IA, IIA, greatest improvement initially observed in patients receiving manipulation, no significant differences at long term follow-up. IB, best results with physiotherapy (short term) and back school (long-term). IIB, best results (short- and long-term) with physiotherapy patients. IC, greatest improvement observed at 3 wk in physiotherapy points, and at 6 months in back school patients.
Rasmussen, 1979 (37)	24, selected outpatients referred to rheumatology department	Low back pain	1. Short wave treatment 2. Manipulation therapy*	Before each treatment (3 times per week for 14 days), 1 yr	Manipulation does have some effect. Manipulation abbreviates the duration of acute low back pain. 97% of patients in manipulation treatment were free of symptoms within 14 days, while there were 25% of patients in the short wave treatment free of symptoms. In the manipulation group, all patients' mobility were improved, whereas in the other group, only half showed improvement.

Author(s)	n, Sampling	Presenting Condition	Type of Treatment	Reassessed	Conclusions/ Comments
Sims-Williams et al., 1978, part I (38)	94, general practitioner referrals	Nonspecific lumbar pain	1. Mobilization and manipulation of the spine* 2. Placebo physiotherapy (microwave radiation at lowest possible setting)	1 and 3 months, l yr	Results suggest that most sufferers from back pain obtain relief without any specific treatment and that mobilization and manipulation may hasten this improvement but make no difference to the long term prognosis. Immediately following treatment, most patients improved with physiotherapy, but improvement was more noticeable in the group who had received active treatment. In retrospect, patients failed to distinguish active from placebo physiotherapy.
Sims-Williams et al., 1979, part II (39)	94, patients referred to hospital rheumatology and orthopedic clinics	Nonspecific lumbar pain	1. Mobilization and manipulation* 2. Placebo physiotherapy	1 and 3 months, l yr	Many patients showed improvement, but in contrast to the study on general practitioner patients with nonspecific back pain, no definite advantage could be associated with mobilization and manipulation. The benefits of mobilization and manipulation for low back pain are probably restricted to hastening recovery in patients likely to rapidly improve spontaneously.
Waagen et al., 1986 (40)	19, selected patients presenting to a college chiropractic clinic	Mild to moderate low back pain less than 3 wk duration	1. Full spine SMT † 2. Sham adjustment and soft tissue massage	2 week	Significantly greater improvement in pain relief and spinal mobility in manipulation group. Considered preliminary because of small sample size.

(Continued.)

Author(s)	n, Sampling	Presenting Condition	Type of Treatment	Reassessed	Conclusions/ Comments
Waterworth and 112, selected general Hunter, 1985 (41) practitioner patients	Acute mechanical low back pain less than 1 month duration	1. Nonsteroidal anti-inflammatory drug (diflunisal) 2. Conservative physiotherapy (heat, short-wave diathermy, exercises ultrasound) 3. Manipulation of the lumbar spine and mechanical therapy	3-4 days, 10-12 days	Serial assessments of pain and spinal mobility showed similar response rates in all three treatment groups and no significant difference between therapies. Treatment failures occurred in all groups highlighting the need for a variety of therapeutic approaches in managing the patient with low back pain.	
Zylbergold and Piper, 1981 (42)	28, selected from a waiting list of hospital physical therapy outpatients	Nonspecific low back pain	1. Lumbar flexion exercises 2. Manual therapy* 3. Home care	1 month	No statistically significant differences were demonstrated between the 3 groups in measurements of pain, forward, right side and left side flexion or functional activity. However, the mean performance of groups suggests that manual therapy may be more likely to relieve pain and immobility in forward flexion than a home exercise program.

* Not distinguishable or both methods applied at discretion of treating doctor or therapist.
† Manipulation.
‡ Mobilization.
(Courtesy of Anderson R, Meeker WC, Wirick BE, et al: *J Manipulative Physiol Ther* 15:181-194, 1992.)

TABLE 2.—Cohen's D Effect Size

Outcome Variable	Time Periods 1	2	3	4	5	6	7	8	Overall	SD	n
Subjective measures											
Pain	0.32	0.55	0.40	0.22	0.47	0.10	0.48		0.38	0.38	25
Global assessment											
Clinician	0.30	0.68	0.44	0.25					0.38	0.14	5
Patient		0.10	0.31	0.21	0.28	0.21	0.10	-0.26	0.18	0.09	6
Objective measures											
Flexion	0.24	0.44	0.19	0.14		0.30			0.34	0.39	9
Extension	0.24	0.41	0.03	0.03		0.02			0.17	0.34	6
Straight leg raise	-0.27	0.64		-0.22	-0.39	-0.17			-0.01	0.52	5
Functional measures											
Work				0.15		0.22		-0.03	0.40	0.38	4
Daily activities	0.21	0.47	0.59	0.25					0.30	0.23	8
Work/activities	1.07	1.00		0.30		0.34			0.70	0.51	4

(Courtesy of Anderson R, Meeker WC, Wirick BE, et al: *J Manipulative Physiol Ther* 15:181–194, 1992.)

Objective.—The literature was searched for studies of spinal manipulative therapy (SMT) completed through mid-1989.

Methods.—Twenty-three randomized controlled clinical trials of SMT were found; all included concurrent controls managed by methods other than SMT. The trials totaled 34 mutually exclusive and discrete samples.

Coding methods were verified by a blinded research assistant who independently extracted data from a subset of the studies. Effect sizes were calculated for 9 outcome variables at 8 time points after the start of treatment.

Findings.—The studies are individually summarized in Table 1. Thirty-eight of 44 effect sizes indicated SMT to be superior to the comparison treatment (Table 2). True no-treatment control groups, however, were rare. The quality of the trials correlated positively with differences in reported effect sizes, but not to a marked degree.

Interpretation.—Spinal manipulative therapy is consistently more effective than comparison treatments in the management of low back pain. If no-treatment controls were more often used, the effect would probably be more evident. Researchers should attempt to use more consistent measures for describing SMT and evaluating outcomes. The impression that manipulation is more effective than mobilization is based on very limited data.

▶ Meta-analysis is becoming a more popular methodology for the evaluation of the literature base. This procedure is more specific than a simple literature review because it provides objective measures of effect size. Manipulation was shown to be more effective using 9 outcome variables. The authors believe the evidence of effectiveness might have been more definite if there had been more studies involving no-treatment control groups. This is difficult to accomplish because it is not ethical to ask patients experiencing pain to forgo treatment for research purposes. Of the 23 trials included in this study, chiropractic was a player in only one.—R.B. Phillips, D.C., Ph.D.

A Blinded Randomized Clinical Trial of Manual Therapy and Physiotherapy for Chronic Back and Neck Complaints: Physical Outcome Measures

Koes BW, Bouter LM, van Mameren H, Essers AHM, Verstegen GMJR, Hofhuizen DM, Houben JP, Knipschild PG (Univ of Limburg, The Netherlands; Univ Hosp Maastricht, The Netherlands; Inst of Higher Education in Heerlen, The Netherlands)

J Manipulative Physiol Ther 1:16–23, 1992 1–3

Background.—The randomized clinical trials done on the efficacy of manipulation and mobilization for back and neck complaints have yielded inconsistent results. Interpretation is often difficult because of methodologic flaws. A trial comparing manual therapy, physiotherapy, treatment by the general practitioner, and placebo was reported.

Methods and Findings.—Two hundred fifty-six patients with chronic nonspecific back and neck complaints were enrolled in the randomized clinical trial. Placebo treatment consisted of detuned ultrasound and detuned short-wave diathermy. The physical outcome measures assessed

TABLE 1.—Baseline Characteristics of the Study Population

Characteristic	Manual therapy	Physio-therapy	Placebo therapy	General pract.	All subjects
No. of subjects	65	66	64	61	256
Selected through					
advertisement (%)	75	64	60	62	68
Mean age (yrs)	43	42	43	43	43
Gender(% female)	54	48	52	38	52
Localisation of complaints (%):					
Back	55	54	62	53	56
Neck	20	32	22	26	25
Back and Neck	25	14	16	21	19
Median duration of present episode of complaints (wks)					
patients with back or neck complaints (n = 208)	52	52	52	45	52
patients with back and neck complaints (n = 48)					
back	78	26	92	78	79
neck	91	26	65	52	52
Mean physical functioning					
score (10-points scale)	5.9	5.8	5.7	5.7	5.8
Range of motion (degrees)					
cervical anteflexion	113	112	117	116	115
cervical lateroflexion	60	61	64	62	62
spinal forward flexion (T1)	133	126	129	127	129

(Courtesy of Koes BW, Bouter LM, van Mameren H, et al: *J Manipulative Physiol Ther* 1:16–23, 1992.)

were spinal mobility and physical functioning, which were determined 3, 6, and 12 weeks after treatment. Those patients receiving manual therapy had a faster and greater improvement in physical functioning than did patients receiving the other 3 therapies. Spinal mobility changes among the 4 study groups appeared to be small, showing no consistent pattern (Tables 1 and 2).

Conclusion.—Manual therapy resulted in a faster, greater improvement in physical functioning compared with physiotherapy, treatment by a general practitioner, or placebo. Improvement in physical functioning occurred relatively independently of changes in range of motion of the spinal movements.

▶ Spinal mobility (measured mechanically) and physical functioning (measured by a research assistant) were found to be reliable outcome measures in this controlled clinical trial. Outcome measures are a difficult challenge for any clinical trial. They range from physical function measures to self-reported measures generally collected on a questionnaire.

There is a great need to incorporate the use of outcome measures into the general practice of chiropractic. Pain measures, functional abilities, life-style measures, and physical function measures are all potentially useful outcome measures of chiropractic care.—R.B. Phillips, D.C., Ph.D.

TABLE 2.—Improvement on Physical Functioning and Change in Range of Motion at 3-, 6-, and 12-Week Follow-Up in the Intention-to-Treat Analysis

Outcome measure	3 wks	6 wks	12 wks
Mean (SD) improvement on physical functioning (10-points scale)			
manual therapy (n=53) *	2.3 (2.1)	3.5 (1.9)	4.0 (2.3)
physiotherapy (n=54)	1.6 (1.9)	3.1 (1.8)	3.2 (2.0)
placebo therapy (n=51)	1.6 (2.2)	2.6 (2.3)	3.4 (2.3)
general practitioner(n=44)	1.7 (2.1)	2.4 (2.6)	3.4 (2.2)
Cervical flexion: patients with neck complaints			
Mean (SD) change of range of motion cervical forward flexion (degrees)			
manual therapy (n=23)	-2 (16)	3 (14)	4 (16)
physiotherapy (n=22)	0 (16)	2 (18)	4 (15)
placebo therapy (n=18)	5 (20)	5 (13)	9 (15)
general practitioner (n=21)	-7 (20)	-11 (23)	-7 (21)
Mean (SD) change of range of motion cervical lateroflexion (degrees)			
manual therapy (n=23)	2 (9)	2 (10)	1 (11)
physiotherapy (n=22)	1 (10)	0 (9)	3 (10)
placebo therapy (n=18)	-3 (8)	- 1 (8)	2 (8)
general practitioner (n=21)	-2 (7)	- 3 (9)	-3 (10)
Spinal flexion: patients with back complaints			
Mean (SD) change of range of motion spinal flexion at T1 (degrees)			
manual therapy (n=36)	0 (10)	- 2 (12)	-2 (15)
physiotherapy (n=31)	-1 (12)	4 (13)	6 (13)
placebo therapy (n=39)	-4 (11)	- 3 (9)	0 (10)
general practitioner (n=30)	3 (10)	0 (14)	0 (18)

* Number of patients after 6-week follow-up. After 3 and 12 weeks, the numbers may vary slightly because of missing values.

(Courtesy of Koes BW, Bouter LM, van Mameren H, et al: *J Manipulative Physiol Ther* 1:16-23, 1992.)

Randomised Clinical Trial of Manipulative Therapy and Physiotherapy for Persistent Back and Neck Complaints: Results of One Year Follow Up

Koes BW, Bouter LM, van Mameren H, Essers AHM, Verstegen GMJR, Hofhuizen DM, Houben JP, Knipschild PG (Univ of Limburg, The Netherlands; Univ Hosp, Maastricht, The Netherlands; Inst of Higher Education, Heerlen, The Netherlands)

BMJ 304:601–605, 1992 1–4

Objective.—A randomized trial was carried out in 256 patients in The Netherlands who were seen with nonspecific neck and back complaints after at least 6 weeks, and who had not received physical or manipulative treatment for at least 2 years (Table 1).

TABLE 1.—Baseline Characteristics of the Study Population

Characteristic	manual therapy	physio-therapy	placebo therapy	general practitioner	all subjects
No. of subjects	65	66	64	61	256
Selected through advertisement (%)	75	64	60	62	68
Mean age (yrs)	43	42	43	43	43
Gender(% female)	54	48	52	38	52
Localisation of complaints (%):					
Back	55	54	62	53	56
Neck	20	32	22	26	25
Back and Neck	25	14	16	21	19
Median duration of present episode of complaints (wks)					
patients with back or neck complaints (n = 208)	52	52	52	45	52
patients with back and neck complaints (n = 48)					
back	78	26	92	78	79
neck	91	26	65	52	52
Mean severity main complaint (10-point scale)	7.0	7.0	6.8	6.8	6.9
Mean physical functioning score (10-point scale)	5.9	5.8	5.7	5.7	5.8

(Courtesy of Koes BW, Bouter LM, van Mameren H, et al: *BMJ* 304:601–605, 1992.)

Management.—Physiotherapy consisted of exercises, massage, and/or physical therapies (e.g., heat, ultrasound, electrotherapy, and short-wave diathermy). Physiotherapy was contrasted with manipulation and mobilization of the spine; ongoing treatment by the general practitioner, which included prescribed analgesia and nonsteroidal anti-inflammatory agents;

TABLE 2.—Mean (Median) Number of Treatments, Length of Session, and Duration of Treatment During the Intervention Period

	Number of treatments	Session time (min)	Duration (wks)
Manual therapy	5.4 (6)	41 (40)	8.9 (9)
Physiotherapy	14.7 (14)	35 (30)	7.8 (8)
Placebo therapy	11.1 (12)	29 (30)	5.8 (6)
General practitioner*	-	-	-

* Treatment by the general practitioner consisted usually of a single visit by the patient at the general practice.
(Courtesy of Koes BW, Bouter LM, van Mameren H, et al: *BMJ* 304:601–605, 1992.)

and a placebo treatment consisting of detuned short-wave diathermy and ultrasound.

Results.—Manual treatment involved fewer sessions than physiotherapy, and the general practitioner group generally paid a single visit (Table 2). Improvement after 1 year was most evident in patients given manipulative therapy (Table 3). Patient ratings of their main complaint, global effect, and physical functioning did not differ markedly, but they consistently indicated superior results from manipulative treatment compared with physiotherapy.

Conclusion.—A 1-year assessment suggested superior results from manipulative treatment of nonspecific pain in this trial. Both manipulative therapy and physiotherapy appear to be better than ongoing treatment by the general practitioner or a placebo condition.

▶ This one of several randomized controlled clinical trials appearing in the literature that have gathered support for the beneficial effects of spinal manipulation for neck and back complaints. This study included long-term follow-up for 1 year and found that manipulation and physiotherapy were better than what the general practitioner was doing, and that manipulation was found to be more effective than physiotherapy over 12 months.

It is imperative that a database of controlled clinical trials continues to grow in support of what chiropractors do most, i.e., spinal manipulation. It would be beneficial to the chiropractic profession if more of these trials included chiropractors and were conducted by chiropractic researchers in conjunction with medical groups.—R.B. Phillips, D.C., Ph.D.

TABLE 3.—Outcome of Therapy at Follow-Up

outcome measure	3 wks	6 wks	12 wks	6 mths	12 mths	difference between manual therapy and physiotherapy[a]
mean (SD) improvement main complaint (10-point scale)						
manual therapy	2.3 (2.1)	3.4 (2.1)	4.0 (2.6)		4.5 (2.2)	0.9 (0.1, 1.7) 12 months
physiotherapy	2.0 (2.3)	3.4 (2.4)	3.8 (2.3)		3.8 (2.3)	
mean (SD) global perceived effect (6-point scale)						
manual therapy	2.5 (1.5)	3.4 (1.7)	3.4 (2.0)	3.5 (1.9)	3.5 (1.8)	0.3 (-0.4, 1.0) 6 months
physiotherapy	2.6 (1.6)	3.3 (1.6)	3.7 (1.7)	3.5 (1.8)	3.2 (1.9)	0.4 (-0.3, 1.4) 12 months
mean (SD) improvement on physical functioning (10-point scale)						
manual therapy	2.3 (2.1)	3.5 (1.9)	4.0 (2.3)		4.2 (2.1)	0.6 (-0.1, 1.3) 12 months
physiotherapy	1.6 (1.9)	3.1 (1.8)	3.2 (2.0)		3.7 (2.0)	

[a] The group differences (95% confidence intervals) were calculated with a linear regression model.
(Courtesy of Koes BW, Bouter LM, van Mameren H, et al: *BMJ* 304:601–605, 1992.)

Differences in Treatment History With Manipulation for Acute, Subacute, Chronic and Recurrent Spine Pain

Triano JJ, Hondras MA, McGregor M (Natl College of Chiropractic, Lombard, Ill)

J Manipulative Physiol Ther 15:24–30, 1992 1–5

Objective.—Case management of spine disorders is based more on clinical judgment than an understanding of the underlying pathology. With the recent emphasis on standards of care and cost-containment strategies in health-care delivery, there is an increasing need for quantitative data to make rational policy decisions. The clinical characteristics of patients with spine pain seeking treatment at a private, teaching chiropractic clinic were examined.

Methods.—During a 14-week period, 241 patients seeking treatment for spine pain were asked to enter the study. All patients were paying for their own treatment. The patients were divided into 3 groups based on their willingness to complete a set of questionnaires and come in for a follow-up evaluation at the end of the treatment period. The records of all 3 groups were tracked prospectively until each case was resolved. Based on duration of symptoms, the chief complaint was classified as acute, subacute, chronic, or recurrent. Based on clinical findings, the patients were classified as having entrapment syndromes, mechanical spine pain, or muscular spine pain.

TABLE 1.—Analysis of Treatment Frequency During 6 Weeks by Chronicity and Group

Type of Patient	Acute	Subacute	Chronic	Recurrent	Grand Range
Participants					
Compliers	5.3 (4.7)	5.6 (3.1)	8.2 (5.0)	7.1 (4.6)	1-22
n	29	23	37	29	118
Non-compliers	3.6 (2.4)	1.3 (0.6)	5.3 (3.3)	3.3 (4.9)	1-11
n	11	3	13	3	30
Nonparticipants	5.0 (4.7)	4.7 (4.7)	5.4 (3.8)	4.9 (3.4)	1-21
n	27	21	27	15	90

(Courtesy of Triano JJ, Hondras MA, McGregor M: *J Manipulative Physiol Ther* 15:24–30, 1992.)

TABLE 2.—Analysis of Treatment Frequency During 6 Weeks by Descriptive Classification and Group

Type of Patient	Pain Type Entrapment	Mechanical	Muscular	Grand Range
Participants				
Compliers	6.7 (4.9)	7.0 (4.8)	4.8 (2.6)	1-22
n	6	100	12	118
Noncompliers	1.5 (2.1)	4.4 (3.0)	4.0 (3.8)	1-11
n	2	24	4	30
Nonparticipants	6.9 (6.6)	5.2 (4.3)	3.9 (2.5)	1-21
n	9	57	26	92

(Courtesy of Triano JJ, Hondras MA, McGregor M: *J Manipulative Physiol Ther* 15:24–30, 1992.)

Results.—Of 241 patients invited to enter the study, 149 agreed and 118 (79.2%) of them completed all questionnaires. The range for the number of treatment sessions associated with case resolution was 1–22. Chronic disorders required more treatment to resolve symptomatic episodes than did the other 3 categories (Table 1). The number of treatments was not related to the descriptive classifications for entrapment, mechanical, and muscular spine pain (Table 2). Complaints of the thoracic spine responded more quickly to treatment than did complaints of the cervical, lumbar, or lumbosacral areas (Table 3). Of the 241 patients, 216 (89.6%) reached clinical resolution within 6 weeks of starting treatment. The 24 patients for whom care beyond 6 weeks was required received a mean of 3.8 additional treatments (Table 4).

TABLE 3.—Number of Treatment Sessions to Resolution by Region of Chief Complaint

Spinal region contrasts	Mean Number of Treatments	F	p
Thoracic vs. cervical	3.0 vs. 5.9	4.655	0.032
Thoracic vs. lumbar	3.0 vs, 6.7	9.136	0.003
Thoracic vs. lumbosacral	3.0 vs. 7.0	8.410	0.004

(Courtesy of Triano JJ, Hondras MA, McGregor M: *J Manipulative Physiol Ther* 15:24–30, 1992.)

TABLE 4.—Treatment Sessions Beyond 6 Weeks by Group

Type of patient	n	Mean	Range
Participants			
Compliers	11	5	2-10
Noncompliers	3	2	1-3
Nonparticipants	11	3.1	1-11

(Courtesy of Triano JJ, Hondras MA, McGregor M: *J Manipulative Physiol Ther* 15:24-30, 1992.)

▶ This is a prospective study of patients with acute, subacute, chronic, or recurrent low back pain. It demonstrates a good method with which to measure length and the effectiveness of care rendered by chiropractors. The conclusions support the fact that spinal manipulation is most effective for acute back pain but requires more extended care for chronic conditions. The number of treatments was not in excess of what has been reported in numerous studies, and it is not inconsistent with the recommended frequencies published in the RAND reports. The authors' conclusion that the number of treatments had little relation to the descriptive classifications for entrapment, mechanical, and muscular spine pain is interesting.—R.B. Phillips, D.C., Ph.D.

Spinal Manipulation for Low-Back Pain

Shekelle PG, Adams AH, Chassin MR, Hurwitz EL, Brook RH (Univ of California, Los Angeles; VA Med Ctr, West Los Angeles; Consortium for Chiropractic Research, Los Angeles; et al)

Ann Intern Med 117:590–598, 1992 1–6

Background.—Although spinal manipulation has been used in the treatment of musculoskeletal complaints for centuries, the modern medical community has labeled it an unorthodox treatment, in part because it has been equated with the practice of chiropractic for the past 50 years. The use of lumbar spinal manipulation of all types in treating low back pain was examined.

Methods.—Fifty-eight articles on the use and complications of spinal manipulation, including 25 reports of controlled trials of the efficacy of spinal manipulation, were identified and analyzed. The controlled trials were appraised critically, and data on the use and complications of spinal manipulation were summarized. Data from 9 studies were combined using meta-analysis techniques to estimate the effect of spinal manipulation on pain and functional outcomes.

Findings.—Chiropractors provide most of the manipulative treatment for low back pain given in the United States. Lumbar manipulation has been associated with serious complications, including paraplegia and death. Although the occurrence rate of these complications has not been established, it is probably low. The difference in the probability of recovery for patients with uncomplicated, acute low back pain at 3 weeks favoring spinal manipulation was .17. For those with low back pain and sciatic nerve irritation, the 4-week difference in probabilities of recovery is .098.

Conclusion.—Spinal manipulation benefits some patients in the short term, especially those with uncomplicated, acute low back pain. The efficacy of this treatment for patients with chronic low back pain has not yet been determined.

▶ This is a meta-analysis of the literature dealing with manipulation in the treatment of low back pain. The authors are confident in their position that spinal manipulation is an effective form of treatment for acute low back pain. The need for further study on the role of spinal manipulation in the treatment of chronic low back is also stated by the authors. Two meta-analytic studies of such treatment bring strong support to the efficacy of this form of care. The challenge lies in establishing the credibility of practitioners of manipulation in the public's eyes. Studies of this nature by chiropractic researchers will go a long way toward accomplishing this need.—R.B. Phillips, D.C., Ph.D.

Mechanical Low-Back Pain: A Comparison of Medical and Chiropractic Management Within the Victorian WorkCare Scheme

Ebrall PS (Phillip Inst of Technology, Melbourne)

Chiroprac J Aust 22:47–53, 1992 1–7

Background.—Low back injury and mechanical low back pain (MLBP) are a significant medical problem in the Western world. Chiropractors have historically promoted their management of such injury as more cost-effective than that provided by other health-care professionals. Cost and time outcomes for patients treated with different management strategies of chiropractors and medical practitioners for work-related MLBP were studied.

Methods.—All work-related MLBP claimants in Victoria, Australia, in a 12-month period were studied retrospectively. Two matched samples were identified—1 treated solely by chiropractic methods and 1 treated by medical methods. The 2 groups each contained 998 patients aged 15 to more than 60 years.

Findings.—Comparisons of costs and outcomes between groups showed that a significantly lower number of claimants in the chiropractic management group required compensation days, and fewer compensation days were taken by individuals receiving chiropractic management. A higher number of patients progressed to chronic status when medical management was given. In addition, the average payment per claim was higher with medical management. The average practitioner payment was higher with chiropractic management, suggesting a more intense level of practitioner/patient interaction chiropractors.

Conclusions.—Chiropractic participation in the Victorian compensation scheme for work-related low back pain significantly benefits the community. Chiropractors must report and critically analyze the components of their management for MLBP to determine what they do that achieves such significant effectiveness.

▶ This study is another example of the cost-effectiveness of chiropractic care in the management of work-related back injuries. Chiropractic patients consistently show less compensation for loss of work time. Generally, chiropractic patient care is less costly than medical care but this finding is not consistent across all studies. This study does show that cases under medical management are more likely to progress to a chronic condition, an interesting finding deserving of further investigation.

There is also a great need for chiropractic cost-effective analysis to progress beyond the worker's compensation arena, which is where most studies are currently based. There is need for cost-effective analysis in the areas of private insurance, personal injury, Medicare, and cash-paying patients.—R.B. Phillips, D.C., Ph.D.

Chiropractic Treatment of Patients in Motor Vehicle Accidents: A Statistical Analysis

Dies S, Strapp JW (King City, Ont, Canada; Atmospheric Environmental Service, Downsview, Ont, Canada)

J Can Chiroprac Assoc 36:139–145, 1992 1–8

Objective.—Motor vehicle accidents (MVAs) are a common cause of spinal injury, and chiropractors treat many such patients. There is little information, however, on the use of spinal manipulation for these types of injuries. Treatment outcome for patients with MVA injuries for whom spinal manipulation was the main treatment modality was examined retrospectively.

Methods.—Review of the records of a single chiropractor during a 10-year period revealed 149 patients treated for MVA injuries. Treatment consisted primarily of manipulation, which was begun immediately after examination and/or radiography. Analysis of variance was performed to calculate the effect of age, sex, vehicle damage, symptoms, and concurrent physiotherapy on the dependent variables of number of treatments, improvement, and need for ongoing treatment.

Findings.—Fifty-nine percent of the sample were females, and the average patient age was 35 years. Forty percent of patients had persistent pain requiring ongoing treatment. The average number of treatments was 14. Eighty-three percent of patients were much improved, and 12% were somewhat improved. Thirty-one percent of the patients sought treatment within 1 week, whereas 16% delayed longer than 1 year. A greater number of treatments was required by patients complaining of headache or low back pain. Delay in seeking treatment, presence of uncomplicated nausea, and advancing age all decreased the level of improvement. However, no factor studied had a significant effect on the need for ongoing treatment.

Conclusion.—Treatment by spinal manipulation, when continued periodically, seems to help control persistent pain resulting from MVAs. Seeking treatment early appears to improve the outcome of treatment. The results of this study are comparable to those of previous studies.

▶ This is an interesting retrospective analysis of chiropractic management of patients who have had a motor vehicle accident. One of the more fascinating findings of this study is the 40.2% of patients requiring ongoing treatments for the management of chronic pain. Although patients responded well to the chiropractic care received, chronic pain appeared to be a persistent problem and may well have been related to the type and/or severity of the injury.

The challenge associated with a retrospective study is the recall of information or the abstracting of data from the historical record. This type of information is more susceptible to errors of interpretation than data obtained in a prospective fashion. Restrospective studies are needed to provide access to information that often would take years to collect.—R.B. Phillips, D.C., Ph.D.

Effects of Joint Mobilization on Joint Stiffness and Active Motion of the Metacarpal-Phalangeal Joint

Randall T, Portney L, Harris BA (Reynolds Army Hosp, Ft Sill, Okla; MGH Inst of Health Professions, Boston; Massachusetts Gen Hosp, Boston)

J Orthop Sports Phys Ther 16:30–36, 1992 1–9

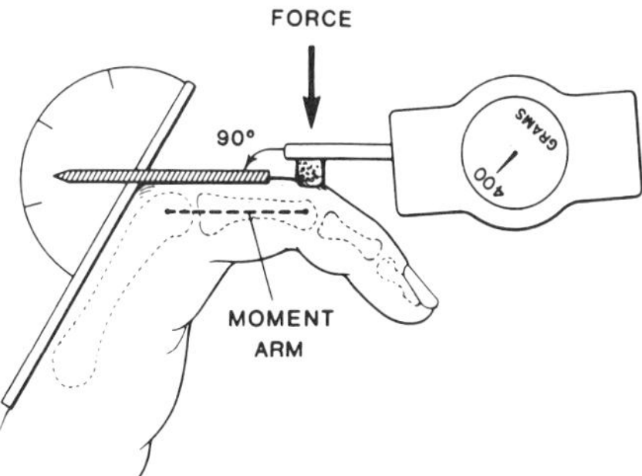

Fig 1–4.—Procedure for measuring flexion torque range of motion. (Courtesy of Randall T, Portney L, Harris BA: *J Orthop Sports Phys Ther* 16:30-36, 1992.)

Objective.—Although joint mobilization is widely used for the restoration of joint motion, there is sparse documentation of its effectiveness. Metacarpal fractures are commonly treated by immobilization, which has documented ill effects on joint mobility. Whether joint mobilization can effectively increase active range of motion (AROM) and decrease joint stiffness after immobilization of the metacarpophalangeal joint was determined.

Methods.—The study sample comprised 18 patients who had been followed for treatment of a metacarpal fracture and who had been treated by hand immobilization for at least 2 weeks. The patients were randomized to receive either joint mobilization treatment with traction and palmar/dorsal glide techniques or no treatment. Three treatments were given during 1 week. Before and after each session, the subjects were measured for both AROM and torque range of motion (TROM), a noninvasive method of measuring the mechanical qualities of tissues that resist motion. This technique uses standard goniometric methods while the joint is positioned by a known force (Fig 1–4).

Findings.—Within each session, the treatment group achieved a significantly greater change in both AROM and TROM than did the control group. As expected, both groups had a significant change in AROM and TROM between sessions. Initial stiffness was not a useful indicator of treatment response.

Conclusion.—Joint mobilization increases AROM and decreases joint stiffness in subjects whose metacarpophalangeal joints had been immobilized after metacarpal fracture. Thus, joint mobilization does appear to alter joint mechanics and increase excursion, measured both actively and with controlled force. Although this study does not find initial stiffness to be a good predictor of treatment response, a larger sample representing the full spectrum of joint stiffness might do so.

▶ More and more professions are using joint mobilization as part of their therapeutic armamentarium; as a result, there are more studies examining the use of the procedure. This particular study comes from the physical therapy profession, and it will not come as a surprise to any chiropractor that the authors were able to show an increase in joint flexibility beyond that of a control group for a set of patients who had had immobilization of the carpal-metacarpal joint after fracture. I do note that the authors fail to cite any specifically chiropractic research surrounding the effects of manipulation on joint motion, something I hope they will rectify in their future work.—D.J. Lawrence, D.C.

The Effects of Early Mobilisation and Immobilisation on the Healing Process Following Muscle Injuries

Järvinen MJ, Lehto MUK (Univ of Turku, Finland Univ Hosp, Tampere, Finland)
Sports Med 15:78–89, 1993 1–10

Purpose.—Muscle injury is followed by 2 competitive events, muscle fiber regeneration and production of granulation tissue. Early mobilization, usually preceded by a short period of immobilization, has become favored over immobilization for the treatment of muscle injuries. Rats were studied to determine the effects of early mobilization and immobilization of direct muscle injuries similar to those seen in athletes.

Methods.—A standard contusion injury was produced in the left calf of anesthetized rats. The injury induced only a partial rupture of the gastrocnemius muscle, preserving some functional capacity. One group of animals received no treatment but was left to move freely, and another group was immediately immobilized in a plaster cast. There were 4 mobilization groups: 1 was mobilized immediately and the others were mobilized after 1, 2, or 5 days of immobilization.

Findings.—Immobilization limited the size of the area of connective tissue at the injury site. There was prominent penetration of muscle fi-

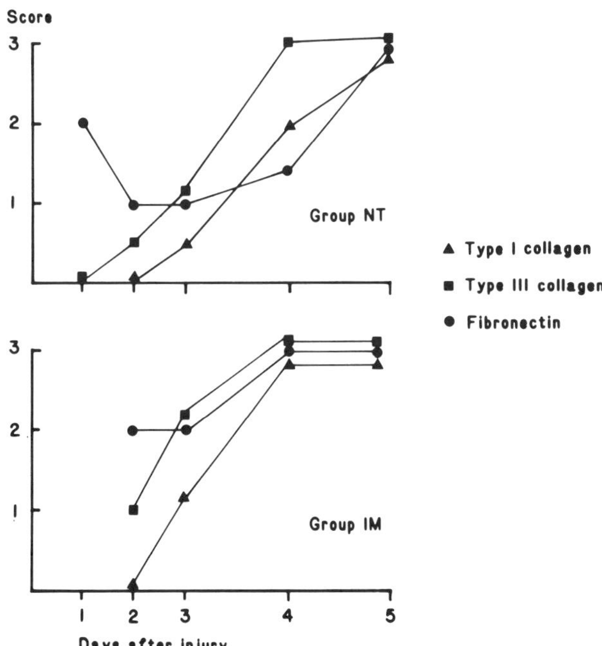

Fig 1–5.—Schematic presentation of accumulation of connective tissue components in the site of injury in rats receiving no treatment (NT) or immobilized (IM) after trauma. The scoring system is presented in detail in the original article (Lehto et al. 1985a). (Courtesy of Järvinen MJ, Lehto MUK: *Sports Med* 15:78–89, 1993.)

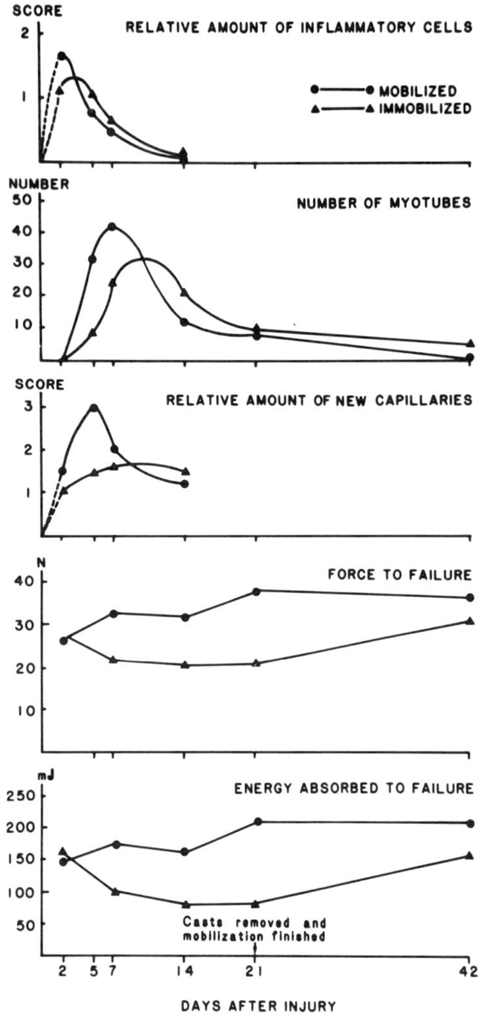

Fig 1–6.—Schematic presentation of results with pronounced differences observed in healing muscle treated by mobilization or immobilization. Scoring systems are presented in detail in the original articles (Järvinen 1975, 1976a). (Courtesy of Järvinen MJ, Lehto MUK: *Sports Med* 15:78–89, 1993.)

bers through the connective tissue, but these fibers had a complex orientation that was not parallel with the uninjured fibers. The muscle showed marked atrophy after more than 1 week immobilization. The untreated group had fibronectin, which acts as a primary matrix by cross-linking with fibrin, in the injured area as early as 24 hours after the injury (Fig 1–5). When mobilization was begun immediately after the injury, a dense scar formed, prohibiting muscle regeneration. There was better penetration of muscle fibers through the connective tissue when mobilization was begun after a brief period of immobilization. The regenerated tissues were aligned with the uninjured fibers. There was some delay in morphological signs of healing with mobilization after brief immobilization, but their gains in strength and energy absorption capacity was similar to that of muscles treated by early mobilization alone.

Conclusions.—In muscle injuries, early immobilization and mobilization have major effects on the production of connective tissue components and on the rate and intensity of muscle fiber regeneration (Fig 1-6). Connective tissue scarring can hinder the regeneration of muscle fibers; immobilization reduces the size of the connective tissue area, but prolonged immobilization leads to muscle atrophy. When mobilization is preceded by a brief period of immobilization, there is good penetration of muscle fibers through the connective tissue layer in alignment with the uninjured muscle fibers.

▶ Because muscle healing is inhibited by the formation of scar tissue, procedures that limit the formation of scar tissue will have a positive impact on tissue regeneration. The authors describe a 3-stage muscle injury repair process: an inflammatory phase with hematoma formation, necrosis and degeneration, and inflammation; a repair stage with phagocytosis, regeneration of tissue, and production of scar tissue; and a remodeling phase, in which the muscle regeneration proceeds, the scar tissue reorganizes, and the function of the muscle returns. The best response to muscle injury repair is for the chiropractor to initiate mobilization procedures not immediately after injury, because that may promote scar formation; rather, a short period of immobilization will allow for the mobilization procedures to work to far better effect.—D.J. Lawrence, D.C.

The Effect of Training on Physical Therapists' Ability to Apply Specified Forces of Palpation

Keating J, Matyas TA, Bach TM (La Trobe Univ, Bundoora, Victoria, Australia)
Phys Ther 73:38–46, 1993 1–11

Background.—The purpose of intervertebral joint palpation is to provide valuable information about joint behavior. The task of applying force to the joint and evaluating the many aspects of its reponse is obviously a complex one to perform as well as teach. Whether postgraduate physical therapy students studying manipulation could learn to accurately produce specific forces during intervertebral joint palpation was determined.

Methods.—The subjects were 12 physical therapists enrolled in a 12-month postgraduate course in manipulative therapy. All were graduates of a 4-year degree course in physical therapy and had 3–10 years of clinical experience. Practicing 10 minutes per day for 30 days, 6 of the therapists were trained to apply specific forces of 1, 5, 10, 15, 20, and 25 kp; the other 6 had no training. Before training, immediately afterward, and

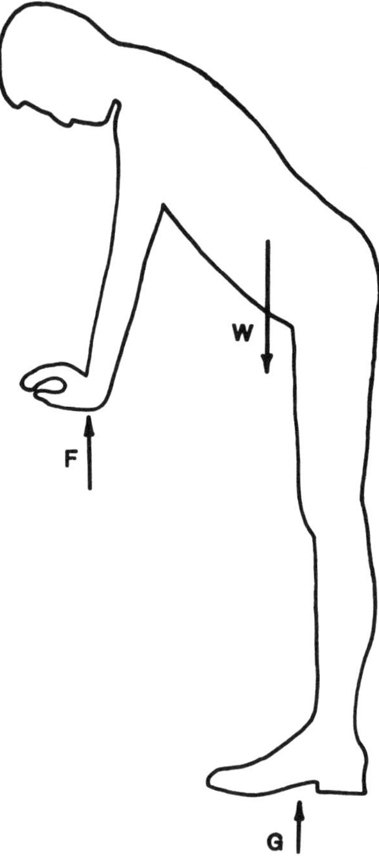

Fig 1–7.—The forces that act on a therapist performing spinal mobilization or palpation are body weight (W), the ground reaction force (G), and the reaction to the force applied to the patient (*F*). (From Keating J, Matyas TA, Bach TM: *Phys Ther* 73:38–46, 1993. Courtesy of Wong M: Postgraduate diploma dissertation. Melbourne, Victoria, Australia, La Trobe University, 1981.)

1 month afterward, the subjects were tested for their ability to produce these forces to the lumbar spines of healthy subjects on command, as measured by a force platform (Fig 1–7).

Results.—The trained group showed reduced error in force production at both post-training assessments (Fig 1–8). At the latter assessment, they were also more accurate in applying specific forces to the scales used in training.

Conclusion.—Physical therapists can be trained to produce specified forces during lumbar passive accessory intervertebral movement. They can also produce selected forces from a spectrum of 1–25 kp. The training described in this experiment can develop an appreciation of the external scale associated with the forces they apply.

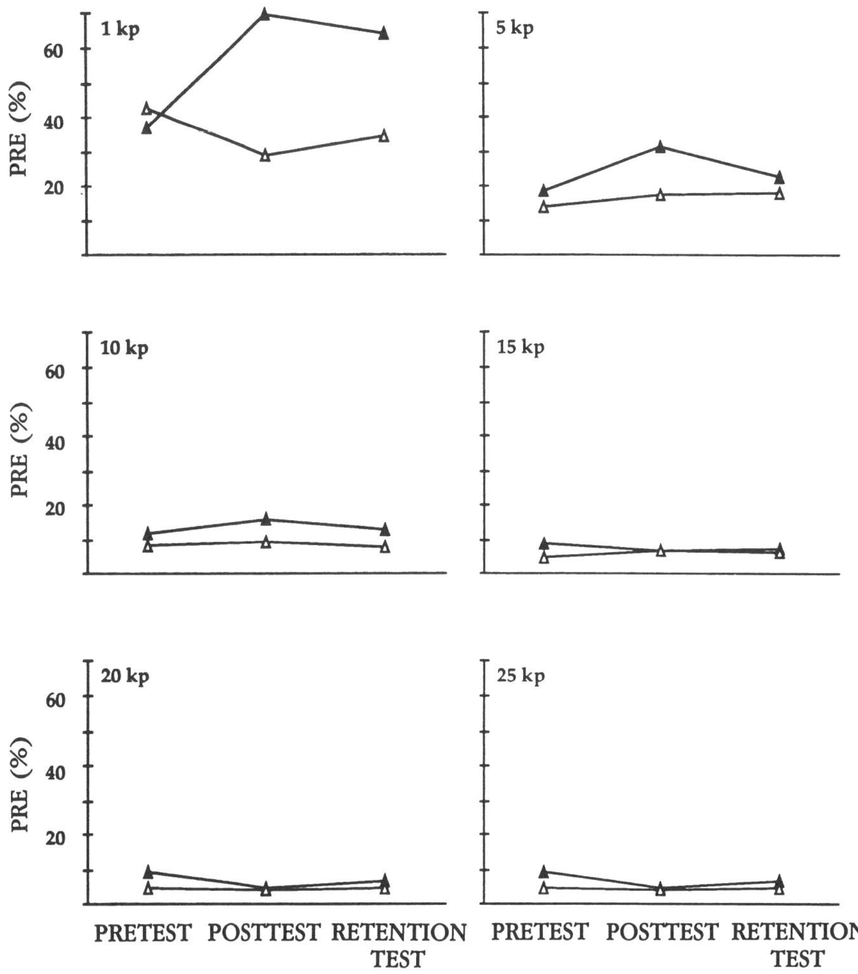

Fig 1–8.—Percentage random error (PRE) score at each force for control group (*filled triangles*) and experimental group (*open triangles*) at pretest, post-test, and retention test of performance on the lumbar spine. (Courtesy of Keating J, Matyas TA, Bach TM: *Phys Ther* 73:38–46, 1993.)

▶ One of the very real problems facing researchers investigating manipulative technique is how to accurately reproduce forces during palpatory or adjustive procedures. Research is made more difficult when the forces generated by a participant in these studies cannot be reliably repeated. One could never properly assess the effect of the procedure, because the question of force would also be a bias, i.e., if we alter the force, would that create a different outcome? Training and practice thereby becomes one means to decrease that bias.—D.J. Lawrence, D.C.

The Effect of Manipulation on Pain and Range of Motion in the Cervical Spine: A Pilot Study

Cassidy JD, Quon JA, Lafrance LJ, Yong-Hing K (Royal Univ Hosp, Saskatoon, Sask, Canada; Canadian Mem Chiropractic College, Toronto)

J Manipulative Physiol Ther 15:495–500, 1992 1–12

Objective.—Although different types of therapy, including spinal manipulation, are used for neck pain, there are insufficient clinical studies into their efficacy and effects. The number of patients needed for a randomized, controlled trial of spinal manipulation for neck pain was ascertained, and whether there is a relationship between pain and range of motion in the cervical spine was determined.

Methods.—The study sample comprised 50 consecutive outpatients with unilateral neck pain and radiation into the trapezius muscle. All subjects were otherwise in good health with no neurologic deficit. Before and after a single spinal manipulation treatment, the patients underwent measurement of cervical range of motion on a goniometer and rating of pain intensity on a 101-point numeric scale.

Results.—Thirty-seven patients had improvement in pain after spinal manipulation. The mean pain score decreased from 43.7 to 31.1. Range of motion increased in all planes, particularly in ipsilateral rotation. The decrease in pain was significantly related to the increase in ipsilateral and contralateral rotation.

Conclusion.—Although this noncontrolled study cannot prove the efficacy of spinal manipulation for neck pain, it does show a correlation between increased cervical rotation and decreased pain. The outcome measures used may be useful in the design of the future controlled studies.

▶ Although this is only a pilot study, the authors have addressed an area in need of additional study. The literature has become quite supportive of the benefits derived from manipulation for the management of low back pain. Chiropractic needs to demonstrate the efficacy of spinal manipulation for the treatment of conditions other than low back pain. Addressing the cervical area would be a natural extension of the work on the low back and would also be consistent with the types of conditions commonly seen in chiropractic practice.

A pilot study is not designed to formulate definitive answers to research questions but, rather, the presence of meaningful correlations may point the direction for fruitful future research efforts. This study certainly indicates the potential value for future clinical controlled studies in the management of cervical spine problems.—R.B. Phillips, D.C., Ph.D.

Soft Tissue Effects of Sacroiliac and Lumbosacral Joint Manipulation
Schneider MJ (Pittsburgh, Pa)
Chiroprac Tech 4:136–142, 1992 1–13

Background.—Within the chiropractic profession, it is generally believed that specific adjustments are more effective than nonspecific manipulations. Variables, including doctor and patient positioning, torque, and speed and depth of thrust, among others, are considered during chiropractic manipulation. Through modification of these variables, the chiropractor attempts to deliver a manipulative thrust over a specific joint in a specific direction. However, the force of any manipulative thrust must first pass through several layers of muscles and ligaments before affecting the deeper joint surfaces. These tissues absorb a great deal of the manipulative force, altering the force vectors before the joint surface is reached. Despite this, limited information is available regarding the role

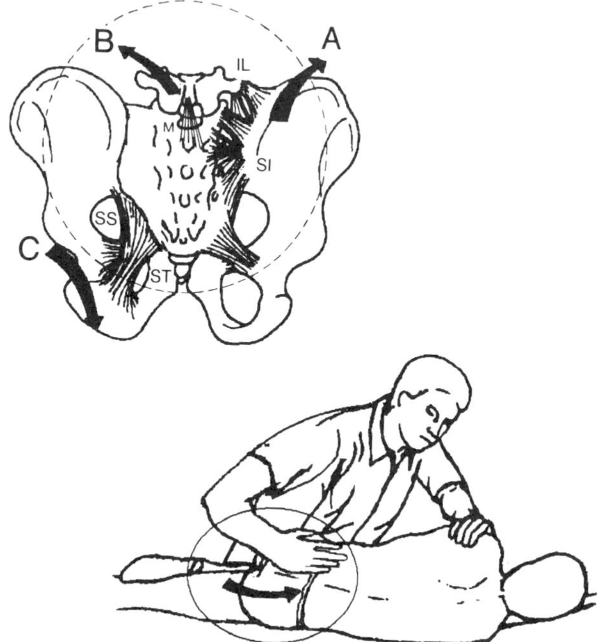

Fig 1–9.—Analysis of various side posture manipulations. The common "lumbar roll" position, which is used for manipulations of the lumbrosacral and sacroilial joints. The *circular inset* depicts the various sites for manipulative thrusts and the associated soft tissue effects. **A,** thrust on the PSIS or iliac crest may cause motion in the lumbrosacral joint through tension on the iliolumbar ligament (*IL*). **B,** thrust on the spinous or mamillary process will pull on the contralateral multifidus muscle (*M*). **C,** thrust on the ischial tuberosity may cause motion in the lumbrosacral joint through tension in the sacrotuberous (*ST*) and sacrosiatic (*ST*) or sacrosiatic (*SS*) ligaments. Note that if the sacroiliac ligament (*SI*) or sacroiliac joint itself has undergone fibrosis, any force applied to the innominates may move the pelvis as a unit upon the lumbrosacral joint, rather than cause motion in the sacroiliac joint. (Courtesy of Schneider MJ: *Chiroprac Tech* 4:136–142, 1992.)

of muscles and ligments during spinal manipulation. Some possible biomechanical effects on the paravertebral soft tissues during spinal manipulation were described.

Discussion.—The side posture lumbar roll is a commonly used technique for manual manipulation of the lumbar facet and sacroiliac joints. Many variations and modifications of side posture are available that permit the chiropractor to specifically direct the manipulative thrust over certain joints. For example, when specifically adjusting the right upper sacroiliac joint, the thrust would generally be on the right posterior superior iliac spine (PSIS) or right sacral base. When the right L4–5 or L5–S1 facet joints are specifically adjusted, a spinous or mamillary thrust would be used. Alternate methods of adjusting the sacroiliac joint include thrust on the PSIS or ischial tuberosity, instead of the sacral base. However, these techniques may also cause concurrent motion in the lumbar facet joints. During PSIS contact, the force of the thrust can cause tension in the iliolumbar ligament and lower fibers of the quadratus lumborum muscle. As a result, motion in the lower lumbar facet joints may be created, because of their attachments to the L4 and L5 transverse processes. During thrusts to the ischial tuberosity, the sacrotuberous and sacrosciatic ligaments may be tensed, causing the sacral apex to be pulled anteriorly along with the ischium. As the sacral apex moves anteriorly, the sacral base moves posteriorly, creating motion at the L5–S1 facet joint (Fig 1–9).

Implications.—Most joint manipulation is probably not as specific as was once believed. It cannot be determined whether a manipulative thrust delivered over the right sacral base or PSIS is actually causing motion in the right sacroiliac joint, rather than the lower lumbar spine, or whether a therapeutic effect is achieved by stretching the ligaments and muscles that traverse the region. After adjustment, the patient may experience great relief from acute low back pain. However, this does not necessarily mean the clinician moved the right sacroiliac joint.

Conclusion.—Further studies on the role of paravertebral soft tissues in joint manipulation are suggested.

▶ Dr. Schneider questions whether a specific or nonspecific adjustment is more clinically effective, and while he prefers to be as specific as possible, he notes that any adjustment must affect several layers of muscular and ligamentous structures before it can affect bone. That muscular and ligamentous anatomy is discussed here, and Dr. Schneider offers several procedures that create differing effects on those structures. Here we have a reminder of the import of those structures in the overall adjustive process.—D.J. Lawrence, D.C.

The Immediate Effect of Manipulation Versus Mobilization on Pain and Range of Motion in the Cervical Spine: A Randomized Controlled Trial

Cassidy JD, Lopes AA, Yong-Hing K (Royal Univ Hosp, Saskatoon, Sask, Canada; Canadian Mem Chiropractic College, Toronto)
J Manipulative Physiol Ther 15:570–575, 1992 1–14

Background.—Neck pain with limited mobility affects 40% to 50% of the general population at some point in their lives. Two common manual methods used to treat neck pain include mobilization and spinal manipulation. Typically, mobilization consists of assisted passive or active maneuvers applied by the active and passive range of motion of the spine. Spinal manipulation involves a high-velocity, low-amplitude thrust directed beyond the spine's passive range of motion. Manipulation is also associated with an audible crack, caused by cavitation of the underlying facet joint, and is considered by some to be a more traumatic intervention than mobilization. The immediate effects of mobilization and

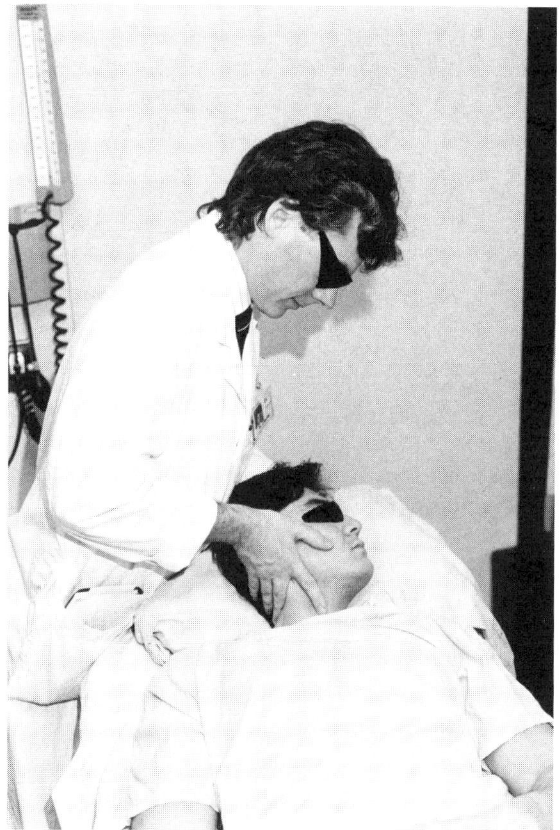

Fig 1–10.—A demonstration of cervical manipulation. (Courtesy of Cassidy JD, Lopes AA, Yong-Hing K: *J Manipulative Physiol Ther* 15:570–575, 1992.)

spinal manipulation on pain and range of motion were compared in patients with neck pain.

Patients and Methods.—A total of 100 consecutive outpatients experiencing unilateral mechanical neck pain with radiation into the trapezius muscle were studied. Of these, 48 participants received mobilization in the form of a muscle energy technique, and 52 received a single rotational manipulation (Fig 1–10). The mean patient ages were 37.7 and 34.5 years, respectively, for the mobilization and manipulation groups. No significant between-group differences were noted in terms of neck pain history or disability levels, as measured by the Pain Disability Index. Cervical spine range of motion was recorded in 3 planes both before and immediately after the treatment, and pain intensity was assessed using the 101-point numerical rating scale.

Results.—Range of motion was increased after both mobilization and manipulation treatment. However, manipulation had a significantly greater effect on pain intensity. Pain improvement was reported immediately after treatment by 85% of the manipulated patients and by 69% of those who were mobilized, although the decrease in pain intensity was more than 1.5 times higher in the manipulated group.

Conclusion.—In patients with mechanical neck pain, a single manipulation treatment is more effective in decreasing pain than mobilization. However, further studies are necessary to determine if there are any long-term benefits from spinal manipulation therapy.

▶ Patients who received manipulation responded better than those who were mobilized. The contrast between manipulation and mobilization was that the former involved a high-amplitude thrust, whereas the latter was a more generalized movement procedure. One point to note is that only a single manipulation or mobilization was provided the patient, so it is not possible to determine long-term effects through this study. The authors postulate that the manipulation exerts its effect via reflex mechanisms involving joint proprioceptors and muscle spindle, but this remains subject to debate.—D.J. Lawrence, D.C.

A Rationale for the Treatment of Back Pain and Joint Pain by Manual Therapy

Twomey LT (Curtin Univ of Technology, Perth, Western Australia, Australia)

Phys Ther 72:885–892, 1992 1–15

Background.—Insufficient pathogenic knowledge and diagnostic uncertainty make the treatment of back pain a largely empirical proposition. Recent advances, however, have increased understanding of the effects of physical and manual therapy on the spine. The current rationale explaining the success of manual therapy was studied.

Effects of Movements and Exercise.—Exercise has been shown to be essential for maintenance of muscle bulk and bone mass. Back and joint pain respond positively and negatively to rest. The experience with physical therapy treatment of athletes has led to the development of aggressive physical therapy and work conditioning for the treatment of chronic back pain. The therapist must understand the effects of exercise on all parts of the musculoskeletal system to optimize the benefits of manual therapy for back pain and dysfunction.

The health of the spinal joints relies on repeated, low-stress movements, as the intervertebral disks and facet joints require movement for the transfer of fluid and nutrients. Although exercise does not reduce the number of episodes of back pain, it makes sure the patient can cope with the problem, recover more quickly, and have an improved quality of life.

Effects on Bone and Muscle.—Some controlled studies have documented the lifelong need of bone and muscle for exercise. Exercise has been shown to increase bone mineral content and total body calcium in elderly women. In other studies, the bone gain of exercise has been shown to be specific for site and type of exercise, with weight lifters having the greatest bone density and swimmers having the least. Although regular exercise helps maintain skeletal health in both sexes, it is especially important in women after menopause, when involutional bone loss occurs as the result of hormone deficiencies.

Spinal Manipulation of Spinal Lesions.—In most cases of back pain, the cause of the spinal lesion and the mechanism of the effect of spinal manipulation are unknown. Spinal manipulation does not appear to work by reducing subluxations, correcting vertebral alignment, adjusting nuclear prolapse, or tearing joint adhesions. In certain cases of acute, painful locked back syndrome, spinal manipulation does appear to have a truly mechanical effect. Some neurophysiologic explanations for the success of spinal manipulation have been offered, including an inhibitory effect on reflex muscle spasm. The same author posits the presence of a hysteresis or delayed effect of neural discharge in joint afferents after repetitive end-range passive movement. Another hypothesis suggests that the effects of manipulation may be related to a mechanical compromise of neural tissue and axoplasmic flow.

Summary.—Movement and exercise are central to the lifelong maintenance of the musculoskeletal system. Manual therapy uses movement, stress, and loading to the body toward the goal of functional improvement and pain reduction. The mechanisms of its effects are largely a matter of speculation, but increasing evidence suggests a possible biomechanical explanation. Most of the recent advances in the management of back pain are based on intensive, aggressive physical therapy. Customary postures may play an important role in back and regional pain problems.

▶ Dr. Twomey provides ample evidence supporting his contention that movement and exercise comprise the principal tools for treating musculoskeletal complaints. He rejects the concept of subluxation reduction as a means of relieving low back pain, and he notes that this hypothesis has never been proven scientifically. He also rejects the concept of aligning vertebrae, reducing nuclear prolapse, or tearing joint adhesions. I must note that none of his 69 references come from the chiropractic literature, so his rejection may not be supportable. His point, however, is well taken; chiropractors need to do more research to ever hope to establish these concepts, and it may very well be that they will not withstand this testing. So be it.—D.J. Lawrence, D.C.

Treatment of Bell's Palsy by Mechanical Force, Manually Assisted Chiropractic Adjusting and High-Voltage Electrotherapy
Frach JP, Osterbauer PJ, Fuhr AW (Activator Methods, Inc, Phoenix, Ariz)
J Manipulative Physiol Ther 15:596–598, 1992 1–16

Introduction.—Bell's palsy is a relatively common, unilateral facial paralysis of sudden onset. The cause is unknown, but the mechanism probably includes swelling of the facial nerve as a result of immune deficiency or viral disease. It must be differentiated from other disorders of the facial nerve or its nucleus. Two cases of Bell's palsy were treated by chiropractic methods and high-voltage electrotherapy.

Case 1.—Woman, 18, was seen with a 10-day history of left-sided Bell's palsy, which her medical physician told her would resolve without treatment. She had temporomandibular joint syndrome, soreness of the neck, and loss of taste within a few days after having some cold symptoms. She was unable to raise the eyebrow, her face was sagging, and she had no expression and diminished hearing on the left side. Because the patient was pregnant, no radiographic studies were obtained. She was treated with mechanical force, manually assisted (MFMA) adjustment, and modified high-voltage therapy. She noted improvement within 3 days of her first treatment and was asymptomatic after 5 treatments.

Case 2.—Man, 37, had a 3-week history of Bell's palsy, along with moderate low back pain beginning about 2 weeks previously. He had pain behind the right ear, temporomandibular joint syndrome, neck pain, headache, and cold sensitivity. His expression was flaccid, with inability to close the right eye and moderate atrophy of the right side of the face. He had a positive foraminal compression and shoulder depression and the results of Weber's tests were positive. Radiographic findings were unremarkable except for moderate cervical hypolordosis and rotation of the C2 vertebra. Treatment was with MFMA adjustment, high-voltage therapy, and facial muscle exercises. After 9 treatments, the patient reported 60% to 70% improvement, although he still had some facial pain and right-sided paralysis of the orbicularis oris. He ceased treatment against advice.

Discussion.—Two cases of Bell's palsy managed with MFMA adjustment and high-voltage electrotherapy are presented. This report, rather than representing a rule for chiropractic treatment, provides an initial time-treatment baseline with which to compare the same and other treatment methods.

▶ Use of the Activator Adjusting Instrument remains controversial, although many chiropractors do use it. Its general use is in managing musculoskeletal conditions, although practitioners have broadened it to other, organic, disorders. Many of the procedures need to be tested; few such trials currently exist. Efforts are under way at Activator Methods, Inc., to perform research studies, and several have already been completed. These 2 cases of Bell's palsy treated by the Activator Adjusting Instrument can help to form the basis for a future clinical trial.—D.J. Lawrence, D.C.

The Use of an Eclectic Approach for the Treatment of Low Back Pain: A Case Study

Beattie P (Univ Hosp, Albuquerque, NM)
Phys Ther 72:923–928, 1992 1–17

Introduction.—It is difficult to establish the effectiveness of manual therapy techniques that are widely used on patients with low back pain (LBP). Previous efforts have focused on identifying movement positional faults, or quality of movement rather than identifying impairments and their link to disability by testable hypotheses. An examination approach that met this goal was presented, and eclectic treatment approach to a patient with LBP was described.

Case Report.—Man, 22, who competed as a pole vaulter on the international level, complained of chronic central midlumbar pain and stiffness that impaired his performance during the take-off phase. The pain had recently forced him to stop training. He also complained of pain when sitting for longer than 45 minutes.

On physical examination, he appeared to have stiffness or hypomobility of spinal motion segments of L2–3 and L3–4, and it was hypothesized that this hypomobility and pain were preventing the patient from achieving an adequate active range of trunk motion to perform the take-off phase. To restore lumbar backward bending without pain or stiffness, posterior-anterior pressure was applied to the spinous processes of L2–4 in an oscillating fashion, as described by Maitland. This was done for 2 repetitions of about 90 seconds each, to the maximum pressure that did not elicit pain. Lumbar extension exercises, or prone press-ups, were also prescribed. To modify the patient's habit of frequent, prolonged, unsupported sitting, he was given a lumbar roll to use behind his lower back whenever he was seated.

Reexamination and reapplication of oscillations resulted in full, pain-free lumbar extension at the end of a second physical therapy session. Although it is difficult to determine the relative efficacy of the various treatments used, and the joint mobilization procedures may have been useful, the key factor was probably his reported behavioral changes. These included frequent performance of extension exercises and correction of his habitual sitting posture. Failure to address this posture may have accounted for his inability to achieve symptom reduction during a previous course of chiropractic treatment.

Discussion.—The examination process described in this athlete identified his impairments and related them to his disabilities. Treatment was based on a qualitative assessment, and outcome was judged by the patient's disability. This eclectic approach achieved the treatment goals in 2 physical therapy sessions.

► Even though physical therapists acknowledge that research lags behind practice in the use of manipulative procedures, they are using them more and more often in handling their patients. The examination procedures used in this case are similar to those used by chiropractors, but there was failure to use any motion palpation procedure. Static palpation for pain was done, as was assessment of active range of motion and leg length. Interestingly, the diagnosis offered by the physical therapist here was "hypomobility" of L2–L4 (with the use of the quotation marks printed in the text). This diagnosis may be hard to confirm without the necessary motion testing that most chiropractors would perform. The patient in this case had previously seen a chiropractor but failed to respond to therapy. The reason for this response failure, as suggested by the author, was that the patient sits in a position of spinal flexion for long periods, which McKenzie believes predisposes to chronic spinal stiffness. We are not provided any information about the chiropractic workup. Given the amount of research now available, motion testing should be a standard part of a disgnostic workup for spinal conditions.—D.J. Lawrence, D.C.

Intertester Reliability of Judgments of the Presence of Trigger Points in Patients With Low Back Pain

Nice DA, Riddle DL, Lamb RL, Mayhew TP, Rucker K (Virginia Commonwealth Univ, Richmond)

Arch Phys Med Rehabil 73:893–898, 1992 1–18

Background.—Trigger points, hyperirritable areas in soft tissue that produce a predictable pattern of pain when palpated by the examiner, have been proposed as one of the sources of pain symptoms reported by some patients with low back pain. The patterns of pain and body diagrams defined by Travell and Simons are frequently used by clinicians

Intertester Reliability for Judgments of the Presence of Trigger Points When Therapists Used Correct Technique and Patients Reported Pain Immediately Before Examination

Trigger Point	n	Kappa (SE)	Percent Agreement	Ppos	Pneg
A	23	.25 (.24)	70	.46	.79
B	25	.42 (.23)	80	.56	.87
C	20	.38 (.21)	70	.62	.75

(Courtesy of Nice DA, Riddle DL, Lamb RL, et al: *Arch Phys Med Rehabil* 73:893–898, 1992.)

examining patients with low back pain for the presence of trigger points. The intertester reliability of assessments of the presence of trigger points was determined in 50 patients with low back pain who were examined by 12 physical therapists.

Method.—Randomly paired therapists examined the patients for 3 of the trigger points described by Travell and Simons. A total of 197 trigger point examinations were considered appropriate for study based on the zones of reference described by Travell and Simons. The Kappa coefficient, percent agreement, the observed proportion of positive agreement (Ppos), and the observed proportion of negative agreement (Pneg) were used to describe reliability.

Findings.—Low Kappa coefficients demonstrated poor intertester reliability even though a high percentage of agreement between raters was found for most measurements. The percent agreement of .79 was considered high but chance agreement is also high at .69. The low Kappa and Ppos values suggest that therapists cannot reliably determine when a trigger point is present in a patient with low back pain. Incorrect patient positioning or incorrect palpation techniques, varying amounts of force or amounts of time at a trigger point, or the presence of pain may have contributed to poor reliability (table).

Conclusion.—An assessment of intertester reliability of judments of the presence of trigger points found poor reliability evidenced by low Kappa and Ppos values. On the basis of this poor reliability, the usefulness of examining for the presence of trigger points in patients with low back pain should be questioned.

▶ Several therapists were unable to reliably locate a number of trigger points in a series of patients. A number of explanations can be offered: (1) the level of therapist training may have varied; (2) patient positioning may have been incorrect; (3) pain levels may have varied; and (4) even trigger points may not have been present where the researchers thought they were. In any clinical diagnostic procedure, the levels of concordance and reliability will not be close to perfect; therefore, the authors' recommendation to not use trigger point assessment procedures in patients with low back pain cannot be supported. No single experiment should lead to the wholesale deletion of a widespread clinical assessment tool.—D.J. Lawrence, D.C.

The Reliability of Lumbar Motion Palpation

Panzer DM (Western States Chiropractic College, Portland, Ore)

J Manipulative Physiol Ther 15:518–524, 1992 1–19

Background.—Spinal motion palpation is used by practitioners of manipulation and mobilization as a means of diagnosing intervertebral joint dysfunction. Significant palpable hypomobility is a key component of identifying a motion segment appropriate for treatment with manipulation. However, findings based on motion palpation techniques have not been shown to correspond to specific clinical syndromes, and clinical trials of manipulation have not used palpatory findings to monitor spinal changes. Furthermore, a survey of the literature on reliability studies of lumbar motion palpation has revealed marginal-to-poor interexaminer reliability.

Method.—Studies pertaining to intraexaminer and interexaminer reliability of lumbar motion palpation identified from database and manual searching were reviewed along with relevant articles identified through the bibliographic references of the retrived articles. Of particular interest in the literature review were statistical analysis, subject selection, method of palpation, and sources of error.

Findings.—Multiple variations in type of palpation, the subjects examined, statistical analysis, and experience of the examiners were noted (table). Most studies demonstrated marginal to poor interexaminer reliability and good-to-moderate intraexaminer reliability.

Recommendations.—In a 1983 review of motion palpation, Alley cited 3 requisites for the validation of motion palpation: (1) accurate techniques of motion palpation offering interexaminer reliability exist; (2) such techniques are related to underlying motion abnormalities; and (3) the underlying movement abnormalities may be associated with pathologic changes and not simply normal variation. There are several suggestions for future research: (1) using representative chiropractic patients; (2) applying motion palpation to clinical decision making and patient monitoring; (3) further developing of multiple diagnostic test regimens; (4) identifying any association between palpatory findings and specific clinical syndromes or pathologic change; (5) identifying the most reliable motion palpation test(s); and (6) improving standardization of palpatory techniques and established threshold values.

▶ Dr. Panzer reviews the literature on motion palpation and finds that it comes up short in measures of reliability. Because motion palpation is one of

Summary of Lumbar Motion Palpation Reliability Studies

Author/date	Type of exam	Examiners	Subjects	Statistical Analysis	Reliability reported
Gonella et al (1982)	Side-lying passive ROM	5 PTs, 3-20 yr experience	5 pts students	None	Intertherapist poor Intra - "reasonably good"
Larsson (1984)	Sitting passive	3 DC students 1 new DC	32 asymptomatic students	% agreement only	Inter - 56% agreement Intra - 74% agreement
Grant & Spadon (1985)	Prone passive laterna flexion joint play	4 DC interns	60 DC students	% agreement only	Inter - 67% agreement Intra - 88% agreement
Bergstrom & Courtis (1986)	Sitting passive laterna flexion joint play	2 DC students	100 DC students	% agreement only	Inter - 82% agreement Intra - 95% agreement
Love & Brodeur (1987)	Sitting "scanning" for most hypo-mobile	8 senior DC students	32 DC students	Pearson's	Inter - not significant beyond chance Intra-significant ($p < .05$)
Jull & Bullock (1987)	Side-lying passive ROM prone joint play	2 PT manipulative therapists	inter-10 intra-20 asymptomatic adults	Pearson's	Inter - significant $r = .82$ to $r = .94$ intra - significant $r = .81$ to $r = .98$

(Continued.)

Table *(continued)*

Boline et al. (1988)	Sitting end-feel	1 DC intern 1 new DC	50: 23 symptomatic 27 asymptomatic	Kappa	Inter - significant only at T12-L1 (K = 0.031, $p < .005$) and L3-4 (K = 0.31, $p < .01$)
			23 back pain patients only	Kappa	Inter - significant only at T12-L1 (K = 0.32, $p < .05$) and L3-4 (K = 0.33, $p < .05$)
Mootz et al. (1989)	Sitting end-feel	2 DCs 7 and 10 yr experience	60 DC students mostly asymptomatic	Kappa	Inter - not significant Intra - significant L1-2, L4-5 only
Leboeuf et al. (1989)	Passive ROM	4 DC students	45 chronic low back pain (mean duration 11.05 $\pm$ 2.1 years)	Z-test	Inter - "generally good" ($p < .05$) Intra - significant ($p < .05$)
Keating et al. (1990)	Sitting end-feel	3 DCs, 10, 5 and 2.4 yr experience	21 symptomatic patients 25 asymptomatic DC students	Kappa	Inter - not consistently significant

(Courtesy of Panzer DM: *J Manipulative Physiol Ther* 15:518–524, 1992.)

the most common chiropractic procedures, this gives chiropractors pause. There are only a limited number of studies that examine motion palpation, and a much greater amount of work has to be done to establish its use in the clinical setting. Although there is an impressive body of theoretical knowledge surrounding motion palpation, its clinical support is lagging. Until it has better foundational support, its use should be in conjunction with other, more established procedures.—D.J. Lawrence, D.C.

MASSAGE

Massage Reduces Anxiety in Child and Adolescent Psychiatric Patients

Field T, Morrow C, Valdeon C, Larson S, Kuhn C, Schanberg S (Univ of Miami, Fla; Duke Univ, Durham, NC)
J Am Acad Child Adolesc Psychiatry 31:125–131, 1992 1–20

Background.—Emotional disturbances, such as depression and adjustment disorder, are typically associated with anxiety, muscle tension, increased cortisol levels, and sleep disturbances. The independent effects of massage on the behaviors and physiology of children and adolescents hospitalized for depression or adjustment disorder were assessed.

Methods.—Forty boys and 32 girls, 7–18 years of age, were enrolled in the study. Massage was chosen as an intervention because of concern about touch deprivation in hospitalized children. The intervention consisted of a 30-minute back massage daily for 5 days. The control group viewed a relaxing videotape during the same periods.

Findings.—Children in the massage group were less depressed and anxious than children in the control group. The massage group also had lower saliva cortisol levels after massage. In addition, nurses rated these children as being less anxious and more cooperative on the final day of the study. Nighttime sleep also increased during this period. In depressed children, urinary cortisol and norepinephrine levels were reduced.

Conclusion.—The findings, consistent with those of other relaxation therapy studies, suggest that anxiety and depression are reduced just after treatment sessions. Patients' self-reported anxiety and depression scores dropped significantly after massage sessions. Massage treatment also produced longer term effects.

▶ Chiropractic has long held that physical contact is an important part of the healing process. This study supports this premise by demonstrating how 30-minute massage, applied to depressed and adjustment-disordered children, resulted in a decrease of anxiety levels and decreased levels of urinary cortisol and nonepinephrine production. These results would directly support the use of massage as an adjunct to regular chiropractic care.—R.B. Phillips, D.C., Ph.D

Physical Procedures

EXERCISE

Cost-Effectiveness of a Back School Intervention for Municipal Employees

Brown KC, Sirles AT, Hilyer JC, Thomas MJ (Univ of Alabama, Birmingham; City of Birmingham, Ala)

Spine 17:1224–1228, 1992 1–21

Background.—Workers who lack sufficient strength or fitness for their jobs are most likely to experience low back injury. Among workers in the U.S., this type of injury is the leading cause of compensable injury (at a cost of $16 billion annually); it also is the major cause of job-related absenteeism. Because of the escalating costs associated with low back injuries, several previous cost-related studies have been conducted. However, they have been flawed by a lack of randomization and small sample sizes. Thus, pre- and post-test studies were conducted to investigate the costs of a back school intervention for municipal employees.

Methods.—One hundred forty municipal employees who had low-back injuries participated in this study. Of these, 70 received mandatory back school treatment, and 70 randomly selected injured employees served as a comparison group. The back school treatment consisted of 6 weeks of strength and flexibility exercises and 30-minute classes held 4

Preintervention Differences Between Back School Participants and Comparison Groups

	Mean+			
	Back School n=70	Comparison n=70	t	P
Lost work time	.63	.36	3.07	.003 †
Lost time cost	2.10	1.75	2.46	.015 *
Medical cost	2.09	1.82	1.70	.091
Total cost	2.34	1.10	2.06	.042 *
No. of injuries	.57	.54	.34	.737

* $P < .05$.
† $P < .01$.
Cost variables transformed to logarithms.
Number of injuries transformed to square root.
(Courtesy of Brown KC, Sirles AT, Hilyer JC, et al: *Spine* 17:1224–1228, 1992.)

days per week on topics related to back care. The educational classes covered such topics as the function of the spine, ergonomics, control of pain, relaxation, and weight control.

Results.—Although the distribution between treatment and comparison groups was similar, street and sanitation workers not only comprised the largest group of participants, but they historically had the largest number of back injuries. Independent tests were performed on the dependent variables to evaluate equivalence before intervention. Medical costs and the number of injuries were equivalent between the 2 groups. However, the groups differed significantly in lost work time and lost-time costs (table). The greatest time loss and lost-time costs were found among the group that received the back school treatment. Its costs were almost 4 times as great. A 1-tailed analysis of covariance revealed that the back school group had significantly fewer injuries. Paired t tests on pre-post differences among the back school group showed that pre-post differences were significantly decreased for all the dependent measures and that no significant pre-post differences existed on any dependent measures for the comparison group. These findings indicate the effectiveness of the back school intervention.

Conclusion.—A key finding was that reinjury among the back school participants was half that of nonparticipants. This reduction in injuries benefited the city in actual dollars saved, while it increased the quality of life for the treatment participants. Research is still being conducted, and methodology problems are being resolved by randomly assigning employees who are injured to either the treatment group or the control group.

▶ Back schools represent increasingly successful means to manage costs and care in treating low back pain. The procedures used by the back school in this study consisted of 6 weeks of exercises for strength and flexibility, along with a series of educational programs covering all aspects of back care. This study involved a variety of municipal workers, such as streets and sanitation workers, police, parks and recreation workers, etc. A comparison group was also studied as a control. Implementation of back schools in the municipal setting helps to decrease the incidence of injury as well as keep costs down. In the current environment of health-care reform, such savings carry health policy implications.—D.J. Lawrence, D.C.

Psychobiologic Responses to Exercise at Different Times of Day

O'Connor PJ, Davis JC (Arizona State Univ, Tempe)

Med Sci Sports Exerc 24:714–719, 1992 1–22

Background.—Behavioral and biological rhythms (e.g., the circadian rhythm) have implications for health and disease ranging from the occurrence of life-threatening events to the effectiveness of therapeutic regimens. Although data are available on circadian variation in athletic performance and its physiologic concomitants, the potential overall health consequences of exercising at different times of the day have not been investigated as fully. Whether selected psychological responses to acute submaximal running exercise depend on the time of day that exercise is initiated was determined.

Method.—Twelve volunteer adult males were evaluated with the Eysenck Personality Questionnaire, Morningness-Eveningness Questionnaire, Spielberger's State-Trait Anger Expression Inventory and State-Trait Anxiety Inventory. All 12 volunteers scored within the normal range on the traits assessed and were not classified as either "morning" or "evening" types based on the Morningness-Eveningness Questionnaire. The 12 men were randomly assigned to 4 bouts of submaximal exercise at 8 AM, noon, 4 PM, and 8 PM on 4 subsequent days. State anxiety, state anger, blood pressure, and heart rate were assessed 10 minutes before and 10 and 20 minutes after exercise bouts.

Findings.—The mood improvements and cardiovascular changes were independent of the time of day that exercise was performed, with adjustments for differences in initial values across the 4 time-of-day conditions. Multivariate analyses of variance demonstrated significant main effects for the trial factor for state anxiety, state anger, systolic blood pressure, and heart rate. State anxiety, state anger, and systolic blood pressure were all significantly reduced at 10 and 20 minutes post exercise. At 20 minutes post exercise, the heart rate was lower than at 10 minutes post exercise, but it was still higher than preexercise values.

Conclusion.—The selected affective benefits of acute exercise were independent of the time of day that the exercise bout was completed. There is no optimum time of day to engage in exercise.

▶ Should our patients exercise in the morning or in the evening? Which is more beneficial? This study addressed that question by having 12 adult male volunteers exercise at 4 different times during the day on 4 subsequent days. Using a series of personality questionnaires, all 12 subjects were shown that they were neither a "morning" person nor an "evening" person. The questionnaires were administered and blood-pressure measures taken after the exercise periods. The authors were unable to show that exercising during any particular time of the day had any optimum benefit. One must wonder how the results might have looked if the 12 subjects had been shown to be either a "morning" or an "evening" person.—R.B. Phillips, D.C., Ph.D.

Exercise-Induced Analgesia: Fact or Artifact?

Padawer WJ, Levine FM (Lenox Hill Hosp, NY; State Univ of New York, Stony Brook)

Pain 48:131–135, 1992 1–23

Background.—Anecdotal evidence and the theory that exercise releases endorphins that in turn reduce pain have led to the belief that exercise-induced analgesia (EIA) is an established phenomenon. However, anecdotal reports are no substitute for carefully controlled experiments. The experimental support for EIA is surprisingly weak. Exercise-induced analgesia was tested for, controlling both the effects of exercise and of pain testing.

Methods.—The 2-part study was designed to test whether previous findings of analgesia were induced by the exercise procedures or by the stress of the pain testing procedures themselves. In part 1, post-test cold pressor pain ratings were obtained from college student volunteers after exercise on a bicycle and 2 control tasks—minimal and no exercise. There were no significant between-group differences. In part 2 of the study, exercise and nonexercise groups preexposed to cold pressor pain testing were compared with subjects without such preexposure. Exercise had no significant effects. However, there were significant analgesic effects for pain test preexposure.

Conclusion.—No analgesic effect for exercise was found, but such an effect for the pain testing itself occurred. Pain pretesting, regardless of subsequent activity, resulted in significantly lower post-test pain ratings.

▶ It is not uncommon to hear the phrase: "We need to work through our pain threshold." This study questions the validity of such a statement. Exercised and nonexercised groups were compared for pain thresholds measured by lengthy immersion of the hand in cold water. There were no significant differences between the 2 groups. When pain testing was done before and after exercising, there was an increased analgesic effect for all groups. The authors believe the pre-post testing procedures affected pain perceptions, not exercise. One may question the extent of similarity between how painful it is to put your hand in a cold bucket of water and how painful it is to experience a decrease of pain in a muscle during rigorous exercise.—R.B. Phillips, D.C., Ph.D.

Passive Exercise System: Effect on Muscle Activity, Strength, and Lean Body Mass

Nafziger NA, Lee SB, Huang SQ (MetroHealth Med Ctr, Cleveland, Ohio; Case Western Reserve Univ, Cleveland, Ohio)

Arch Phys Med Rehabil 73:184–189, 1992 1–24

Background.—Little is known about the effects of passive exercise training in healthy individuals. Muscle activity and the associated changes in strength and lean body mass resulting from a passive exercise program were investigated.

Methods.—Twenty-eight healthy volunteers aged 26 to 44 years participated in the study. Ten volunteered for the control group and 18 were assigned to the experimental group for the 6-week study. Changes in lean body mass were assessed by tetrapolar bioelectric impedance measurements; strength changes were measured by isokinetic strength assessment; and muscle activity was evaluated by surface electromyographic methods.

Findings.—Twenty-four of the 28 subjects completed the study. Reproducible muscle activity was documented in all 3 muscles studied in 2 of 3 preselected exercises. Fusimotor and postural reflexes appeared to explain this involuntary muscle activity. However, there were no significant changes in muscle strength or lean body mass at 6 weeks.

Conclusion.—Involuntary active muscle contractions occurred during passive exercise in this study, but they did not induce a measurable change in lean body mass or strength. Individuals wishing to increase muscle strength or lean body mass should perform activities other than passive exercise.

▶ Getting patients to do their exercises is always a challenge. They often ask whether some machine could do the exercises for them while they sit back and allow the machine to function. This study has shown that, as part of a passive exercise program, involuntary muscle contractions had no effect on changing lean body mass or muscle strength. Sorry, but to obtain the benefit of exercise, we must work. No pain, no gain! This finding is not to be confused with the demonstrable benefit gained from continuous passive movement in the rehabilitation of cartilage in an injured joint.—R.B. Phillips, D.C., Ph.D.

The Effects of a Wobble Board Exercise Training Program on Static Balance Performance and Strength of Lower Extremity Muscles

Balogun JA, Adesinasi CO, Marzouk DK (Obafemi Awolowo Univ, Ile-Ife and Ilesa, Osun State, Nigeria; Texas Woman's Univ, Houston)

Physiotherapy Can 44:23–30, 1992 1–25

Introduction.—There have been several anecdotal reports suggesting that the wobble, or rocker, board can increase ankle range of motion, decrease chronic and recurrent ankle injuries, and strengthen the muscles of the lower extremities. The effects of a 6-week program of wobble board exercise on static balance performance and lower extremity strength were assessed.

Methods.—The study sample comprised 30 healthy young men. The patients were randomized to an experimental group, which performed a graduated wobble board exercise program 3 times a week for 6 weeks, and a control group, which performed no exercise. A cable tensiometer was used to assess maximal isometric contraction of the right knee extensor and flexor and right ankle dorsiflexor and plantar flexor muscles, and the static balance test was performed with the eyes open and closed.

Both assessments were done before training and at the end of the second, fourth, and sixth weeks.

Results.—At the end of 6 weeks, the training group had isometric strength increases of 56.3% in the knee extensors, 58.6% in the knee flexors, 133.1% in the ankle dorsiflexors, and 97.3% in the ankle plantar flexors. Static balance performance also improved, by 201.2% with the eyes open and 58.8% with the eyes closed. No change in either measure was observed in the control group.

Conclusion.—A 6-week program of wobble board exercise can improve the performance and strength of the muscles of the lower extremities in young, healthy subjects. Further studies of patients with musculoskeletal injuries and balance dysfunction are needed. However, the use of wobble board exercise in sedentary subjects is recommended.

▶ Use of a wobble board is becoming increasingly more popular in chiropractic. This study demonstrates impressive gains in isometric contraction of the knee extensors (56%), knee flexors (59%), ankle dorsi flexors (133%), and ankle plantor flexors (97%). Static balance also improved. These changes, in contrast to the lack of change seen in a control group, speak strongly in favor of the effectiveness of this procedure. There is some concern when a 6-week exercise program demonstrates a ± 33% increase in strength in what was a normal healthy male respondent at the beginning of the exercise program. Further research is needed to evaluate the use of this procedure in the population with low back pain.—R.B. Phillips, D.C., Ph.D.

The Use of Thermal Agents to Influence the Effectiveness of a Low-Load Prolonged Stretch

Lentell G, Hetherington T, Eagan J, Morgan M (California State Univ, Fresno; Gulf Coast Physical Therapy Group, Gulfport, Miss; Fresno Community Hosp, Calif; et al)

J Orthop Sports Phys Ther 16:200–207, 1992 1–26

Background.—Increased flexibility is an important goal of physical therapy. The effectiveness of low-load prolonged stretch (LLPS) to promote long-lasting connective tissue elongation is well known. The temperature of the connective tissue has also been determined to influence the amount of stretching that can occur. However, the use of thermal agents to enhance stretching has not been well investigated. Therefore, the clinical effect of superficial application of heat and cold to a shoulder joint during LLPS (Fig 1–11) to increase flexibility was examined.

Study Design.—Ninety-two healthy men were assigned to LLPS, LLPS with heat in the initial phase, LLPS with cold applied in the final phase, LLPS with initial heat and final cold application, or no intervention. The subjects received 3 40-minute treatments in a 5-day period. A follow-up measurement was taken 3 days after the final treatment.

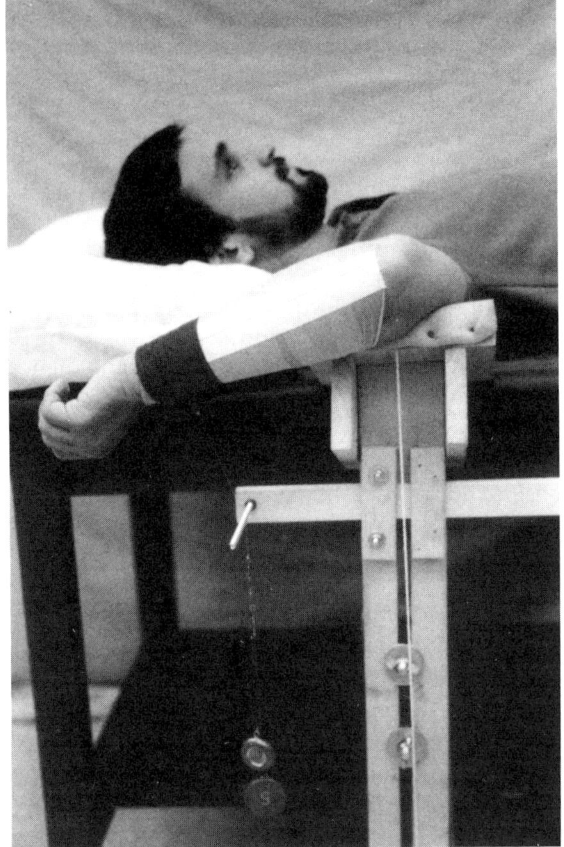

Fig 1–11.—Application of low-load prolonged stretch into shoulder external rotation. (Courtesy of Lentell G, Hetherington T, Eagan J, et al: *J Orthop Sports Phys Ther* 16:200–207, 1992.)

Outcome.—Low-load prolonged stretch treatment, whether associated with heat, ice, both, or nothing, facilitated greater long-term improvements in flexibility compared to those controls with no intervention (table). Only those subjects receiving the LLPS with heat in the initial phase had a significant improvement over those receiving LLPS alone.

Conclusion.—The use of superficial heat in the initial phase of LLPS is a superior method for obtaining lasting improvement in joint flexibility.

▶ Joint stiffness and loss of muscular flexibility are commonly involved in shoulder pathology. Chiropractors will frequently provide patients of such injuries and pathologies a series of exercises to help increase the flexibility of shoulder muscles, which then helps to increase joint motion. Are there ways to augment the action of these exercises? In this study, the use of heat was

Short-Term Gains of ROM by Treatment Sessions

GROUP	SESSION 1	SESSION 2	SESSION 3
A: Stretch Alone	5.6 ± 5.4	8.1 ± 5.4	8.5 ± 5.5
B: Moist Heat + Stretch	10.6 ± 7.1†	11.7 ± 7.3	11.2 ± 5.7
C: Stretch + Ice Pack	6.7 ± 6.2	8.7 ± 6.0	8.9 ± 4.7
D: Moist Heat + Stretch + Ice Pack	8.4 ± 5.6	12.8 ± 6.9 †	11.1 ± 8.0

* Mean ± SD.
† Significant $P \leq .05$ differences found compared to stretch alone group.
(Courtesy of Lentell G, Hetherington T, Eagan J, et al: *J Orthop Sports Phys Ther* 16:200–207, 1992.)

shown to augment the effects of a low-load prolonged stretch to shoulder musculature. For those involved in providing stretching exercises to patients, particularly those in athletics, the combined use of hot moist packs while performing the exercises may be worthy of consideration.—D.J. Lawrence, D.C.

PHYSICAL THERAPY REHABILITATION

Controlled Trial of Balneotherapy in Treatment of Low Back Pain

Konrad K, Tatrai T, Hunka A, Vereckei E, Korondi I (Natl Inst of Rheumatology and Physiotherapy, Budapest, Hungary)

Ann Rheum Dis 51:820–822, 1992 1–27

Introduction.—Low back pain often is a devastating problem, in part because it usually affects individuals in their most productive years. The effects of balneotherapy, underwater traction bath, and underwater massage were assessed in a prospective series of 158 patients with lumbosacral pain, with or without radiation to the thigh. Patients had to have pain for at least 1 month but no longer than 3 months. All had been free of pain for a year before the current episode began.

Treatments.—Balneotherapy involved immersing the group A patients in thermal water. Other patients were massaged by a stream of hot water (group B) or underwent underwater traction (group C) by grasping a bar under the arms, using either their own weight or a traction belt carrying 3 kg on either side.

Results.—Pain scores were significantly reduced in all treatment groups, with no significant difference among the groups. Less analgesia was prescribed after treatment, but there was no significant change in spinal motion. The only effect still evident after 1 year was less analgesic consumption.

Conclusion.—Most patients with low back pain improve without specific treatment. Balneotherapy may speed improvement, but it does not alter the long-term outlook.

▶ Treating patients with low back pain by immersing them in water is a novel approach. This study looked at the effects of being immersed in water, receiving water massage, and receiving traction underwater. This study found underwater therapy to be beneficial as measured by the reduction in the consumption of analgesics. After one year, there was no difference between these patients and similar patients treated in a more typical fashion. If facilities are available, water therapy is generally enjoyed by patients, but investing in the necessary facilities to use this form of therapy may not be justified.—R.B. Phillips, D.C., Ph.D.

The Effect of Local Heat and Cold Therapy on the Intraarticular and Skin Surface Temperature of the Knee

Oosterveld FGJ, Rasker JJ, Jacobs JWG, Overmars HJA (Hosp Medisch Spectrum Twente, Enschede, The Netherlands; Univ Hosp, Utrecht, The Netherlands)

Arthritis Rheum 35:146–151, 1992 1–28

Objective.—The effects of ice chips, ligno-paraffin, short-wave diathermy, and nitrogen-cold air on the skin and intra-articular temperatures were assessed in 42 healthy subjects without a history of knee injury.

TABLE 1.—Changes in Skin Surface Temperatures in the 4 Treatment Groups

Treatment	Baseline * temperature	Minimum/ maximum temperature†	Temperature after 3 hours	Change, minimum/ maximum versus baseline†	Difference from change produced by comparable procedure‡
Cold					
Ice chips	27.9 ± 0.4	11.5 ± 1.1§	25.2 ± 0.3§	−16.4 ± 1.2	1.4
Nitrogen	28.8 ± 0.7	13.8 ± 1.3§	27.5 ± 0.9	−15.0 ± 1.2	
Heat					
Short-wave diathermy	27.6 ± 0.5	30.0 ± 0.5§	27.0 ± 0.5	2.4 ± 0.5	6.5¶
Ligno-paraffin	28.8 ± 0.6	37.7 ± 0.5§	28.8 ± 0.9	8.9 ± 0.4	

* Values are the mean ± SEM degrees centigrade.
† Minimum refers to results with cold treatments; maximum refers to results with heat treatments.
‡ Ice chips compared with nitrogen, or short-wave diathermy compared with ligno-paraffin.
§ $P < .01$.
¶ $P < .001$.
(Courtesy of Oosterveld FGJ, Rasker JJ, Jacobs JWG. et al: *Arthritis Rheum* 35:146–151, 1992.)

TABLE 2.—Changes in Intra-Articular Temperatures in the 4 Treatment Groups

Treatment	Baseline * temperature	Minimum/ maximum temperature†	Temperature after 3 hours	Change, minimum/ maximum versus baseline†	Difference from change produced by comparable procedure‡
Cold					
Ice chips	31.9 ± 0.5	22.5 ± 1.1§	27.5 ± 0.5§	−9.4 ± 0.7	5.3¶
Nitrogen	32.9 ± 0.5	28.8 ± 0.7§	31.0 ± 1.0#	−4.1 ± 0.3	
Heat					
Short-wave diathermy	32.5 ± 0.3**	33.9 ± 0.4§	30.8 ± 0.4§	1.4 ± 0.4	2.1§
Ligno-paraffin	32.5 ± 0.7	36.0 ± 0.4§	32.3 ± 0.9	3.5 ± 0.4	

* Values are the mean ± SEM degrees centigrade.
† Minimum refers to results with cold treatments; maximum refers to results with heat treatments.
‡ Ice chips compared with nitrogen, or short-wave diathermy compared with ligno-paraffin.
§ $P < .01$.
¶ $P < .001$.
|| $P < .05$.
** Calculated as the mean in the other 3 groups.
(Courtesy of Oosterveld FGJ, Rasker JJ, Jacobs JWG. et al:*Arthritis Rheum* 35:146–151, 1992.)

Methods.—A temperature probe was placed in the knee joint cavity, and another was placed on the overlying skin. Temperature changes were recorded over 3 hours in conjunction with application of ice chips for 30 minutes; cooling with nitrogen-cold air at −160°C; 15 minutes of short-wave diathermy to produce a mildly warm feeling; and treatment with ligno-paraffin for 10 minutes.

Results.—The mean skin surface temperature fell more after ice application than with cold air (Table 1), and it increased much more with ligno-paraffin than with short-wave diathermy. Intra-articular temperatures followed the same pattern (Table 2).

Conclusion.—Synovitis might be exacerbated by measures that raise the intra-articular temperature, and controlled by lowering joint temperature through physiotherapy. Local ice or nitrogen-cold air probably is a better treatment for inflammatory joint disease than short-wave diathermy or the use of ligno-paraffin.

▶ This study compared different ways of raising and lowering intra-articular temperatures of the knee. Such procedures are commonly used in the treatment of arthritic joints. Temperatures were measured with a surface and intra-articular temperature probes. Ice was more effective than short-wave diathermy in changing temperatures. The clinical application of these procedures is advocated with cautious concern regarding the underlying etiology and the extent of the pathology at the affected joint.—R.B. Phillips, D.C., Ph.D.

A Physical Approach to the Rehabilitation of Patients Disabled by Chronic Low Back Pain

Edwards BC, Zusman M, Hardcastle P, Twomey L, O'Sullivan P, McLean N (Brian C Edwards & Associates; Perth, Western Australia; Curton Univ, Shenton Park, Western Australia; Royal Perth Rehabilitation Hosp, Shenton Park, Western Australia)

Med J Aust 156:167–172, 1992 1–29

Background.—Although most episodes of acute back pain are self-limiting and respond well to a wide range of treatments, a significant number of individuals eventually become chronically disabled by low back pain. The outcome of a multidisciplinary, physically based program for such patients was investigated.

Methods.—The Spinal Injury Rehabilitation Programme (SIRO), operating in Western Australia since 1987, consists of mobilizing physiotherapy, isokinetic testing, physical reconditioning, work hardening, and psychological testing. Rehabilitation was carried out 7 hours a day, 5 days a week for 4 weeks. Fifty-four patients, all medically referred, participated in the program. Although no specific exclusion criteria were used, all participants were not working and had not responded previously to therapy.

Findings.—Thirty of the 54 patients, or 55%, who completed the program in its first year returned to work, and they were still working at the 1-year follow-up. No firm indicators of successful outcome for participants on study entry could be identified. Participants who returned to work had a marked improvement in the physical parameters measured and a substantial reduction in low back pain.

Conclusion.—A rehabilitation program such as SIRP has an important role in rehabilitating patients with chronic low back pain. Selection criteria for successful rehabilitation have to be established.

▶ The role of rehabilitation in the management of low back pain is becoming more popular. Research-based evidence supporting the rehabilitation approach is becoming more common. Concerns include the process of patient selection, indicating that some causes of back pain will be more receptive than others. Defining what is included in the rehabilitation program is also important. There is a wide variety of machines, exercises, and various programs that are all included under the ruberic of rehabilitation. The methods described in this study are well within the chiropractic approach to health care.—R.B. Phillips, D.C., Ph.D.

Limited Range-of-Motion Lumbar Extension Strength Training

Graves JE, Pollock ML, Leggett SH, Carpenter DM, Fix CK, Fulton MN (Univ

of Florida, Gainesville)
Med Sci Sports Exerc 24:128–133, 1992 1–30

Background.—Little information is available on limited range-of-motion (ROM) dynamic resistance training on muscle groups other than the knee extensors. Thus, the effects of variable resistance lumbar extension strength training through a 36-degree ROM on the development of lumbar extension strength through 72 degrees of lumbar motion were assessed.

Methods.—Twenty-five women and 33 men (mean age, 30 years) were assigned randomly to 1 of 3 training groups or a nontraining control group. Training, conducted once a week for 12 weeks, consisted of 1 set of 8–12 repetitions of variable resistance lumbar extensions until volitional fatigue. Group 1 trained from 72 degrees to 36 degrees of lumbar flexion; group 2, from 36 degrees to 0; and group 3, from 72 degrees to 0. Isometric lumbar extension torque was evaluated at 72, 60, 48, 36, 24, 12, and 0 degrees of lumbar flexion before and after training.

Findings.—Analysis of covariance demonstrated that the 3 training groups increased lumbar extension torque at all angles compared with the control group. Groups 1 and 2 had the greatest gains in their respective ranges, but groups 1 and 2 did not differ from group 3 at any angle.

Conclusion.—Limited ROM lumbar extension training through a 36-degree ROM is effective for developing strength through 72 degrees of lumbar extension, findings which may have important clinical implications.

▶ This article describes a specific training procedure that was used in a study to determine its effectiveness in treating low back pain. This study involved a small cohort of individuals divided into 4 groups, making the determination of statistical significance difficult. The description of the exercise is well explained and may have valuable application to those in practice who have access to the kind of equipment used. Further application of the study results resides in the awareness that muscle conditioning is closely related to the presence of back pain.—R.B. Phillips, D.C., Ph.D.

Stretching in the Rehabilitation of Low-Back Pain Patients

Khalil TM, Asfour SS, Martinez LM, Waly SM, Rosomoff RS, Rosomoff HL (Univ of Miami, Fla)
Spine 17:311–317, 1992 1–31

Background.—Chiropractors commonly use stretching, mobilization, and manipulation in the rehabilitation of low back pain. The efficacy of one university's physical conditioning program in restoring certain elements of the functional abilities of individuals with chronic low back pain was investigated. Also, the effectiveness of a systematically applied, aggressive stretching maneuver as an add-on therapy in such patients was studied.

Methods.—Twenty-eight patients with chronic low back pain were assigned randomly to 1 of 2 groups. The control group underwent a multimodal rehabilitation program. In addition to this multimodal treatment, the patients in the experimental group underwent a systematic stretching maneuver.

Findings.—Patients who were undergoing multimodal rehabilitation with and without the stretching maneuver significantly improved in their functional abilities, as determined by the significant increase in the static strength of the back extensors, with corresponding significant increases in back muscle myoelectric (ME) signals. After 2 weeks of continuous therapy, there was also a significant reduction in pain levels. The systematic stretching maneuver enhanced the functional gains of these patients.

Conclusion.—For patients with chronic low back pain, muscle stretching results in an immediate and a cumulative gain in ME activity, muscle force produced, and ranges of motion. It also helps reduce pain levels. Patients in a comprehensive physical conditioning program—with and without stretching—significantly improve in terms of physical ability. The systematic use of a stretching maneuver enhances the restoration of physical ability in these patients.

▶ This study examines the effectiveness of muscle stretching as an addition to a multimodal physical therapy approach to the management of low back pain. The stretching procedure is well described in this article and follows the methods taught by Travell. The group who received the stretching in addition to the other modalities did demonstrate a significant improvement over the other group. This study would support the hypothesis that muscle stretching is a beneficial adjunct to the management of low back pain.—R.B. Phillips, D.C., Ph.D.

Auricular Acupuncture in the Treatment of Female Infertility

Gerhard I, Postneek F (Univ of Heidelberg, Germany)

Gynecol Endocrinol 6:171–181, 1992 1–32

Background.—In cases of female infertility, hormonal disturbances are a major contributing factor. Antiestrogen and gonadotropin therapy can produce adequate ovogenesis, although the conception rate trails far behind the ovulation rate. In addition, hormonal treatment may cause such side effects as ovarian cysts and multiple pregnancies, and the hormonal disturbance is never permanently normalized. Several previous studies have reported successful results using auricular acupuncture to treat orthopedic problems, migraine, mastopathy, and chronic pain. Therefore, whether hormone-induced female infertility could be treated with auricular acupuncture was determined.

Pregnancy Rate and Outcome of Pregnancy in the Acupuncture and Control Group

Groups of patients	*Pregnancy induction*	*First pregnancy under observation*			*Second pregnancy*
		Patients	*Abortion*	*Delivery*	
Acupuncture (n = 45)	acupuncture	11	1	10	1 abortion
	spontaneous	4	0	4	1 delivery
	medical treatment	7	3	4	1 abortion
	total	22	4	18	
	no pregnancy	23	—	—	
Control group (n = 45)	spontaneous	5	2	3	1 abortion
	medical treatment	15	2	13	1 delivery
	total	20	4	16	
	no pregnancy	25	—	—	

(Courtesy of Gerhard I, Postneek F: *Gynecol Endocrinol* 6:171–181, 1992.)

Patients and Methods.—After a complete gynecologic and endocrinologic examination, auricular acupuncture was performed once a week for 3 months in a total of 45 infertile women. Of these, 27 had had oligomenorrhea diagnosed, and 18 had had luteal insufficiency diagnosed. If pregnancy was not achieved after 3 months, all therapy was suspended for 6 months, and hormone substitution was then offered. The results were compared with those of 45 women who had been treated with hormones. Age, infertility duration, body mass index, previous pregnancies, menstrual cycle, and tubal patency were well matched between groups.

Results.—The pregnancy rates were similar in both groups. A total of 11 pregnancies occurred during the acupuncture treatment trial. In addition, 4 pregnancies occurred spontaneously more than 3 months after treatment and another 7 after hormonal therapy had been initiated in patients treated with acupuncture. Patients who received hormones experienced a total of 20 pregnancies. Of these, 15 occurred as a result of therapy, and 5 occurred spontaneously. Four women in each group had abortions (table). In patients who achieved pregnancy after acupuncture or hormone treatment, only 4% had endometriosis, and normal cycles were noted in 7%. In addition, higher body mass indices and testosterone values were noted in patients who continued to be infertile after hormone therapy, when compared with therapy responders within this same group. Patients who achieved pregnancies after acupuncture experienced menstrual abnormalities and luteal insufficiency with lower estrogen, thyrotropin, and dehydroepiandrosterone sulfate more often than women who became pregnant after hormone treatment. In addition, adnexitis, endometriosis, out-of-phase endometria, and reduced postcoital tests were noted more frequently in eumenorrheic patients treated with acupuncture, when compared with patients receiving hormones. Although hormonal disorders were more frequent in the acupuncture group, continued infertility after acupuncture treatment was noted in 12 of 27 patients with menstrual disorders as compared with 15 of 27 control patients treated with hormones. Side effects were noted during hormone treatment only.

Conclusion.—Based on these results, auricular acupuncture may be a valuable treatment alternative in infertile women with hormonal disorders.

▶ Acupuncture is used by many chiropractors, primarily for pain control but certainly for the management of a wide range of other problems. In the past, acupuncture has been advocated for use in childbirth and dysmenorrhea; this study examines its use in treating infertility. The standard medical therapy for infertility involves the use of hormone therapy, which carries with it certain known risks. Because this was considered standard therapy, women receiving hormone therapy comprised the control group for this study. With matched groups, the results were similar between groups, showing that auricular acupuncture may represent a viable method for treating infertility by conservative means.—D.J. Lawrence, D.C.

Acupuncture Fails to Improve Treatment Outcome in Alcoholics

Worner TM, Zeller B, Schwarz H, Zwas F, Lyon D (Long Island College Hosp, Brooklyn, NY)

Drug Alcohol Depend 30:169–173, 1992 1–33

Introduction.—Acupuncture has been applied as treatment for chemical dependency with mixed results. The efficacy of acupuncture as a treatment for alcoholism in another population was measured in a randomized, prospective study.

Methods.—Of the 56 alcoholic subjects enrolled in the study, there were 49 men and 7 women who had ingested alcohol 10 days before the beginning of the trial period. The subjects came from the lower socioeconomic class, and one third had a history of additional drug use. They received 1 of 3 treatments: point-specific acupuncture, sham transdermal stimulation, or standard care (control). A licensed acupuncturist performed the treatment 3 times a week for 30 minutes each session for 3 months.

Results.—The study populations of the 3 treatment groups were similar. All 3 groups demonstrated a similar number of previous detoxification or inpatient rehabilitation hospitalizations. No significant differences resulted for attendance of Alcoholic Anonymous meetings, the number of outpatient sessions attended, the number of weeks in the study, the number of individuals completing the treatment program, or relapse rate. Neither the sham procedure nor the acupuncture procedure increased the number of subjects completing the treatment.

Conclusion.—Acupuncture appeared not to improve patient outcome among this small, urban, racially mixed group with alcoholism. The beneficial effects for acupuncture previously reported may actually be classified as a placebo effect. The routine use of point-specific acupuncture should be avoided until large, randomized, controlled studies of this treatment demonstrate a beneficial outcome.

▶ Alcoholism is one of the most common and troubling of societal problems, with more than 1.5 million patients seeking some form of treatment during 1987. Standard therapies for alcoholics include 12-step programs such as Alcoholics Anonymous, counseling, and hospitalization. Acupuncture has been postulated as a means to treat the alcoholic, but it has the limitation of little controlled testing. Based on this study, which was limited by its small number of participants and a lack of blinding by the acupuncturist (who obviously was aware of the therapy he or she was rendering), acupuncture appears to be ineffective for treating chronic alcoholism.—D.J. Lawrence, D.C.

An Integrated Therapy for Peripartum Pelvic Instability: A Study of the Biomechanical Effects of Pelvic Belts

Vleeming A, Buyruk HM, Stoeckart R, Karamursel S, Snijders CJ (Med Univ of Istanbul, Turkey)

Am J Obstet Gynecol 166:1243–1247, 1992 1–34

Objective and Methods.—Pelvic belts have been used in peripartum women to lessen pelvic instability, although the specific biomechanical effects are uncertain. Sagittal rotation was induced in the sacroiliac joints of 6 human pelvis-spine specimens through bidirectional force directed at the acetabulum, and a compressive force was applied to the spine to mimic weight-bearing. Measurements were repeated with a pelvic belt at 50 newtons or 100 newtons of tension.

Findings.—The pelvic belt significantly reduced sagittal rotation in the sacroiliac joint when compressive force was applied to the spine. The 50-newton and 100-newton belts were comparably effective, reducing rotation by nearly one fifth.

Implications.—Along with muscle training, use of a pelvic belt in the peripartum period can enhance pelvic stability even with only a relatively small load. The belt apparently acts by reducing sacroiliac joint motion. A belt should not be used without also training the internal pelvic muscles and gluteus maximus. The lithotomy position must be used cautiously if there is hypermobility at the symphysis.

▶ Back pain related to the sacroiliac joints in pregnant females and postpartum patients is very common in chiropractic practice. Successful management of these types of patients has been reported anecdotally. For those cases in need of supportive care, this article suggests that a pelvic belt may be helpful. Results of studies on cadaveric specimens may not always be applicable to live patients. In this case, the procedure is noninvasive, and the research provides justification for its use when indications are appropriate.—R.B. Phillips, D.C., Ph.D.

Effect of Lumbar Orthosis on Intervertebral Mobility: A Roentgen Stereophotogrammetric Analysis

Axelsson P, Johnsson R, Strömqvist B (Lund Univ Hosp, Sweden)

Spine 17:678–681, 1992 1–35

Background.—External lumbar supports reduce the overall load on the lumbar spine by restrictions of upper body gross motions, but the effect on actual intervertebral mobility has been hard to evaluate. Three-dimensional roentgen stereophotogrammetric analysis (RSA) was used to determine the effect of external lumbar supports on intervertebral mobility.

Method.—Four men and 3 women who underwent posterolateral fusion without internal fixation were examined with RSA 1 month after surgery. The 1-month timetable was after soft tissue healing but before fusion consolidation. Each patient was evaluated in the erect and supine positions without external lumbar support, with a molded, rigid orthosis made of a lightweight thermoplastic material, and with a canvas corset splinted with thin metal ribbons and a molded posterior plastic reinforcement.

Findings.—In all 7 patients, neither the rigid nor the soft lumbar support had any stabilizing effect on the sagittal or vertical intervertebral translations. In 6 of the 7 patients, external lumbar supports increased the translations. The mean sagittal translation without support was 3.8 mm; with molded rigid orthosis, 4.7 mm; and with canvas corset, 5.1 mm.

Conclusion.—Using RSA provides a 3-dimensional image of human skeletal kinematics and can be used to measure intervertebral movements with a high degree of accuracy. Neither the rigid nor soft types of lumbar support had any stabilizing effect on the sagittal, vertical, or transverse intervertebral translations measured with RSA, compared with no external support. Although external lumbar support had no stabilizing effect on the intervertebral mobility of the lower lumbar spine, it does have an effect on restricting gross motions of the trunk. For this reason, lumbar support is useful during lumbar fusion healing to remind the patient to keep the trunk straight.

► This article provides an interesting approach to evaluating spinal motion. Through the implantation of tantalum markers during surgery, postsurgical x-ray films are able to depict the relative position of those metallic markers. The findings of this study should be very meaningful to the practice of chiropractic. The failure of both soft and rigid devices to restrict spinal motion should come as no surprise. Restraining devices such as corsets have been used for the support of the musculature and ligaments, and primarily to prevent patients from using their backs in a fashion that may further aggravate the condition.—R.B. Phillips, D.C., Ph.D.

Treatment of Limited Shoulder Motion: A Case Study Based on Biomechanical Considerations

McClure PW, Flowers KR (Hahnemann Univ, Pa)

Phys Ther 72:929–936, 1992 1–36

Causes of Limited Motion.—The optimal treatment of limited shoulder motion requires a distinction between structural changes, which generally result from inflammation and/or immobilization, and nonstructural changes in the periarticular tissues, such as pain or a loose body in the joint space. When structural changes limit passive range of motion, attempts should be made to apply tension to elongate the restricting tissues. Findings indicating structural change include a history of trauma followed by immobilization; limited motion for longer than 3 weeks; a capsular pattern of loss of passive motion; a capsular end-feel; and a lack of pain on resisted isometric contractions with the shoulder in neutral position.

Management.—Kaltenborn proposed an indirect method of determining how to apply gliding mobilization termed the "concave-convex rule." The humeral head slides in the direction opposite humeral motion. The head should, for example, slide inferiorly with abduction, and anteriorly during lateral rotation or horizontal abduction. In addition to gliding-type mobilization, other forms of stretching, such as active and passive range of motion, continuous passive motion, and splinting, may be used to treat limited range of motion.

Case Report.—Woman, 57, sustained a 2-part Neer fracture when falling on the ice, with avulsion of the greater tuberosity of the right humerus and, possibly, an anterior dislocation. Her husband, a physician, reported reducing the dislocation manually, and the arm was immobilized in a sling and swathe for 6 weeks, after which time limited motion was described, creating problems in dressing and household activities. Passive flexion and abduction were limited to 80 and 60 degrees, respectively, and pain was elicited at the end-ranges of all passive motions. No muscle atrophy was apparent.

Initially, hydrocollator packs were applied along with ultrasound, and pendulum exercises were performed. Low-grade anterior and inferior gliding movements followed the pendulum exercise. More forceful gliding movements ensued, as tolerated, and the patient was taught to exercise at home. Modest improvement was noted 8 weeks after injury. Improvement continued when the home program was augmented with a static, end-range, abduction splint. Desired gains were reached 12 weeks after injury. The splint was continued, and a strengthening program undertaken for the rotator cuff. The patient was discharged at 25 weeks.

Summary.—Limited shoulder motion caused by adaptive shortening of the periarticular tissues is best managed by methods that hold the joint at —or near —the end-range of motion for prolonged periods. Applying tension to restricting structures is more helpful than attempting to restore translatory gliding motion of the humeral head.

▶ The authors offer a prudent course of therapy for treatment of restricted shoulder motion in a patient who had had fracture/dislocation. They classify the causes of limited shoulder motion as those from structural changes and those from nonstructural changes, and they suggest that these are best treated in different manners. In this study, the therapy involved hot packs, ultrasound, pendulum exercise, and manual therapy that did not attempt to enter an end range. This was not done until much later. This is a significant departure from the chiropractic approach, where the therapy would undoubtedly involve articular adjusting past end range, into the paraphysiologic space. Although the overall approach is fine, the addition of the high-velocity thrust may prove quite beneficial.—D.J. Lawrence, D.C.

Resolution of a Groin Injury in a Professional Hockey Player by Soft Tissue Mobilization: A Case Report

Horrigan JM (Soft Tissue Ctr, Los Angeles)

Chiroprac Sports Med 6:151–154, 1992 1–37

Background.—With the increasing popularity of ice hockey at all levels of competition has come an increase in associated injuries, especially of the groin. Groin pull or strain includes microscopic and macroscopic lesions of muscle, periosteum, and tendons; the most commonly injured muscles are the adductor longus, rectus abdominis, and rectus femoris. Injury and inflammation may occur along the adductor origin, particularly the adductor magnus, and may radiate into the rectus abdominis and symphysis pubis. A case of groin injury in a professional hockey player, which was managed by soft tissue mobilization, was reported.

Case Report.—A professional hockey player, 34, complained of a left groin pull that had caused him to miss several games. He had a mild swelling in the midmedial thigh with no ecchymosis, as well as a tight feeling with pain at the site of the injury, which he sustained by rapid hip abduction. Physical therapy did not improve the disability. When subjected to dynamic muscle testing, pain occurred on resisted hip flexion, hip adduction, and medial rotation, but not with extension and lateral rotation with extension. Mild pain was felt at the maximum passive hip abduction. There was no apparent tear of the adductor muscle.

Fibrosis and adaptive shortening of the myofascial structures around the hip were treated by dynamic soft tissue mobilization, followed by pulsed ultrasound, 1 w/cm^2 × 4 min. The adductor longus and the anterior aspect of the adductor magnus showed the greatest amount of fibrosis and tenderness. After 2 treatments over 72 hours, the patient was able to return to competition, scoring a hat trick in his second game back.

Conclusion.—Proper management of groin strain depends on correct identification of the specific injury. Soft tissue manipulation may be used for strains of the adductor group, whereas tears of the rectus abdominis or internal oblique require surgical repair. Peripheral neuropathies require electrodiagnostic studies. Conditioning, specifically flexibility and strengthening, can prevent groin pulls; however, unfamiliarity with progressive resistance training may put the patient at risk of injury.

▶ Dr. Horrigan suggests that chiropractic manipulation is not indicated in hip adductor strain, preferring instead to use soft tissue mobilization coupled with pulsed ultrasound. Given the fact that "groin pulls" represent a broad spectrum of muscular injuries, it may be premature to rule out adjustive procedures. His point that the injury may be career threatening (as it might have been in this hockey player) does indicate a need for caution and precision in diagnosis.—D.J. Lawrence, D.C.

Counseling and Behavior

The Prevention of Chronic Pain and Disability: A Preliminary Investigation

Philips HC, Grant L, Berkowitz J (Univ Hosp, Vancouver, BC, Canada; Berkowitz & Assocs, Vancouver, BC, Canada)

Behav Res Ther 29:443–450, 1991 1–38

Objective.—Preventing chronic pain by "tagging" patients in the acute phase might effectively prevent chronic disability and, thereby, reduced health-care costs. Two commmon approaches to acute back pain, letting pain guide the return to normal activity and graded reactivation regardless of pain were compared.

Series.—A total of 117 patients seen within 15 days of the onset of acute back or neck pain, who had no signs of neural or disk damage, were paid to remain in the study. The average patient age was 32 years, and the patients were first seen an average of 8 days after the onset of pain. The second visit was an average of 14 weeks after the onset, and the third was at 6 months.

Measures.—In addition to a structured interview dealing with the pain itself, subjects completed the Beck Depression Inventory, the State-Trait Anxiety Inventory, the Pain Behavior Checklist, the Pain Evaluation Questionnaire, the Sickness Impact Profile, and the Pain Quality Questionnaire.

Management.—Either patients were encouraged to return to their previous level of function when lessening pain permitted, or they built back to normal functioning without reference to the degree of pain. An incremental activity schedule was used for the latter group.

Results.—At 6-month evaluation, about 40% of patients still had the pain thought to have begun at the time of the acute episode. Behavioral counseling appeared to be more effective than discussions with a counselor, but these approaches did not significantly affect the course of pain itself. The relationship between chronic pain and litigation was unaffected by either method of rehabilitation. Logistic regression analysis was able to define a group at increased risk based on the quality of pain and psychological reactions to the acute injury.

Implications.—The type of rehabilitation used shortly after acute back injury may be less important than providing behavioral counseling. Patients who are unlikely to have continuing problems from pain or to become disabled can be predicted quite accurately 3 months after the acute event.

▶ The incidence of chronic pain problems is rising, costing an estimated 60 billion dollars per year in the United States alone. It is currently difficult to predict which patients with acute pain will ultimately have these chronic problems develop, although estimates range from 10% to 40% of patients with acute back pain. Behavioral counseling, not typically the province of chiropractors, is one method that may help to decrease the incidence of chronic pain. Efforts toward implementation of behavioral counseling shortly after injury may prove cost-efficient and effective in limiting the development of chronic pain. Chiropractors may want to consider developing professional relationships with these practitioners for the best overall treatment of their patients.—D.J. Lawrence, D.C.

The Evolution of Chronic Pain Among Patients With Musculoskeletal Problems: A Pilot Study in Primary Care

Potter RG, Jones JM (Univ of Keele, Staffordshire, England)

Br J Gen Pract 42:462–464, 1992 1–39

Introduction.—Few studies have addressed the pathogenesis of chronic pain in primary care. Chronic pain might be preventable if factors associated with chronicity could be identified. The 6-month outcome of acute musculoskeletal pain was described, and assessment data were assessed for patients in whom chronic pain does or does not develop.

Methods.—The study sample included 45 adult patients who saw their general practitioners with a new episode of musculoskeletal pain lasting approximately 4 weeks. The patients were seen by 8 physicians during a 10-month period. After baseline assessment, including evaluation of pain by a visual analogue scale, the patients were followed up for 26 weeks by a research nurse using a structured interview and formal assessment instruments.

Findings.—Pain continued at 26 weeks in 20 patients who were considered to have chronic pain and resolved within 12 to 26 weeks. At baseline, the chronic pain group had a higher score on the visual analogue scale, 59 vs. 34, and a higher prevalence of depression, 85% vs. 36%. Scores for both present pain and pain during the past week decreased over time, although the average score was higher than the present score. There was an association between pain intensity scores and the use of passive coping strategies, which became more strongly positive with duration of pain.

Conclusion.—The development of chronic pain may be associated with initial high pain intensity scores, depression, and increasing use of passive coping strategies. Average pain scores are higher than present scores, and both decrease over time. This may result from the patient's wish to accurately represent his or her pain, even if it is not intense at that moment. Further, more definitive research is planned.

▶ Again we look at the development of chronic pain and the use of psychological inventories as a means to predict future pain patterns. These psychological issues may be overlooked by conservative practitioners, particularly those who take a mechanistic view of the patient's problems. In particular, depression at entry seems an important predictor of future chronic pain; this may be assessed using the Goldberg questionnaire. This opens the intriguing possibility of adding interdisciplinary associations to best manage patients with chronic pain.—D.J. Lawrence, D.C.

Mind-Body Health: Research, Clinical, and Policy Applications

Pelletier KR (Stanford Univ, Calif)

Am J Health Promot 6:345–358, 1992 1–40

Background.—Clinicians and scientists have long tried to relate emotions, behaviors, and mental attitudes to the onset and course of illness. In a critical review, an overview of the development of mind-body medicine in the past decade was presented.

Method.—Clinical and experimental medical literature related to the interaction between mind and body was reviewed thoroughly. New and complex research in the field of psychoneuroimmunology was analyzed.

Findings.—Although current findings are mixed and sometimes conflicting, increasingly compelling evidence indicates that mind and body interact inextricably. Data from psychoneuroimmunology and related fields increasingly indicate this mind-body interaction, discrediting Cartesian dualism. Concepts and models from quantum physics and theoretical speculations from key researchers suggest that human consciousness is not reducible to neural or biochemical events but may, in fact, exert a superordinate organizing function over biological events. An alternative to the biological determinism or the quantum mechanical models of the mind is aspects of consciousness emerging as irreducible, organizational, irremovable, and causal principles in the mind-body system. Although biological substrates and the lawful functions of the electric and biochemical mediations of brain activities are acknowledged, human consciousness may not be limited to such laws.

Conclusion.—Psychological factors appear to play a causal role in the onset and course of many chronic disorders. Psychological, emotional, psychosocial, and behavioral interventions have at least as much proof of efficacy as many purely medical treatments.

▶ The Office of Alternative Medicine of the National Institutes of Health devotes an entire section of its coverage to mind-body interactions. Many who are involved in studying this area are convinced that it may represent the next major health-care breakthrough. There are aspects of chiropractic that interface well with the developing mind-body science: a break with Cartesian dualism, such as that demonstrated by the effect of prayer on sick individuals when the subjects were unaware that they were being prayed for, and emphasis on holism and homeostasis (and immune function). The study of psychology will take on increasing importance during the next decade, as the psychological and psychosocial aspects of pain and disease are integrated in standard medical and chiropractic practice.—D.J. Lawrence, D.C.

Powerlessness, Empowerment, and Health: Implications for Health Promotion Programs

Wallerstein N (Univ of New Mexico, Albuquerque)

Am J Health Promot 6:197–205, 1992 1–41

Background.—The words "powerlessness" and "empowerment" appear with increasing frequency in public health literature. Casual use of these terms has resulted in a lack of theoretical clarity and measurement problems. Relevant social science and public health literature was synthesized to clarify the terminology and to demonstrate the importance of these concepts for promoting good health.

Methods.—Health and social science research on the role of powerlessness as a risk factor for disease and the role of empowerment as a health-enhancing strategy was reviewed. Articles came from the fields of social epidemiology, occupational health, stress research, social psychology, community psychology, social support and networks, community competence, and community organizing.

Findings.—Powerlessness, or a feeling of lack of control over destiny, appears to be a broad-based risk factor for disease. Although it is more difficult to assess, empowerment can be demonstrated as an important health promoter. A model of empowerment education is proposed for health practitioners. Measuring empowerment raises issues for researchers on how to assess the multiple personal and community changes that may result from an educational intervention designed to empower.

Implications.—Powerlessness can be thought of as a broad risk factor for disease, and empowerment is an important strategy for improving a population's health. If these preliminary findings hold, health practitioners should adopt an empowerment education approach. Researchers must measure more accurately the psychological, interpersonal, organizational, and community changes that may occur as people participate in their communities to improve health status.

▶ "Empowerment" has gained wide acceptance within business management circles, and it is beginning to integrate into health-care practice. To empower someone is to give them the power to make decisions on their own, to take responsibility for their actions. In health care, that means shifting the burden of healing from the doctor (which fosters a feeling of powerlessness in many) to the patient (empowering him or her). The more control individuals feel they have over life events, the better able they are to cope with negative events. In social science research, powerlessness has been found to bring a negative impact on healing and sickness. The chiropractic profession should work toward improving patient education, cultivating more patient responsibility in the healing process, and studying the personal and cultural changes that occur in illness and healing. In this way, we can optimize the healing response and better understand the psychological issues that are involved in illness.—D.J. Lawrence, D.C.

Living With Fibromyalgia: Consequences for Everyday Life

Henriksson C, Gundmark I, Bengtsson A, Ek A-C (Univ Hosp, Linköping, Sweden)

Clin J Pain 8:138–144, 1992 1–42

Background.—Little information on how fibromyalgia influences everyday life for patients and their families has been published. How fibromyalgia symptoms affect activities of daily living was investigated in detail.

Methods.—Fifty-five women and 3 men with fibromyalgia (mean age, 45 years) were included in the study. A questionnaire with a 2-day diary was mailed to the patients to elicit information on each patient's social background, employment status, symptoms, physical training habits, experience of general health, physical condition, and problems in performing motor tasks. In the diary, patients were asked to report every half hour on their degree of pain and fatigue, whether the activities were hard to do, and whether the activities were enjoyable, valuable, and meaningful.

Findings.—Fifty-five percent of the patients had jobs; however, most worked shorter hours and had changed work tasks. Motor tasks, such as carrying, holding, and running, were harder to perform than before symptom onset. Half of the patients felt that most of their activities were strenuous to perform. Sixty-seven percent reported very short or no pain-free periods during the 2 days recorded in the diary.

Conclusion.—The symptoms of fibromyalgia affect daily life considerably. Almost all patients had changes in habits and routines as a result of their condition. Assessing patients' total life situation provides valuable information for understanding their ability to handle daily activities.

▶ Fibromyalgia remains a controversial illness, with some doctors not admitting it as a legitimate diagnosis. With symptoms of pain and fatigue and few discrete physical findings, it can be difficult to authenticate its existence. Notwithstanding this controversy, for those who are given a diagnosis of fibromyalgia, it can have profound effects on their daily existence. Those consequences include perceived poor health, difficulty in household and leisure tasks, difficulty in sleeping, and poor motor function. These deficiencies need to be taken into account when designing a rehabilitation and treatment plan for patients with primary fibromyalgia, and chiropractors should be sensitive to the difficulties these patients face in everyday life.—D.J. Lawrence, D.C.

Key Factors in Health Counselling in the Consultation

Arborelius E, Krakau I, Bremberg S (Natl Inst for Psychological Factors and Health, Stockholm; Uppsala Univ, Sweden; Karolinska Inst, Huddinge, Sweden)

Fam Pract 9:488–493, 1992 1–43

Objective.—Counseling in life habits can help enhance health activities such as quitting smoking and cutting down on alcohol. Health counseling appears to be more effective if it is related to the patient's symptoms, is concrete, emphasizes the short-term advantages, and includes a follow-up visit. Obstacles to effective counseling include lack of training, lack of time, pessimism about the effectiveness of counseling and the patient's ability to change, and fear of alienating the patient, as well as the clinician's own health habits. The health belief model holds that the clinician's ability to discuss perceived barriers is a major factor in health-enhancing behavior.

Methods.—In this qualitative study, 16 general practitioners and 14 general nurses at 2 health-care centers were interviewed regarding their procedures for health counseling and the perceived barriers to prevention. The clinicians were asked about their frequency and technique of health counseling, attitude toward prevention, patient vs. clinician-centered style, ideas about the patient's attitude toward preventive counseling, perceived efficacy of prevention, and possible conflicts with their own life-style.

Findings.—Most of the clinicians thought that health counseling was important and believed that they had time and space for counseling. However, most voiced disappointment about their perceived ability to effect behavioral change. Half the clinicians were regarded to have a patient-centered style, whereas most of the rest could be identified as having a clinician-centered or mixed style.

Conclusion.—In regard to health counseling, many clinicians appear to lack an effective method of handling the issues raised. Most do not subscribe to an educational theory in which the patient is the starting point. This impedes their ability to be role models from whom the patient learns and supports the idea that patients fail to change mainly because of psychologic reasons, with little importance ascribed to the role of differing values. Education of clinicians in patient-centered pedagogy is advocated.

▶ The best prevention programs will never be successful if there is a lack of commitment on the part of the physician or others involved in the prevention program. In addition, how often do we give mixed messages—asking patients to stop smoking when continuing to smoke ourselves, or asking them to lose weight when overweight ourselves? The obstacles that interfere with the effectiveness of prevention programs include a lack of physician training, pessimism regarding the effect our advice will have on our patient and fear of alienating the patient. The health-belief model of health counseling posits that the doctors ability to discuss barriers to prevention is the determining factor in their success. How can we optimize health counseling? By studying the best counseling method and coupling that with methods to enhance our overall belief in the effectiveness of what we do. Chiropractors tend to bring a positive "spin" to our clinical intervention, which, if coupled to the appropriate counseling methodology, should make our prevention efforts more successful.—D.J. Lawrence, D.C.

Cognitive Functioning After Common Whiplash: A Controlled Follow-Up Study

Radanov BP, Di Stefano G, Schnidrig A, Sturzenegger M, Augustiny KF (Univ of Berne, Switzerland)

Arch Neurol 50:87–91, 1993 1–44

Background.—After whiplash injury, impaired cognitive functioning, including poor concentration and attentional deficit, has frequently been reported. Although impairment of higher cognitive functions, such as memory, has not been revealed by global testing, altered attentional processing may play an important role in the common whiplash syndrome. Cognitive function and possible factors affecting cognitive ability were investigated in a group of randomly selected patients after trauma.

Symptoms at Baseline and Follow-Up Examinations

	No. (%)		
	Baseline		
Symptoms†	**Asymptomatic Group (n=67)**	**Symptomatic Group (n=31)**	**Follow-up Examination, Symptomatic Group (n=31)**
Neck pain	59 (88)	30 (97)	25 (81)
Headache	34 (51)	21 (68)	25 (81)
Shoulder pain	29 (43)	19 (61)	17 (55)
Back pain	24 (36)	12 (39)	11 (36)
Blurred vision	10 (15)	13 (42)	11 (36)
Dizziness	9 (13)	9 (29)	3 (10)
Finger paresthesia	3 (5)	5 (16)	7 (23)
Difficulty in swallowing	7 (10)	1 (3)	0 (0)
Fatigue‡	34 (51)	21 (68)	19 (60)
Anxiety§	29 (43)	15 (48)	10 (32)
Sleep disturbances‖	20 (30)	23 (74)	13 (43)

Sensitivity to noise	19 (28)	12 (39)	9 (29)
Irritability	11 (16)	10 (32)	13 (42)
Poor concentration	14 (21)	11 (36)	15 (48)
Forgetfulness¶	4 (6)	10 (32)	10 (32)

Note: There were significant differences between the groups in respect to finger paresthesia ($P < .05$) and blurred vision, sleep disturbances, and forgetfulness ($P < .01$).
† A combination of symptoms should be considered.
‡ Although no chronic fatigue was assessed, subjects reported increasing levels of fatigue during the day with involvement in different activities.
§ Phobic reaction as a consequence of being a driver or passenger in congested traffic. No post-traumatic stress disorder was diagnosed in any of the groups.
|| Difficulties in falling asleep and/or sleep interruption exclusively because of pain.
¶ When interviewed about forgetfulness, patients reported difficulties in acquiring information because of impairment in following the information flow. No real memory inpairment was assessed.
(Courtesy of Radanov BP, Di Stefano G, Schnidrig A, et al: *Arch Neurol* 50:87–91, 1993.)

Patients and Methods.—A total of 98 patients with common whiplash syndrome were included in this study. All were examined shortly after trauma, at a mean of 7.3 ± 3.9 days, and again 6 months later. Both examinations included complete physical and neurologic evaluations, medication screening (coded according to its possible influence on cognitive ability), semistructured interviews (with an emphasis on subjective complaints), attentional functioning assessments, and self ratings of well-being and cognitive ability. In addition, baseline examinations included cervical spine roentgenograms and neuroticism assessments. The timing of initial neck pain or headache onset and the restriction of neck movement early after trauma were also evaluated as possible indicators of injury severity.

Results.—At baseline, the most frequently noted symptoms in all patients included neck pain and headache (table). At 6-month follow-up, the symptoms had fully resolved in 67 patients (asymptomatic group), whereas the remaining 31 continued to experience symptoms (symptomatic group). A greater variety of symptoms, higher neck pain intensity, and greater subjective cognitive impairment were noted in symptomatic patients who were older at baseline. The average onset of initial neck pain was 7 ± 15.1 and 11.9 ± 16.9 hours in the symptomatic and asymptomatic groups, respectively. The average onset of headache was 9 ± 16.2 and 10.3 ± 13.2 hours in the symptomatic and asymptomatic groups, respectively. Restricted neck movement at baseline was noted in 77% of symptomatic patients compared with 48% in the asymptomatic group. In tests requiring complex attentional processing, both groups scored poorly at baseline. At 6 months, all neuropsychological functions had returned to normal in each group. A delayed recovery in complex attentional functioning was noted in the symptomatic group, although this may have been the result of adverse effects of medication.

Conclusion.—Although the existence of major cognitive impairment after common whiplash was not supported by these results, some change in cognitive equilibrium was indicated. This may be caused in part by the type of medication used and should remain a consideration during whiplash treatment.

► We tend to view whiplash injuries from a mechanistic viewpoint, asking ourselves what tissues have been damaged and how severely. One less frequently considered complication of the whiplash injury is impaired cognitive functioning. This study used a series of interviews and cognitive assessment techniques to examine the extent of cognitive dysfunction. A number of task-oriented cognitive procedures were used, such as the Number Connection Test (essentially a dot-to-dot test) and the Paced Auditory Serial Addition Test (asking the patient to add consecutive numbers). Indeed, patients with whiplash showed decreased processing times compared with normal but, importantly, the effect seems to be a result of the effects of medication. Obviously, if the medication could be eliminated, the cognitive dysfunction would clear much quicker. Chiropractic intervention uses no medication and is effective in whiplash cases; therefore, it would appear that it offers one of the best methods for managing whiplash cases while, at the same time, decreasing negative cognitive effects.—D.J. Lawrence, D.C.

The Effect of Graded Activity on Patients With Subacute Low Back Pain: A Randomized Prospective Clinical Study With an Operant-Conditioning Behavioral Approach

Lindström I, Öhlund C, Eek C, Wallin L, Peterson L-E, Fordyce WE, Nachemson AL (Univ of Göteborg, Sweden; Volvo Co, Göteborg, Sweden; Univ of Washington, Seattle)

Phys Ther 72:279–293, 1992 1–45

Purpose.—Few randomized studies have investigated the effectiveness of any treatment for lower back pain (LBP) lasting more than 8 weeks. Restored function has been reported with comprehensive programs for patients with LBP, but these programs have been of differing types and directed at patients with differing durations of pain. A graded activity program with an operant-conditioning behavioral approach in restoring function in industrial workers with LBP was reported.

Methods.—The graded-activity program was part of a randomized study comparing traditional medical care with traditional care plus a graded activity program. The subjects were 103 workers sick-listed for 8 weeks with subacute, nonspecific, mechanical LBP. All were examined by an orthopedic surgeon and a social worker before randomization, and those with defined orthopedic, medical, or psychiatric disorders were excluded. The activity program included functional capacity measurements; a workplace visit; back school training; and a submaximal, gradually increased exercise program, based on an operant conditioning approach, using the test results and the patient's work requirements. This system was based on Fordyce's model of exercise to quota rather than pain (table). Outcome was assessed by records of sick leave during 3 years.

Results.—The activity group had a significantly quicker return to work than the control group. Their median number of physical therapy appointments was 5, and the average number of appointments was 11. In the second year of follow-up, the average sick leave attributable to LBP was 12 weeks vs. 20 weeks for controls. The outcome was permanent disability pension in 1 worker in the acitivity group vs. 4 in the control group.

Conclusion.—The graded activity program described can restore occupational function, as measured by return to work and reduced sick leave, in industrial workers with subacute, nonspecific, mechanical LBP. With graded activity, patients learn that it is safe to move while they regain function. This approach requires no intensive or "work-hardening" exercises nor any expensive equipment.

▶ Operant conditioning is a behavioral process that uses positive and negative reinforcement. It was used in this study to enhance a graded exercise program that ultimately led to a faster return to work. The exercise programs recommended in this study are those based on each individual's functional

Exercise Performance and Quota-Setting in the Activity Group

BACK MUSCLES

Extension exercises were performed with the patient lying prone, arms along the trunk. The trunk was raised until there was no contact between the male patients' chest and the support surface or until there was no pressure on the breasts of the female patients; this amount of back muscle extension was never to be exceeded. The exercises were increased by adding arm or leg support in different combinations when performing back muscle extension. One exercise was to hold that upper position 75% of the tested endurance time. For example, if the tested endurance time was 16 seconds, then the quota of exercise endurance time was 12 seconds. If the tested frequency was 12 repetitions, then the quota of exercise frequency was 9. Increased quota could mean increased number of endurance seconds or increased number of repetitions.

ABDOMINAL MUSCLES

Exercises were performed with the patient lying supine, knees flexed, feet unsupported, hands stretched toward the knees, and trunk curled until the angulus inferior of the scapula had no support. Increase of abdominal muscle exercises were activated by repositioning the arms when performing the exercises. The quota was set in the same way as for back muscle exercises.

FITNESS EXERCISES

The exercise on a stationary bicycle was set to quota by recording the number of minutes and the load on the bicycle. If the test showed a capacity of 12 minutes of 150 W, the quota could be 5 minutes at 50 W followed by 9 minutes at 100 W and then 5 minutes at 50 W. Increased quota could mean either increased number of minutes or increased load. Fitness exercise could also include stepping up and down on a stool, climbing stairs, swimming backstroke, walking, or jogging.

SWIMMING BACKSTROKE

The patient swam 8 laps backstroke in the initial trials. The quota for swimming backstroke was set at 6 laps. Increased quota meant increased number of laps or shorter time per lap.

LEG MUSCLES

Exercises were carried out standing and shifting the body weight between the legs while lifting the heels or bending the knees. Sitting in a chair or on the floor, unilateral lifting of one straight leg was also performed.

ARM MUSCLES

Exercises were carried out by lifting the arms in different directions while holding dumbbells. The arm exercises were performed lying prone, lying supine, sitting, or standing. Increase of arm exercises meant addition of heavier dumbbells or further lifting positions.

LIFTING

Exercises were carried out by lifting dumbbells in different directions while standing. Increase of lifting exercises meant addition of further directions or heavier dumbbells.

(Courtesy of Lindström I, Öhlund C, Eek C, et al: *Phys Ther* 72:279–293, 1992.)

capacity, generally including low back and abdominal procedures. These were done in quotas, which were rewarded or unrewarded as necessary by a physical therapist. It would be interesting to add manipulation as part of the experimental group; however, the authors have shown how behavioral science can mesh with therapeutic intervention.—D.J. Lawrence, D.C.

Pain Complaint and the Weather: Weather Sensitivity and Symptom Complaints in Chronic Pain Patients

Shutty MS Jr, Cundiff G, DeGood DE (Western State Hosp, Staunton, Va; Univ of Virginia, Charlottesville)

Pain 49:199–204, 1992 1–46

Background.—Patients with chronic pain frequently report that weather conditions influence their pain, but the clinical literature has not reported any reliable and standardized instruments to measure self-report of weather sensitivity. The development of a brief, internally consistent, and reliable self-report weather sensitivity index was described for use with patients who have chronic pain with musculoskeletal disorders.

Method.—Seventy patients, male and female, who were undergoing outpatient treatment for chronic pain, completed a Weather and Pain Questionnaire (WPQ) to assess their sensitivity to meteorologic variables (e.g., temperature or precipitation defined by the National Weather Service). Average patient age was 43.2 years. The most common complaint was low back pain, followed by upper back, neck, arm, and shoulder pain. The Weather and Pain Questionnaire was revised using factor analysis to produce a Weather Sensitivity Index with high internal consistency and test-retest reliability. The patients were classified as being high or low weather sensitive based on scores on the WPQ.

Results.—Nearly three fourths of the sample reported that temperature, humidity, precipitation, and sudden weather changes affected their pain to some degree; however they were unable to reliably identify specific symptoms consistently influenced by the weather. Temperature and humidity were the most frequently reported metorologic variables that affected pain complaint; joint and muscle aches were the physical complaints associated most frequently with the weather. "Weather-sensitive" patients reported significantly greater pain intensity, greater chronicity of pain problems, and more difficulties sleeping than patients with low scores on the WPQ. There were no differences in gender, education level, disability status, or global psychological distress between the high and low "weather-sensitive" groups. The effect of the weather may be mediated by psychological factors including unreliability of observation, beliefs and expectations, and mood state.

Conclusion.—Despite the factors that may bias patient judgments regarding the influence of weather on pain, patients could reliably identify which meteorologic variables influenced their pain, although they could not reliably determine which physical symptoms were consistently affected.

▶ Although patients with chronic pain frequently describe weather-related pain patterns, this is not a very-well-understood or well-studied phenomenon. The Weather and Pain Questionnaire provides a first major tool to examine weather-related pain factors, lending proof to patients' perceptions of the effect of weather on their symptoms. It will be interesting to study this phenomenon as it relates to subluxation or joint dysfunction, particularly as barometric pressure may correlate to spinal joint motion or pain as well as extravertebral pain.—D.J. Lawrence, D.C.

Pain-Specific Beliefs, Perceived Symptom Severity, and Adjustment to Chronic Pain

Jensen MP, Karoly P (Univ of Washington, Seattle; Arizona State Univ, Tempe)

Clin J Pain 8:123–130, 1992 1–47

Background.—The beliefs of patients with chronic pain as to the cause of pain or one's ability to control pain may determine multidimensional pain adjustment. Several instruments have been developed to assess beliefs hypothesized to be related to adjustment in patients with chronic pain. The connection between pain beliefs and adjustment, or the moderating influence of pain severity on this relationship were examined in a sample of patients with chronic pain.

Method.—Interviews with a sample of 118 patients with chronic pain were conducted by telephone using questionnaires and rating scales to assess pain severity, pain beliefs, adjustment, and social desirability bias.

Findings.—Pain-related attitudes were important predictors of adjustment among chronic patients. Patients who believed themselves to be disabled by their pain had significantly lower levels of activity and psychological well-being and higher levels of professional services utilization. The relationship between disability belief and activity level was strongest among those with low and medium levels of perceived pain. A continuing belief in a medical cure for pain was related to the continued use of medical services. This finding emphasizes the need for educational and clinical experiences that lead to greater self-reliance rather than reliance on continued use of medical services. Patients who believed solicitous responses from others were appropriate, especially those reporting relatively low levels of pain, demonstrated lower levels of well being.

Conclusion.—These findings provide an empirical basis for understanding the relationship between the beliefs about chronic pain and adjustment. Beliefs concerning whether one is disabled by pain were especially important for long-term adaptation. An equally important study finding is that the belief/functioning relationship is not always direct and can be moderated by perceived pain severity.

▶ The general chiropractic approach to chronic pain differs substantially from that of medicine. Chiropractors have traditionally used an approach that is both holistic and patient centered. When patients expect the doctor to take responsibility for curing them of their pain, they can be greatly disappointed when that fails to happen; they may passively respond to the medical advice they receive. As this paper notes, greater self-reliance on the part of the patient can provide a better environment for coping with chronic pain; education and communication can be important factors for the chiropractor to consider in divising coping strategies and expectations for their patients with chronic pain.—D.J. Lawrence, D.C.

Patterns of Normal Personality Structure Among Chronic Pain Patients

Wade JB, Dougherty LM, Hart RP, Cook DB (Virginia Commonwealth Univ, Richmond)

Pain 48:37–43, 1992 1–48

Objective.—Fifty-nine patients seen with chronic pain, most often involving the back or lower extremity, met predefined classification criteria for 1 of the Minnesota Multiphasic Personality Inventory (MMPI) pain subgroups (conversion, hypochondriasis, emotionally overwhelmed, denial/coping).

Method.—Neuroticism was assessed using the NEO Personality Inventory (NEO-PI).

Findings.—High NEO-PI neuroticism scores were ususally found in emotionally overwhelmed patients. Depression, anxiety, vulnerability, and hostility were all relatively prominent in these patients. None of the other NEO-PI domains distinguished between the MMPI-defined subgroups. With the exception of neuroticism in the emotionally overwhelmed group, NEO-PI profile scores were in the average range.

Implications.—Most groups of patients with chronic pain have a relatively normal personality structure. Neuroticism is, however, prominent in emotionally overwhelmed patients.

▶ Of all populations of patients with chronic pain, only those who view themselves as emotionally stressed demonstrate clinical signs of neuroticism. Chiropractors may want to refer such patients for counseling in a multidisciplinary approach to managing the whole patient.—D.J. Lawrence, D.C.

Comparison of Cognitive-Behavioral Group Treatment and an Alternative Non-Psychological Treatment for Chronic Low Back Pain

Nicholas MK, Wilson PH, Goyen J (Univ of New South Wales, Kensington, Australia; Univ of Sydney, Australia; Westmead Hospital, Westmead, Australia)

Pain 48:339–347, 1992 1–49

Background.—Evidence suggests that operant-behavioral and cognitive-behavioral techniques increase activity levels, improve mood, and reduce medication use in patients with chronic low back pain. However, the efficacy of such treatment compared with alternative treatments has not been determined. The relative efficacy of cognitive-behavioral group treatment, including relaxation training, was compared with a control condition in patients with chronic low back pain.

Methods and Findings.—Twenty outpatients were studied. The mean duration of their pain was 5.5 years. Nine patients had had at least 1 operation for their low back pain, and 17 had had some type of physiotherapy. Seven had had at least nerve block. Patients in the 2 conditions received the same physiotherapy back-education and exercise program. The control condition included a control for the therapist's attention in the congnitive-behavioral treatment. Patients receiving the combined psychological treatment and physiotherapy had significantly greater improvement than those in the attention-control and physiotherapy condition after treatment on measures of other-rated functional impairment, use of active coping strategies, self-efficacy beliefs, and use of medication. At 6 months, differences persisted in the use of active coping strategies and, to a lesser extent, self-efficacy beliefs and other-rated functional impairment.

Conclusion.—These findings suggest that cognitive-behavioral treatment for chronic low back pain has a positive effect on daily activity level, medication use, and coping strategies beyond those effects attributable to attention, back-care education, and exercise. Further study is particularly needed to assess the factors affecting long-term improvement on gains derived during cognitive-behavioral treatment.

► The only difference between the 2 groups studied is that one group had a cognitive-behavioral treatment whereas the other was controlled. Otherwise, they both received fairly standard physical therapy interventions, which included physiotherapy, back education, and exercise. In other words, how much effect did just the cognitive therapy have on the experimental group? Apparently, quite a bit, because the experimental group fared much better than the control. Chiropractors should examine methods to add these procedures into their practice; in counseling patients with low back pain, the model suggests that the doctor stress the consequences of inactivity, depression, and helplessness, and repeated failures of therapy as well as the tendency of the patient to focus too much attention on their pain.—D.J. Lawrence, D.C.

Attentional Processing in Cervical Spine Syndromes

Radanov BP, Hirlinger I, Di Stefano G, Valach L (Univ of Berne, Switzerland)
Acta Neurol Scand 85:358–362, 1992 1–50

Background.—"Common whiplash" is widely thought to lead to cognitive problems related to impaired information processing and reduced attentional functioning. A cervical syndrome caused by rheumatism, Barré-Lieou syndrome has a phenomenology similar to that of whiplash. However, studies on cognitive ability in patients with Barré-Lieou syndrome have not been done.

Methods.—Fifty-four patients with common whiplash were compared with 28 patients with Barré-Lieou syndrome. All had clinical interviews and formal testing, which included personality profile, self-ratings of cognitive impairment and well-being, and tasks on divided attention and speed of information processing.

Findings.—Higher relative incidences of adjustment disorder were noted in patients with whiplash. Scoring for divided attention was low in both groups. Patients with Barré-Lieou syndrome indicated hardly any problems on their self-ratings, whereas patients with common whiplash reported significant impairment. This difference was assumed to reflect the different modes of development of the syndromes: in patients with Barré-Lieou syndrome, the condition gradually developed, allowing the patients the opportunity to adapt, whereas the conditions of patients with whiplash occurred abruptly by impact injury. In the latter group, adaptation was inadequate, which explained the appearance of adjustment disorders among patients with common whiplash. Headache from cervical abnormality was probably responsible for impaired attentional functioning in the whiplash group.

Conclusion.—These findings showed no evidence of a specific pattern of attentional impairment in patients with common whiplash. Instead, headache is probably responsible for such patients' impaired attentional functioning.

▶ Patients with whiplash syndrome may have impaired attentional processing, which is believed to be caused by the acute onset of the injury. These types of attentional disturbances may occur in other cervical syndromes, but to differing degrees depending upon acuteness or chronicity.—D.J. Lawrence, D.C.

Relationship of MMPI Cluster Type, Pain Coping Strategy, and Treatment Outcome

Swimmer GI, Robinson ME, Geisser ME (Inst for Medical and Rehabilitation Psychology, Toledo, Ohio; Univ of Michigan, Ann Arbor; Univ of Florida, Gainesville)

Clin J Pain 8:131–137, 1992 1–51

Descriptive Statistics by MMPI Subtype

CSQ scale	Pretreatment Mean	Pretreatment SD	Posttreatment Mean	Posttreatment SD	
Depression/pathological subtype					
Diverting attention	9.7	7.5	18.5	7.6	*
Reinterpreting pain	4.8	6.6	11.3	9.4	*
Coping self statements	18.0	7.6	20.2	5.8	
Ignoring sensations	11.2	7.2	16.9	7.2	*
Praying/hoping	15.6	8.3	10.9	6.2	
Catastrophizing	15.9	8.3	10.0	6.7	*
Behavioral activity	12.6	5.8	17.5	5.9	*
Pain behaviors	17.5	5.5	16.9	5.8	
Control	2.6	1.3	3.2	1.6	
V-type subtype					
Diverting attention	14.5	7.3	18.4	7.6	
Reinterpreting pain	4.1	5.3	11.5	10.1	*
Coping self statements	19.3	9.1	21.6	9.3	
Ignoring sensations	11.5	7.1	14.9	9.1	
Praying/hoping	20.5	6.3	12.0	5.7	*
Catastrophizing	12.8	6.4	4.3	3.7	*
Behavioral activity	14.7	7.1	19.1	7.0	
Pain behaviors	19.6	6.2	14.9	5.9	
Control	2.4	1.4	4.0	0.9	*
Marginal V-type					
Diverting attention	14.5	6.6	23.4	7.7	*
Reinterpreting pain	7.1	9.2	14.3	7.8	*
Coping self statements	19.6	6.9	24.3	5.9	
Ignoring sensations	15.1	9.4	17.7	6.6	
Praying/hoping	13.8	7.4	9.8	6.5	
Catastrophizing	9.4	6.4	4.9	5.2	
Behavioral activity	14.2	6.3	18.3	5.1	
Pain behaviors	18.8	4.6	16.2	4.5	
Control	3.1	1.4	4.1	0.9	
Marginal depression/pathological subtype					
Diverting attention	9.0	8.1	18.0	8.7	
Reinterpreting pain	4.1	7.1	11.4	6.3	
Coping self statements	16.0	5.2	24.9	9.3	
Ignoring sensations	12.3	4.8	17.6	2.5	
Praying/hoping	9.5	4.2	8.4	4.9	
Catastrophizing	12.1	8.5	6.2	5.0	
Behavioral activity	13.7	6.9	18.3	4.1	
Pain behaviors	18.9	5.4	17.3	6.6	
Control	2.2	1.8	3.5	1.0	

* Significant at $P < .005$ (Bonferroni correction).
(Courtesy of Swimmer GI, Robinson ME, Geisser ME: *Clin J Pain* 8:131-137, 1992.)

Background.—Several researchers have studied the relationship between personality style and chronic pain using the Minnesota Multiphasic Personality Inventory (MMPI). Such research has suggested that empirical clustering techniques may be useful for categorizing patients with pain into homogeneous groups. Other studies have examined the differential treatment outcome based on MMPI clusters, with mixed results. Whether cognitive and behavioral coping style is related to personality factors, how coping styles differ across personality types, and how outpatient interdisciplinary intervention influences the coping styles of various personality types in chronic pain patients were assessed.

Methods.—Four clusters—Depression/Pathological, V-type, Marginal Depression, and Marginal V-type—were derived. Seventy patients completed the MMPI and the Coping Strategies Questionnaire before and after 3 weeks of participation in an outpatient pain management program.

Findings.—Pretreatment analysis showed that the Depression/Pathological and Marginal Depression groups used diverting attention less than the V-type groups. The V-type group used praying and hoping strategies significantly more than either of the marginal groups. After treatment, the Depression/Pathological group used catastrophizing significantly more than the marginal groups. Pretreatment and posttreatment analysis showed that the Depression/Pathological group increased their use of diverting attention, reinterpreting pain sensations, ignoring pain sensations, and reduced their catastrophizing. Reinterpretation of pain sensations increased in the V-type group, while praying/hoping and catastrophizing declined. Neither of the marginal groups had significant changes in coping strategies (table).

Conclusion.—Different personality types appear to use different pain-coping strategies before treatment. Those with more severe psychological distress, perhaps related to an underlying personality disorder, exhibited greater changes in coping strategy with treatment but remained more dysfunctional after treatment. Changing coping strategies may be an important treatment effect that needs more individualization to maximize treatment response.

▶ In the treatment of patients with chronic pain, personality types need to be considered. In the workup of patients with chronic pain, the chiropractic physician may want to add psychological inventories such as the MMPI to their assessment tools.—D.J. Lawrence, D.C.

The Effectiveness of Psychological Interventions for the Rehabilitation of Low Back Pain: A Randomized Controlled Trial Evaluation

Altmaier EM, Lehmann TR, Russell DW, Weinstein JN, Kao CF (Univ of Iowa, Iowa City; Humana Suburban Hosp, Louisville, Ky; Soochow Univ)

Pain 49:329–335, 1992 1–52

Background.—A recent meta-analysis of nonmedical treatments for chronic pain found that psychologic treatments were successful compared with no treatment, with the best outcomes for patients who had autogenic training, multicomponent treatments, placebo pills, or biofeedback training. In a randomized clinical trial, a standard inpatient rehabilitation program for chronic low back pain was compared with a standard program plus a psychologically based program.

Methods.—The study sample comprised 45 patients with low back pain—33 men and 12 women with a mean age of 40 years. They were randomized to receive either the standard rehabilitation program, which focused on education and physical reconditioning or the standard program plus a psychologically based program with the added components of operant conditioning, relaxation, biofeedback, and coping-skills training. The psychologic group also received contingent reinforcement for exercise. Reduction of drug usage and a focus on family involvement were emphasized in both programs. Functional status was assessed before the program, at discharge from the 3-week program, and after 6 months.

Results.—Both groups had improvements in overall function at discharge, which were maintained at follow-up. Similar improvements were noted in self-reported pain and interference. Eighty-one percent of patients had either returned to work or begun job retraining by 6 months, and 57% had returned to full-time work at the same or an equivalent job. There was no difference in pain improvement between the 2 groups.

Conclusion.—This controlled clinical trial finds that the addition of psychologic measures does not improve the effectiveness of the standard rehabilitation program for low back pain. This and previous studies suggest that common mechanisms of pain reduction and disability are affected by a number of treatments. Future research should use a multidimensional concept of pain to determine which aspects of pain are affected by specific treatment components.

▶ This is one of the few papers examining psychological interventions in low back pain that fails to report a positive finding. The psychological intervention that was used consisted of relaxation and coping strategies coupled with operant conditioning. It is interesting to note that both the experimental and control groups responded well to the therapy (consisting of rehabilitation procedures); however, the experimental group (which also had the operant therapy) responded no better than the control group. One conclusion: the rehabilitation procedure is worthy of further study. Another conclusion: the rehabilitation program in some way used procedures similar to those being tested. Unfortunately, only more work will answer these question.—D.J. Lawrence, D.C.

Patient Classification, A Key to Evaluate Pain Treatment: A Psychological Study in Chronic Low Back Pain Patients

Talo S, Rytökoski U, Puukka P (Social Insurance Inst, Turku, Finland)

Spine 17:998–1011, 1992 1–53

Objective.—The evaluation of treatment programs for chronic pain has been a continuous problem. Some of this problem results from the heterogeneity of patient samples. The subgrouping of patients with chronic low back pain was emphasized to determine whether this facilitates the evaluation of treatment outcome.

Methods.—A heterogeneous group of patients with chronic low back pain were classified into more homogeneous subgroups. The outcomes produced by 2 pain programs—an active "functioning activation" program and a less active "spa resort" program—were compared by 2 designs. In the first, outcome was compared by groups that were clinically homogenized according to sociodemographic variables and contraindications to heavy physical training. In the second design, response was compared in subgroups homogenized by cluster analysis according to the psychologic profiles of functioning.

Results.—The cluster analysis technique appeared to facilitate outcome evaluation. It provided more specific information on the effects of program quality, patient characteristics, and the interaction of these 2 variables on the improvement resulting from rehabilitation. When the impairment was considered first, mental health improved more in the functioning activation program, especially for "interpersonally distressed" patients. Also in the functioning activation program, belief in chance in disease control increased in interpersonally distressed and dysfunctional patients, whereas it decreased in adaptive copers.

Conclusion.—In the evaluation of pain treatment, subgroup homogeneity must be considered in the outcome analysis. The benefits of treatment appear to depend on the patient's global functional profile. In this study of low back pain, a functioning activation program was more effective for patients with personality disorders and good cognitive abilities, whereas the spa resort program was more effective for cognitively and functionally weaker patients.

▶ On a more technical note, rather than a clinical note, this paper suggests that clinical trails must pay closer attention to subgroup homogeneity in their design. One of the problems of a randomized clinical trial for low back pain is developing matching groups for the study. Because low back pain can be multifactorial in nature, and because the cause may not always be determined, these matched groups can actually be fairly heterogenous. Taking these heterogenous groups and breaking them into more homogenous groups can make a major difference in the final statistical analysis.—D.J. Lawrence, D.C.

The Chronic Illness Problem Inventory as a Measure of Dysfunction in Chronic Pain Patients

Romano JM, Turner JA, Jensen MP (Univ of Washington, Seattle)
Pain 49:71–75, 1992 1–54

Introduction.—In the assessment of physical and psychosocial dysfunction in the patient with chronic pain, the Sickness Impact Profile (SIP) has demonstrated good reliability and validity. A shorter and more easily scored instrument is the Chronic Illness Problem Inventory (CIPI); however, it has yet to be widely applied to the problem of chronic pain. These two measures were compared in 95 patients with chronic low back pain.

Patients and Methods.—There were 49 women and 46 men (average age, 44 years) and the average duration of pain was 13 years. Most had had no previous surgeries for back pain. All patients completed the SIP, CIPI, activity diaries, the McGill Pain Questionnaire, and the Center for Epidemiologic Studies-Depression scale. They then took part in a randomized study of pain control measures. In addition, a standardized assessment protocol was videotaped for recording and coding of overt pain behaviors.

Correlations Between SIP, CIPI, and Other Measures of Pain or Dysfunction

Measure *	Pretreatment †		Post-treatment †	
	SIP (n = 95)	CIPI (n = 95)	SIP (n = 75)	CIPI (n = 74)
MPQ-PRI	0.32 ‖	0.44 ‖	0.49 ‖	0.50 ‖
Total pain behaviors	0.30 ‖	0.21 §	0.19 ‡	0.21 §
Reclining time	0.31 ‖	0.42 ‖	0.35 ¶	0.42 ‖
CES-D	0.54 ‖	0.68 ‖	0.60 ‖	0.62 ‖

* *SIP,* = sickness impact profile total score; *CIPI,* = chronic illness problem inventory total score.

† MPQ-PRI = McGill pain questionnaire-pain rating index; CES-D = center for epidemiologic studies-depression scale.

‡ $P = .05$.

§ $P < .05$.

¶ $P < .01$.

‖ $P < .001$.

(Courtesy of Romano JM, Turner JA, Jensen MP: *Pain* 49:71–75 1992.)

Results.—The measurements were completed after treatment by 75 patients. The SIP and CIPI were significantly correlated both in terms of total score and pretreatment to posttreatment changes in total score. Although they appeared to be measuring similar constructs, there was also considerable unshared variance between them, indicating that they may have addressed somewhat different aspects of dysfunction. Both the SIP and CIPI appeared to be associated with the other pain-related measures in similar ways (table).

Conclusion.—The CIPI appears to be a useful alternative for the assessment of dysfunction in patients with chronic low back pain. It is easy to administer and score and it relates well to the SIP. Further validation is needed.

▶ The Sickness Impact Profile (SIP) is used to determine health status in patients with chronic pain, but it is long and time-consuming in nature and rather difficult to score. The inventory used here is a subset of the SIP known as the Chronic Illness Problem Inventory; it specifically looks at physical limitations, psychosocial impact, marital behavior, and health-care behavior. However, its reliability and validity have not been determined; ergo, this study. It does seem to compare well with the SIP and other inventories of chronic pain, and it may represent a useful outcome measure for research or within a busy practice.—D.J. Lawrence, D.C.

Efficacy of Multidisciplinary Pain Treatment Centers: A Meta-Analytic Review

Flor H, Fydrich T, Turk DC (Univ of Tübingen, Germany; Univ of Marburg, Germany; Univ of Heidelberg, Germany; et al)

Pain 49:221–230, 1992 1–55

Purpose.—Meta-analysis was used to evaluate the relative effectiveness of multidisciplinary treatment of chronic low back pain or heterogeneous pains.

Setting.—Sixty-five studies that used an interdisciplinary treatment approach in a multidisciplinary pain clinic, included empirical data, and were published from 1960 to 1990 were studied. The majority of the 3,089 patients were treated with a combination of medical treatment, physical therapy, and psychological interventions. On the basis of the criteria of Glass et al., the internal validity of the studies was relatively low, with only 8% receiving a high internal validity rating and 86.5% receiving a low validity rating.

Findings.—When compared with no treatment, waiting list, or conventional unimodal treatment approaches, within- and between-group effect sizes showed that a multidisciplinary approach for chronic pain proved to be superior and the effects appeared to be stable over time. In addition to the improvements in pain, mood, and interference, multidis-

Effect Sizes on Specific Behavioral Levels

	Within-group ES			Between-group ES			Treated (% change)			Untreated (% change)		
	Mean	S.D.	N	Mean	S.D.	N	Mean	S.D.	N	Mean	S.D.	N
Work	1.35	0.71	30	0.67	0.55	17	43	28	43	25	32	9
Medication	1.78	1.19	48	0.61	0.63	30	63	27	54	21	21	7
Health care use	0.44	0.29	16	0.47	0.51	15	35	16	21	4	18	3
Activity	0.92	0.66	27	0.63	0.87	16	53	66	49	13	32	14
Pain behavior	0.59	0.44	29	0.61	0.85	13	62	67	34	0	4	8

Note: N, number of variables included in the analysis.
(Courtesy of Flor H, Fydrich T, Turk DC: *Pain* 49:221–230, 1992.)

ciplinary treatment was associated with substantial beneficial effects on behavioral variables such as return to work and use of the health care systems (table).

Conclusion.—Multidisciplinary pain clinic treatment appears to be efficacious. However, the findings should be interpreted with caution because the quality of the study designs and descriptions is marginal.

▶ Meta-analysis is a literature-review process that allows you to collapse the data from past studies to examine them in new ways and therefore draw conclusions. Papers need to be carefully examined; therefore, you might start with 65 papers (as they did here) and ultimately end up being able to use only a handful of them for analysis purposes. While extremely difficult to do, it has yielded significant information regarding therapy in the past. Indeed, the RAND Report is largely a meta-analysis. The main interesting finding in this paper is that approaches to chronic pain that are multidisciplinary in nature have a higher efficacy than a unidisciplinary approach, i.e., physical therapy or chiropractic or medical care alone does not fare as well as when these groups combine and work together. The ramifications are obvious: these differing approaches to health care all have something to offer the patient, particularly in working together as a network.—D.J. Lawrence, D.C.

NUTRITION

Effect of Six Months of Fish Oil Supplementation in Stable Rheumatoid Arthritis: A Double-Blind, Controlled Study

Sköldstam L, Börjesson O, Kjällman A, Seiving B, Åkesson B (Kalmar Hosp, Sweden; Växjö Hosp, Sweden; Univ Hosp, Lund, Sweden)

Scand J Rheumatol 21:178–185, 1992 1–56

Purpose.—Clinical trials suggest that fish oil has weak anti-inflammatory effects in rheumatoid arthritis. Most of these studies have used a duration of treatment of 3 months or less, however. In a randomized, double-blind study, the clinical and biochemical effects of fish oil were documented over a 6-month period.

Methods.—The subjects were 46 patients with rheumatoid arthritis, 34 women and 12 men with a mean age of 57 years. The patients were randomized to receive either fish oil, 10 g/day, or placebo; they were evaluated at baseline and at 3 and 6 months. The nutrient intake of the 2 groups before and after treatment was also studied.

Findings.—Forty-three patients completed the study. There were no significant differences in nutrient intake between the 2 groups. At both 3 and 6 months, the self-reported nonsteroidal anti-inflammatory drug (NSAID) consumption was decreased in the fish-oil group; at 3 months, the physician's assessment of global arthritis activity was also improved. Self-reported global arthritic activity at 6 months was increased in the control group. There were no significant changes in patient assessment of pain, duration of morning stiffness, functional capacity, or biochemical markers of inflammation.

Conclusion.—In patients with rheumatoid arthritis, fish oil appears to lead to modest reductions in disease activity. This effect is first noted at 12 weeks and increases with prolonged use. At best, this is an adjuvant therapy with NSAID-saving potential. Data on the effects of long-term supplementation are lacking.

▶ Fish oil supplementation may reduce the clinical effects of rheumatoid arthritis. These oils are primarily *n*-3 polyunsaturated fatty acids, and they can substitute for arachidonic acid as a precursor for eicosanoids, which are known to mediate inflammation. It remains to be seen what exact dosage will create the best effects, how long such supplementation should last, and whether there are long-term effects (either beneficial or detrimental) for the use of fish oil.—D.J. Lawrence, D.C.

Nutrient Intake and Nutritional Status in Children With Juvenile Chronic Arthritis

Haugen MA, Høyeraal HM, Larsen S, Gilboe I-M, Trygg K (Oslo Sanitetsforening Rheumatism Hosp, Norway; Medstat Research, Stommen, Norway; Univ of Oslo, Norway)

Scand J Rheumatol 21:165–170, 1992 1–57

Introduction.—Nutrient intake has appeared similar in children with both high and low levels of juvenile chronic arthritis (JCA) disease activity. The growth retardation and impaired nutritional status seen in JCA may be explained by an increased nutrient requirement. The relationship of nutritional status and disease activity to dietary intake was examined in children with JCA, and the findings were compared with those of healthy controls.

Methods.—Fifteen children with JCA, 8 with polyarticular and 7 with pauciarticular disease, and 17 healthy controls were recruited into the study. The median age of the 3 boys and 12 girls was about 13 years. One pediatric rheumatologist assessed the disease in all patients, and all had biochemical and anthropometric measurements and completed an extensive dietary record.

Results.—The children with pauciarticular JCA and the controls had similar anthropometric findings. The children with polyarticular JCA, however, had reduced weight and upper arm muscle area. Compared with controls, the children with polyarticular JCA also had reduced concentrations of hemoglobin and serum levels of iron and zinc, but they had increased serum levels of copper. Those with JCA had a negative correlation between concentrations of hemoglobin and serum levels of iron and zinc and the erythrocyte sedimentation rate (ESR), but they had a positive correlation between serum levels of copper and the ESR. In spite of increased energy and protein intake, children with polyarticular JCA had impaired nutritional status. They also had a reduced dietary intake of calcium.

Conclusion.—In children with JCA, there appears to be a relationship between nutritional status and disease severity. In polyarticular JCA, energy and protein intake are increased, suggesting that the inflammatory process increases energy metabolism. Children with high levels of disease activity may need nutritional support to decrease growth retardation.

▶ Children with JCA may require larger nutrient intakes to counter possible growth retardation, and they may benefit from increased calcium intake in particular. It would be wise to optimize the diet in children with JCA, because they additionally have increased energy metabolism. Dietary assessment should be part of the therapeutic process.—D.J. Lawrence, D.C.

The Effect of Ethanol on Fat Storage in Healthy Subjects

Suter PM, Schutz Y, Jequier E (Univ of Lausanne, Switzerland)
N Engl J Med 326:983–987, 1992 1–58

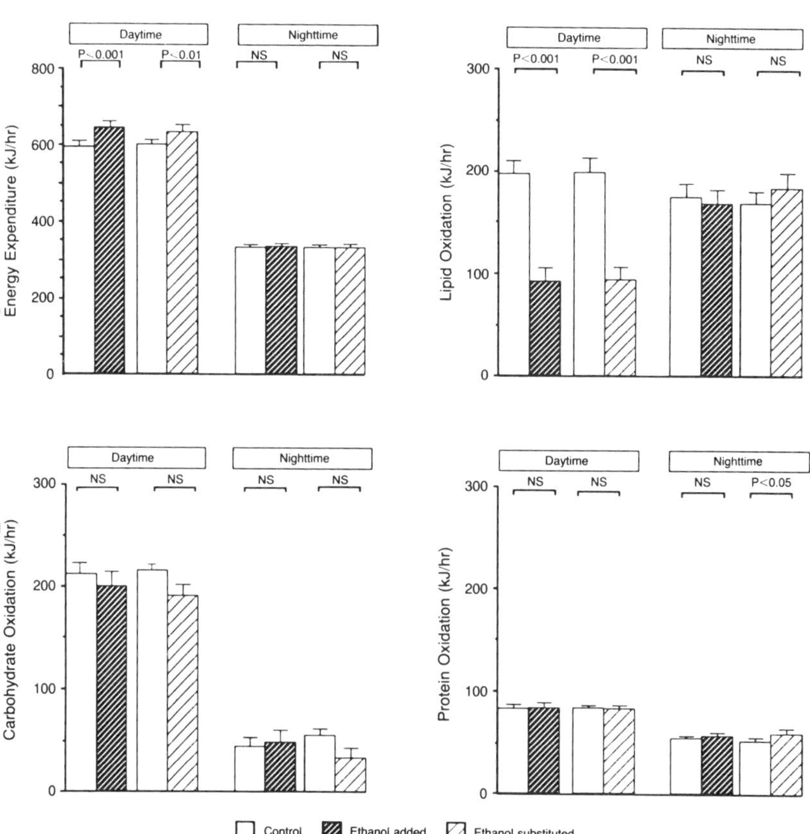

Fig 1–12.—Mean (± SE) energy expenditure and substrate-oxidation rates for the daytime and nighttime periods in 8 men before and during ethanol ingestion. The effects of ethanol were limited to the daytime period (8:30 AM to 11:30 PM), when ethanol was ingested and metabolized. The *T* bars indicate the SE. The *darker hatched bars* indicate days on which ethanol was added to the diet, and the *lighter hatched bars*, the days on which ethanol was substituted for other foods, providing 25% total energy. The *P* values are for comparisons between each day on which ethanol was given and its control day. (Courtesy of Suter PM, Schutz Y, Jequier E: *N Engl J Med* 326:983–987, 1992.)

Background.—Ethanol is an important source of energy, accounting for up to 10% of the energy intake in individuals who consume moderate amounts of ethanol. However, it is not known how this energy is used by the body. Previous studies have shown that ethanol consumption suppresses lipid oxidation. The effects of consumption of moderate amounts of ethanol on substrate oxidation in healthy, nonalcoholic men were assessed.

Methods.—Eight normal, nonalcoholic men with a mean age of 24 years and a mean body weight of 73.8 kg were studied for two 48-hour sessions in an indirect-calorimetry chamber. The interval between the 2 sessions was 5 days. The first day of each 2-day session served as a control day during which no ethanol was ingested. During the second day of one session, an additional 25% of the normal total energy requirement was added as ethanol, yielding a total energy intake of 125%. During the second day of the other session, 25% of the normal total energy requirement was replaced by ethanol, which was isocalorically substituted for lipids and carbohydrates, for a total energy intake of 100%. The order of the 2 sessions was random. Ethanol was given with meals as a 10% solution of 95% pure ethanol diluted with tap water and grape juice. All meals had to be consumed within 15 minutes.

Results.—Both addition of ethanol and the isocaloric substitution of foods by ethanol caused significant increases in 24-hour energy expenditure and significant decreases in whole-body 24-hour lipid oxidation compared with values obtained during the control days. These effects were observed only during the daytime when ethanol was ingested and metabolized (Fig 1–12). Neither the addition of ethanol to the diet, nor the substitution of a part of the diet by ethanol significantly altered the oxidation of carbohydrate or protein.

Conclusion.—Ethanol, when added to the diet or substituted for other foods, increases 24-hour energy expenditure and decreases lipid oxidation. Habitual consumption of ethanol in amounts that exceed normal energy needs probably favors fat storage and weight gain.

▶ Ethyl alcohol may play a role in lipid metabolism in the body by increasing energy use and decreasing oxidation.—D.J. Lawrence, D.C.

Trends in Prevalence and Magnitude of Vitamin and Mineral Supplement Usage and Correlation With Health Status

Bender MM, Levy AS, Schucker RE, Yetley EA (US Food and Drug Administration, Washington, DC)

J Am Diet Assoc 92:1096–1101, 1992 1–59

Objective.—Almost 40% of American adults take regular vitamin and mineral supplements. There are few data regarding the relationship between health status and use of such supplements, however. Two similar surveys on the use of vitamin and mineral supplements were compared to assess its relation to health status.

Methods.—The 2 studies were the 1980 Food and Drug Administration Vitamin and Mineral Supplement Use Survey and the 1986 National Health Interview Survey. They were comparable because they used similar questions and procedures to estimate and identify trends in supplement usage. Both also included self-reports of perceived health, number of physical conditions, and ability to perform major activities.

Results.—The comparison suggested that the prevalence of adult supplement use had slightly decreased, from 42% in 1980 to 38% in 1986. The mean number of supplements decreased form 2.15 to 1.77. The proportion of light supplement users increased from 42% to 57%. Subjects with at least 1 health problem and those who perceived their health as very good or excellent were more likely to use supplements and used them more intensely.

Conclusion.—Use of vitamin and mineral supplements remains a common practice that is associated with popular ideas about good health and well-being. Use of such supplements appears to have moderated in the recent past. It is still an important topic for counseling, especially for patients with chronic health problems. Users will respond to information about the appropriate role of supplements.

▶ Chiropractors have been criticized for their use of nutritional supplements in clinical practice. However, there are no studies that examine usage patterns in chiropractic settings; therefore, such criticisms, although politically useful, may have no basis in fact. This study examines the use of supplements in the entire United States, and it finds that such use is decreasing mildly. This may reflect a great deal of confusion regarding the effects any specific supplement may have; education and standardization, coupled with rigorous testing, should help to better codify the use of the compounds so that in clinical practice they have more active effects.—D.J. Lawrence, D.C.

Malnutrition in Geriatric Patients: Diagnostic and Prognostic Significance of Nutritional Parameters

Volkert D, Kruse W, Oster P, Schlierf G (Krankenhaus Bethanien, Heidelberg, Germany)

Ann Nutr Metab 36:97–112, 1992 1–60

Objective.—Although the frequency of malnutrition in various groups of elderly patients has been well described, there are few data on its poor prognosis. A comprehensive survey of the nutritional status of elderly patients using a variety of assessment methods was presented.

Methods.—The survey included 300 consecutive inpatients aged 75 years or older. There were 73 men and 227 women with a mean age of 82.3 years. Half were housebound before hospital admission. The nutritional assessment included the physician's clinical judgment, anthropometric measurements, and biochemical and immune function tests. Outcome was checked after 18 months, and its relations with the various assessment methods were examined.

Results.—Compared with conventional limits, deficiencies ranged from 10% for prealbumin and vitamin B_6 to 37% for vitamins A and C. Forty-four percent of patients had reduced lymphocyte levels, and 44% were anergic. The clinical diagnosis was undernourishment in 22% of cases. This judgment was associated with low anthropometric measurements and low albumin, prealbumin, transferrin, vitamin A, and vitamin B_1 values. The patients who were dead at follow-up had significantly reduced anthropometric values, plasma proteins, and vitamins A and C. The most significant prognostic factor was the clinical diagnosis of malnutrition.

Conclusion.—Clinical judgment is a useful evaluation of nutritional status in elderly patients and better than other nutritional parameters in estimating risk of long-term mortality. This relationship dictates that intensive efforts be taken to prevent and treat undernutrition.

▶ Nutritional assessment of the elderly should be carefully monitored, because there are great possibilities that the elderly patient may have some degree of malnutrition. One point not addressed by this paper was the exact diagnoses of the intake cohort; it is possible that different disease processes may be seen with different nutritional stresses; this was not addressed, and it might make for an interesting study. Knowing which diseases create which nutritional deficiencies may help in managing the patient. This study uses "generic" classifications such as cardiac disorder, infection, and gastrointestinal disease. Proper nutrition will certainly help in improving quality of life and coping with any disease seen in the elderly patient.—D.J. Lawrence, D.C.

Vitamin and Mineral Status in Physically Active Men: Effects of a High-Potency Supplement

Singh A, Moses FM, Deuster PA (Uniformed Services Univ of the Health Sciences, Bethesda, Md; Walter Reed Army Med Ctr, Washington, DC)

Am J Clin Nutr 55:1–7, 1992 1–61

Introduction.—Vitamin and mineral supplements appear to be unnecessary for individuals who consume a balanced diet, but such high-potency supplements continue to be used as a means of enhancing physical performance. Blood concentrations and urinary excretions were examined in physically active men taking a commercially available high-potency, multivitamin-mineral pill.

Methods.—After collecting baseline dietary records, fasting blood samples, and 24-hour urine samples, researchers assigned 11 subjects to the supplement and 11 to placebo. Two pills were taken each day, in the morning and evening. Dietary records and blood and urine samples were obtained again at 6 and 12 weeks.

Results.—The 2 groups did not differ significantly in their intakes of energy, protein, carbohydrate, fat, and selected vitamins and minerals from food. Only vitamin E and magnesium, of the vitamins and minerals studied, failed to meet or exceed recommended dietary allowances (RDAs). Supplementation significantly increased bold concentrations of thiamin, riboflavin, vitamins B-6, B-12, pantothenate, and biotin. The amounts of these vitamins ranged from 396% to 6,250% of the RDA. No changes were observed, however, in blood concentrations of vitamins A and C measures of zinc, magnesium, and calcium status. Supplementation also increased the urinary excretions of these vitamins.

Conclusion.—The diets of these subjects provided adequate vitamins and minerals without supplementation. Although high-potency supplements raised a number of vitamin and mineral concentrations in blood and in urinary excretions, all values had returned to presupplementation levels approximately 3 months after completion of the study.

▶ Physically active men generally will not require additional nutritional supplementation. Although there were short-term changes in blood concentrations of thiamin, pyridoxine, and vitamins B_6 and B_{12}, these all returned to baseline when the program ceased.—D.J. Lawrence, D.C.

The Case for Using Waist to Hip Ratio Measurements in Routine Medical Checks

Egger G (Univ of Newcastle, Spit Junction, Australia)

Med J Aust 156:280–285, 1992 1–62

Background.—Overweight and obesity have been associated with an increased risk of a number of diseases, including heart disease, diabetes mellitus, hypertension, and gallbladder disease. However, some investigators have not found such associations, especially when using gross measures of obesity, such as skinfold thickness and weight. Growing evidence in the past decade has indicated that a person's level of body fat is less important to health than where the fat is stored. The rationale for using wasit-to-hip ratio (WHR) measures in clinical practice was presented.

Methods and Findings.—The literature on body fat distribution from the mid-1950s to the present was reviewed. Studies showing a clear association between abdominal obesity and a range of ailments—coronary events, hypertension, blood lipid levels, cholecystectomy, diabetes, and gallbladder disease—were analyzed. Data suggest that abdominal fat measured by WHR may be a better single predictor of many diseases than other risk factors, such as overall obesity, hypertension, smoking, or hypercholesterolemia.

Conclusion.—The association between WHR and risk indicators appears to be dose-related and independent of age, race, or sex. However, high WHRs are more characteristic of men in lower socioeconomic groups, and weight control programs are more commonly developed for women. Weight control initiatives should be reoriented according to health rather than aesthetic priorities. Measuring WHR should be done routinely in clinical assessments. When combined with a measure of body mass, the predictability of WHR is improved.

▶ This paper summarizes those studies that examine the regional distribution of body fat as it relates to the presence of many chronic and potentially life-threatening diseases. It concludes that WHRs can be used as the best assessment procedure, but that there can be some pitfalls associated with its use. In practice, the measures are taken at the umbilical midline and at the superior iliac crest. Levels above .9 in men and .8 in women are seen as indicating higher risk.—D.J. Lawrence, D.C.

Treatment of Nocturnal Leg Cramps: A Crossover Trial of Quinine vs. Vitamin E

Connolly PS, Shirley EA, Wasson JH, Nierenberg DW (Veterans Affairs Med Ctr, White River Junction, Vt; Dartmouth Med School, Hanover, NH)
Arch Intern Med 152:1877–1880, 1992 1–63

Objective.—The relative efficacy and safety of quinine sulfate, vitamin E, and placebo in the treatment of nocturnal leg cramps were evaluated in a randomized, double-blind, placebo-controlled crossover trial.

Study Design.—Twenty-seven male veterans, aged 38 to 73 years, who experienced at least 6 leg cramps per month were studied during a period of 28 weeks. In a random fashion, subjects received either quinine sulfate, 200 mg at suppertime and 300 mg at bedtime; placebo at suppertime and 800 U of vitamin E at bedtime; or placebo at suppertime and bedtime for 4-week periods, followed by 4-week washout intervals (table).

Outcome.—Compared with placebo, quinine sulfate significantly reduced the frequency of cramps and sleep disturbance caused by cramps, whereas vitamin E did not. The average severity of cramp did not improve with either quinine or vitamin E. Thirteen subjects demonstrated ≥ 50% reduction in the number of cramps while receiving quinine. Among these quinine responders, the response was usually seen within 3 days of the start of treatment, with a mean percentage reduction of cramps of 85%. There was a slightly increased frequency of side effects while subjects received quinine.

Conclusion.—Quinine sulfate is superior to placebo in the treatment of nocturnal leg cramps, whereas vitamin E is not. In view of the report by Fung and Holbrook on the efficacy of a lower dose of quinine, as

Mean and Median Number of Cramps, Nights With Cramps, Sleep Disturbance, Severity, and Severity Index per 4-Week Period (N = 27)

	Placebo		Quinine Sulfate			Vitamin E		
	Mean ± SD	Median	Median ± SD	Median	P*	Mean ± SD	Median	P †
Cramps, No.	36.6 ± 6.6	28	19.2 ± 5.3	6	.0046	32.3 ± 6.6	20	NS
Nights with cramps, No.	15.4 ± 1.7	15	8.7 ± 1.8	5	.0007	14.4 ± 1.7	13	NS
Sleep disturbance score	36.5 ± 4.8	34	20.5 ± 4.6	11	.0011	33.1 ± 4.5	32	NS
Severity score	38.6 ± 4.6	36	21.4 ± 4.6	12	.0008	37.6 ± 5.4	31	NS
Severity index ‡	2.5	. . .	2.5	. . .	NS	2.6	. . .	NS

* *P* values calculated by repeated measure comparing quinine sulfate or vitamin E with placebo. *NS* indicates not significant.
† One patient did not report data for this period ($n = 20$).
‡ Severity score divided by the number of nights with cramps; reflects average severity during a 4-week period.
(Courtesy of Connolly PS, Shirley EA, Wasson JH, et al: *Arch Intern Med* 152:1877–1880, 1992.)

well as the present evidence of mild increase in side effects with quinine, it may be prudent to start by giving patients a lower dose of 200 mg at bedtime.

▶ Vitamin E cannot be used as therapy for nocturnal leg cramps. Although there had been several uncontrolled studies that indicated it could affect leg cramps, it fared poorly in this study, whereas quinine sulfate fared well. Because the original question for this study dealt with locating a nonpharmacologic intervention, a next step might be to study manipulation as therapy for leg cramping.—D.J. Lawrence, D.C.

Osteoarthritis in Women: Its Relationship to Estrogen and Current Trends

Tsai C-L, Liu T-K (Natl Taiwan Univ, Republic of China)

Life Sci 50:1737–1744, 1992 1–64

Introduction.—Osteoarthritis (OA), a major aging disease of the elderly, affects the non-weight-bearing interphalangeal and other small joints and the weight-bearing knee and hip joints. It is characterized by progressive degeneration of articular cartilage. A review of osteoporosis in women and its relationship to estrogen and current trends was presented.

Discussion.—With increasing knowledge, the concept of OA has been reassessed. It is no longer considered an inevitable disease of aging. Epidemiologic research shows that there is a higher incidence of OA affecting polyarticular joints in women than men of the same age, especially over 55 years. This sex discrepancy highlights the significance of sex hormones and their changes in menopause. These changes may occur early in adult life and persist into menopause. In addition, these hormonal changes are believed to be consequent to obesity in these women. Both in vivo and in vitro studies suggest that estrogen is chondrodestructive through receptor-mediated mechanisms, a hypothesis confirmed by the findings of estrogen receptor in canine, rabbit, and human articular cartilage. Recent studies, showing increased synovial estradiol levels and higher estrogen receptor bindings in human osteoarthritic cartilage, strongly suggest the importance of local uptake of estradiol and the possible up-regulation of estrogen receptors. Like other proposed causes, estrogen is important in the development of OA in women.

Conclusion.—The increased, sustained levels of free estradiol resulting from obesity or other known sources over a long time in young or perimenopausal women may contribute to the OA found frequently among postmenopausal women. The detrimental effect of high levels of unopposed estradiol is not manifest in younger women, possibly in part because of the slow effect of estradiol on cartilage, the protective effects of progesterone, and the active repairing ability of young cartilage resisting the episodes of micro damages from hormonal imbalance.

▶ The risk factors for OA in women include trauma, obesity, hormonal and metabolic imbalances, and genetic factors. With respect to hormonal causes, there is increasing evidence that decreasing levels of sex hormones may be directly related to the onset and development of OA. It may also relate to circulating levels of estrone and estradiol, particularly the latter. (1) This article provides a fine review of the hormonal involvement in OA, and discusses the effect of obesity.—D.J. Lawrence, D.C.

Reference

1. Meldrum DR, et al: *Obstet Gynecol* 57:624, 1981.

2 Evaluation

Orthopedics

Instrumental Straight-Leg Raising: Results in Healthy Subjects

Göeken LN, Hof AL (Univ of Groningen, The Netherlands)

Arch Phys Med Rehabil 74:194–203, 1993 2–1

Background.—Information regarding hamstring and back muscle extensibility (or the ability of a muscle to allow lengthening), elasticity, and electrical activity, as well as pelvic rotation, is provided by instrumental straight-leg raising (ISLR). To date, relevant information on these variables has not been reported. Therefore, ISLR was performed in healthy participants, and the results were described.

Methods.—A total of 24 healthy volunteers, all of whom were similar in age, height, and weight, were studied. Using the toe-touch test, the

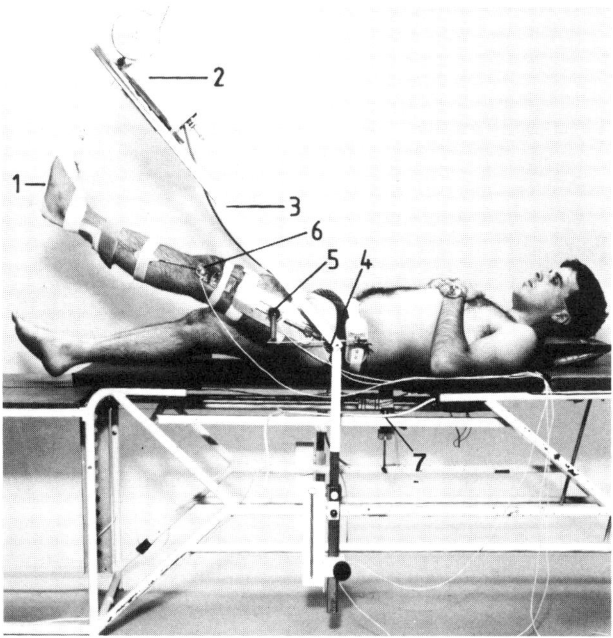

Fig 2–1.—Overview of the instructional setup: polypropylene splint (1), force transducer (2), lift frame (3), electrogoniometer on hip (4) and knee (6), inclinometer on the shank (5), and lordosis meter (7). (Courtesy of Göeken LN, Hof AL: *Arch Phys Med Rehabil* 74:194–203, 1993.)

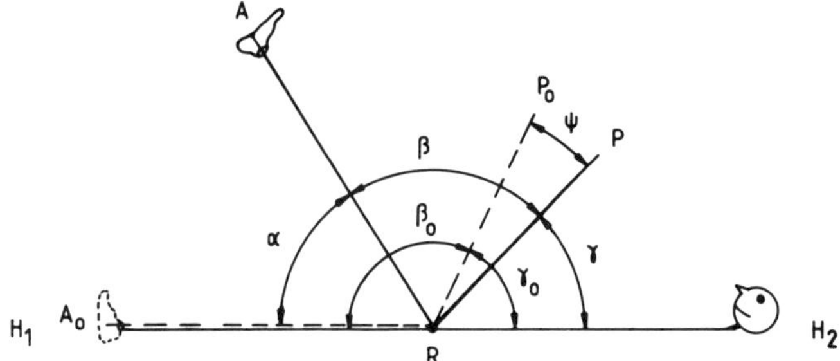

Fig 2–2.—Schematic representation of a sagittal view of the supine subject. *R* represents hip axis; *RA*, leg; *RP*, pelvis; H_1H_2, the horizontal. The initial positions, with the leg lying on the table, are given by RA_0 and RP_0. The angles are defined as follows: α = angle H_1RA, lift angle of the leg with respect to the horizontal; β = angle ARP, angle between leg and pelvis; γ = angle PRH_2, angle between pelvis and horizontal; ψ = angle P_0RP, backward tilt of the pelvis when the leg is raised. (Courtesy of Göeken LN, Hof AL: *Arch Phys Med Rehabil* 74:194–203, 1993.)

participants were assigned to 1 of 3 groups. The flexible group included 8 participants who were able to touch the ground with their hands flat, the median group included 8 participants who were able to touch the ground with their fingertips, and the stiff group consisted of 8 participants who were not able to touch the ground at all. During the ISLR test, each volunteer was placed in a prone position on an examination table, and electromyogram electrodes were applied on the semimembranous, the gluteus maximus, and the erector spinae, all on the ipsilateral side. Next, with the participant in a supine position, electrogoniometers were placed on the hip, upper leg, and knee, and zeroed. The leg was then placed in a polypropylene splint connected through a force transducer to a lift frame and lifted at approximately 3 degrees per second by an electrometer. The depth of the lordosis and, indirectly, pelvic rotation were recorded by a lordosis meter positioned at the level of the maximal lumbar lordosis (Fig 2–1). Lift was terminated at the participant's request, usually because of painful tension in the dorsal part of the thigh, or when an angle α of 90 degrees was achieved. The relative increase in hamstring length was determined from angle θ, which comprised the difference between the shank-hip angle in the supine position and the lift angle of the leg by β_0 and β, respectively (Fig 2–2).

Results.—All participants in the flexible group were able to raise their legs to the vertical position, with a median maximum lift angle of more than 90 degrees. In the medium and stiff groups, measurements were discontinued below a lift angle of 90 degrees because of pain. In the stiff group, considerable muscle pain was noted very soon after the first tension was felt. The median maximum lift angle values were 85 and 65 degrees, respectively, in the medium and stiff groups. A significant difference in hamstring extensibility between groups was revealed, with only a slight difference in back muscle extensibility. Clear between-group differences were also noted for hamstring and back muscle elasticity. Electromyogram activity was most often seen in the stiff group, particularly in the hamstrings.

Conclusion.—In normal participants, the inability to touch the ground during the toe-touch test is primarily caused by poor hamstring extensibility. In addition, positive correlations exist between maximum lift angle values in ISLR and the degree of hamstring extensibility. However, in participants with identical maximum lift angles, hamstring extensibility differs because of interindividual differences in back muscle extensibility.

▶ The straight-leg raise is one of the most common and most reliable of orthopedic tests for low back pain. In clinical use, it can help distinguish between disk and muscular problems; however, its effects have not been well quantified. There are differences in muscular activity in various groups of subjects. The instrumental test used in this study helped to show how the extensibility of the hamstrings can limit the amount of leg lift; this has to be translated into the clinical setting to see how it impacts upon the reliability of the test with injured subjects.—D.J. Lawrence, D.C.

Clinical Measures of Shoulder Subluxation: Their Reliability

Boyd EA, Torrance GM (Rehabilitation Centre, Ottawa, Ont, Canada; Carleton Univ, Ottawa, Ont, Canada)

Can J Public Health 83:24S–28S, 1992 2–2

Background.—This study stems from a larger investigation undertaken to establish an outcome measure for determining whether the use of slings had any effect on reducing shoulder subluxation and/or pain in patients with stroke. A radiologic measure for shoulder subluxation was subsequently developed, and its validity and reliability were tested. The concurrent validity of the x-ray measure with clinical measures of subluxation was found to be only moderate. However, it was suspected that this correlation was more the result of the lower reliability of the 3 clinical measures to which the x-ray measure was compared, rather than a result of the radiologic measure itself. The reliability of these 3 clinical measures used to assess shoulder subluxation changes, including finger breadth, calipers, and a plexiglass jig, was determined.

Patients and Methods.—A total of 36 patients, all of whom had experienced a cerebrovascular accident and all of whom had shoulder subluxation, were studied. Four occupational therapists experienced in stroke rehabilitation were divided into 2 teams of 2 raters each. Each participant was rated independently, and each therapist repeated her assessments on 9 participants to test intrarater agreement. Interrater agreement was also evaluated between members of the same team, with 27 participants per rater pair, as well as between members of different teams, with 18 participants per rater pair. The subacromial space was

Intra-Rater Reliability of 3 Clinical Methods, ICC (2,1) Coefficients, and 95% Lower Bound C.I. ($n = 9$)

	Rater			
	1	2	3	4
CALIPERS (cm)	.806	.889	.949	.952
	(.535)	(.692)	(.852)	(.858)
FINGERS	.909	.901	.938	.938
	(.743)	(.728)	(.832)	(.832)
JIG (cm)	.617	.510	.843	.770
	(.134)	(.024)	(.581)	(.417)

(Courtesy of Boyd EA, Torrance GM: *Can J Public Health* 83:24S–28S, 1992.)

measured using finger breadth, caliper, and plexiglass jig methods. The interclass correlation coefficient, as derived from 2-way variance analysis, was used as the measure of reliability.

Results.—The finger breadth method demonstrated the highest intra-rater reliability, followed by the caliper method, and then the plexiglass jig method (table). In the former 2 cases, the coefficients always exceeded .8, although 1 rater using the jig method only achieved this level. For the finger and caliper methods, agreement between same-team members was above .75, but it was less than .75 for the jig method. However, between different-member teams, reliability exceeding .7 was achieved only with the finger method, and the jig method demonstrated a particularly low reliability.

Conclusion.—Consistent clinical measurements for shoulder subluxation are difficult to achieve. An individual therapist who repeats ratings on the same patient may obtain consistent results. However, when interpreting results from different raters, caution is advised. In research applications, investigators should use more precise x-ray methods or combine within-rater, within-participant results from several raters if clinical methods alone are used.

▶ One thing of which to be mindful when reviewing this study is that the authors are referring to medical subluxation of the shoulder as a clinical entity. They face the same difficulty that chiropractors do in that the diagnosis is open to debate and the methods used to establish its presence remain fairly untested. The analogy to the state of affairs within the chiropractic profession is striking; we have an entity, subluxation, that is defined in many ways and that has not been adequately tested. When we do such testing (and certainly the profession is experiencing a growth in that type of research), I expect we will have results similar to those of these authors; consistent measurement will be hard to achieve. What does that say about the present state of affairs?—D.J. Lawrence, D.C.

The Reliability of Palpation and Other Diagnostic Methods
Breen A (Anglo-European College of Chiropractic, Bournemouth, England)
J Manipulative Physiol Ther 15:54–56, 1992 2–3

Background.—There is a wide gap between the levels of reliability of physical examination techniques and their clinical usefulness. Accurate diagnoses necessitate the reliability of such techniques. Ideally, validating a testing procedure involves calibration against a known standard, test/retest reliability; internal consistency; and observer variability. However, this type of validation is impossible to achieve in reality.

Palpation.—Studies of observer variation in palpating sacroiliac joint fixations have demonstrated that correlations are high, but the results of studies in the lumbar spine have been less promising. One preliminary study with a mechanical spine model has shown that some of the difficulty may lie with simply naming the spinal segmental level involved, which is not a problem with sacroiliac joint palpation.

Provocation Tests.—Only the straight-leg raising test has been found to have any degree of unquestionable reliability in predicting lumbar disk hernias. Interpreting provocation tests will remain a complex problem, despite efforts to develop procedures. If the difficulties of sensitivity and specificity can be overcome, a correct statistical technique for grouping these variables needs to be used to validate the results of test routines.

Conclusion.—Both spinal palpation and provocation tests are relevant to the segmentalization of pathomechanical processes. However, they cannot be considered alone in diagnosis. Future research should focus on how these 2 techniques can be considered as groupings.

▶ Any diagnostic test has less-than-perfect levels of sensitivity and specificity. One of the most common chiropractic diagnostic procedures is palpation, both static and motion. Tests of the reliability of motion palpation have shown that in some patients, it has a low level of inter-rater reliability, i.e., what one examiner finds may not be found by the next examiner. To properly assess this procedure, it is necessary to have criteria against which it can be measured. We have only just begun to do this, and the results of these new research experiments may require us to change our approach to palpation as a diagnostic test.—D.J. Lawrence, D.C.

Straight Leg Raising Test Versus Radiologic Size, Shape, and Position of Lumbar Disc Hernias

Thelander U, Fagerlund M, Friberg S, Larsson S (Univ Hosp, Umeå, Sweden)
Spine 17:395–399, 1992 2–4

Background.—The passive straight-leg raising (SLR) test is widely used in the diagnosis of disk protrusion or disk hernia in the lower lumbar spine. The degree of limitation of SLR at different occasions during conservative treatment of sciatica was correlated with the size, shape, and position of a corresponding lumbar disk hernia assessed on repeated CT scans.

Methods.—Thirty patients with CT-verified lumbar disk herniation were assessed before treatment and 3 and 24 months after nonoperative treatment was begun. Hernia size was expressed as an index relating it to spinal canal size.

Findings.—The limitation of the SLR test was unrelated to size or position of the hernia. Straight-leg raising was equally restricted before treatment in patients with sharply pointed or blunt hernias; however, after 3 months, it was less limited in those with sharply point hernias. After 24 months, SLR was regularly normalized. At all 3 CT scans, the size index was lower for sharply pointed hernias. A reduction in hernia size over time, regardless of shape, was not correlated with a concomitant improvement in SLR.

Conclusion.—The opinion is supported that the limitations of SLR in patients with herniated disks result from tension on an oversensitive nerve root. The amount of limitation of SLR reflects the grade of inflammatory reaction in the dural sheet and nerve root more than the pathoanatomical features of the disk hernia. A positive SLR may also have causes other than an extruded disk.

▶ The SLR test is the single orthopedic test that has been shown to reliably correlate with the presence of lumbar disk herniation. However, its presence does not indicate the size of the prolapsed material, suggesting that positive findings over time may be caused by inflammatory or traction effects on the nerve root.—D.J. Lawrence, D.C.

Electro and Acoustic Myography for Noninvasive Assessment of Lumbar Paraspinal Muscle Function

Lee DJ, Stokes MJ, Taylor RJ, Cooper RG (Univ of Queensland, Brisbane, Australia; Hope Hosp, Salford, England; Univ of Manchester, England)
Eur J Appl Physiol 64:199–203, 1992 2–5

Background.—Acoustic myography (AMG), which records sounds emitted by contracted skeletal muscles, apparently is able to monitor force changes fairly accurately. Acoustic myography activity correlates well with incremental, voluntary, isometric force in different muscles. Before it can be used in studies of paraspinal muscle physiology, AMG must be validated carefully, including the establishment of repeatability. The repeatability of AMG recordings during isometric contractions of the paraspinal muscles in normal subjects and patients with chronic low back pain was examined.

Methods.—Thirty-one healthy men and women, aged 19–48 years, and 8 men and women with chronic low back pain, aged 37–55 years, were studied. Both AMG and electromyography (EMG) were done in the lumbar paraspinal muscles. Five isometric positions were tested. The AMG and EMG signals were full-wave rectified and integrates (iAMG and iEMG), and the variability of the recordings during repeated 5-second isometric contractions was assessed using analysis of variance and the coefficient of variation.

Findings.—With both recording techniques, the most repeatable results were attained during the unsupported, horizontal hold position. The coefficients of variation in healthy individuals were 5.6% for iAMG and 4.9% for iEMG. In the patients, they were 4.4% and 2.6%, respectively. For the other 4 isometric test positions, the coefficients of variation ranged from 15.3% to 29.4% for iAMG and 8% to 15.7% for iEMG.

Conclusion.—A controlled test maneuver for examining AMG and EMG of the paraspinal muscles was vital for repeatable recordings. The standardized, horizontal position would seem to be suitable for physiologic studies of the AMG and EMG activity of the paraspinal muscles in normal subjects and in patients with chronic low back pain.

▶ Acoustic myography is a new procedure that seems to provide more sensitive measurements than surface electromyography does. However, it is expensive, relatively rare, and has not yet been adequately studied. This paper reports a first attempt to use the procedure to examine muscle function in low back pain; it correlated well with the standard EMG procedure. Therefore, although it holds promise, further testing is needed.—D.J. Lawrence, D.C.

School Screening for Scoliosis: Methodologic Considerations: Part 1: External Measurements

Pruijs JEH, Keessen W, van der Meer R, van Wieringen JC, Hageman MAPE (State Univ, Utrect, The Netherlands; Municipal Health Service, Utrecht, The Netherlands)

Spine 17:431–436, 1992 2–6

Background.—School screening of idiopathic adolescent scoliosis has attracted much attention in the past 15 years. The applicability of school screening techniques for scoliosis was determined.

Methods.—A methodologic survey was done within the framework of a school screening project. The accuracy of rib hump height, angle of trunk rotation, and moiré topography assessment was determined by assessing intraobserver and interobserver variation. The validity of the techniques was tested by comparing their results to that of the Cobb angle.

Results.—In intraobserver variation, the Spearman correlation ranged from .46 for the moiré assessment to .75 for the rib hump height. Interobserver variation ranged from .6 for rib hump height to .7 for angle of trunk rotation. Standard deviations show the interobserver range of measures: for rib hump height, 3.7 mm; for rotation, 2.3 degrees; and for moiré, .7 lines. When correlated with the angle of Cobb, the validity of the 3 methods varied from .4 to .53.

Conclusion.—These methods can be used in school screening programs, but they do not allow a sharp distinction between normal and abnormal cases. It would be better to define the borderline in terms of a danger zone instead of a strict single value. These danger zones should be 5–10 mm for rib hump height, 3–7 degrees for the rotation, and 1–3 lines for the moiré topography. Recordings in these zones should be obtained again a few months later.

▶ Standard school screening procedures for scoliosis include rib height measurement, assessment of the angle of trunk rotation, and moiré topography, as well as postural analysis. The practitioner should keep in mind that there is some observer variation in these measures, and that their correlation to Cobb's radiographic procedure is relatively modest. Standards are determined for each procedure; however, because of this variability, a child with suspected scoliosis requires more intensive examination, with a full-spine radiograph likely.—D.J. Lawrence, D.C.

Incidence of Common Postural Abnormalities in the Cervical, Shoulder, and Thoracic Regions and Their Association With Pain in Two Age Groups of Healthy Subjects

Griegel-Morris P, Larson K, Mueller-Klaus K, Oatis CA (The Philadelphia Inst for Physical Therapy; George Washington Univ Hosp, Washington, DC; Beaver College, Glenside, Pa)

Phys Ther 72:425–431, 1992 2–7

Objective.—Postural abnormalities of the thoracic, cervical, and shoulder regions were sought in 88 healthy subjects of both sexes, 58 aged 20 to 35 years and 30 aged 36 to 50 years, and were related to reports of pain.

Methods.—A newly designed questionnaire was used to determine the site, frequency, and perceived severity of pain in the areas of interest.

The subjects stood by a plumb line to evaluate a forward head position, rounded shoulders, and kyphosis.

Findings.—A forward head position was noted in 66% of the subjects, a rounded right shoulder in 73%, a rounded left shoulder in 66%, and kyphosis in 38%. Those subjects with more marked postural abnormalities more frequently had pain. The severity and frequency of pain did not, however, correlate with the severity of postural abnormality. Interscapular pain was more prevalent in those with kyphosis and rounded shoulders. A forward head posture correlated with more frequent cervical, interscapular, and headache pain.

Conclusion.—Some postural abnormalities in the cervical, shoulder, and thoracic regions are associated with the more frequent occurrence of self-reported pain.

A Determination of the Applied Laboratory Error of the Metrecom Computer-Assisted Goniometer

Ebrall PS (Phillip Inst School of Chiropractic and Osteopathy, Victoria, Australia)

Chiroprac Tech 4:46–51, 1992 2–8

Background.—The Metrecom, a relatively new measuring instrument, consists of a link arm connecting a probe tip to a fixed reference point and is the state of the art in computer-assisted goniometry (CAG). The applied laboratory error of the Metrecom CAG was studied and expressed as the coefficient of variation (V).

Methods and Results.—Laboratory-based linear measurement of a short and long distance, for which V ranged from .18% to .26%, was used in assessing the CAG. The V value depended on where the static

TABLE 1.—Data from the Instrument/Operator Combination Measurements of Two Uniplanar Distances in a Controlled Laboratory Environment

	Midrange (mm)		Lower extreme (mm)	
	Short	Long	Short	Long
Data set	1.1	1.2	1.3	1.4
Mean	495.84	998.164	498.354	1001.04
V (%)	0.18	0.13	0.26	0.24
SD	0.891	1.302	1.282	2.43
SEM	0.199	0.921	0.287	0.54
95% CI	495.43-496.26	997.56-998.77	497.42-498.95	991.91-1002.18

(Courtesy of Ebrall PS: *Chiroprac Tech*: 4:46–51, 1992.)

TABLE 2.—Data from the Measurement of Two Common Dimensions Used for Chiropractic Anthropometry

	Static Wooden Frame (mm)		Compliant Human (mm)	
	Upper	Lower	Trunk	Left Leg
Data set	2.1	2.2	3.1	3.2
mean	783.23	968.5	780.69	971.15
V (%)	0.08	0.07	0.35	0.31
SD	0.659	0.656	2.703	2.988
SEM	0.147	0.147	0.855	0.945

(Courtesy of Ebrall PS: *Chiroprac Tech*: 4:46–51, 1992.)

dimension was placed in the acquisition envelope; V was .08% for replicated trunk and .07% for replicated left leg dimensions. Similar dimensions obtained from a human showed V to increase to .35% and .31%, respectively. The major source of the applied laboratory error, the error of the subject, would appear acceptable within clinical anthropometry at V = .35%. However, caution is needed when inferences are to be made about changes or dimensions that approximate the size of this error (Tables 1 and 2).

Conclusion.—These results support the use of the Metrecom for determining leg length and trunk length in the laboratory. Caution must be used for measuring clinical levels of biomechanical dysfunction. A number of questions about the validity of the Metrecom in the clinical situation were raised, including the uncertainty of measuring typical patients in a clinical environment, the validity of nonuniplanar points to generate a singular dimension, and whether the uncertainty level of ± .3% is applicable to the longer dimension of stature.

▶ The use of instrumentation as an analytic tool has long been of interest to the chiropractic profession. The Metrecom is gaining popularity as the state of the art in computer-assisted goniometry. This study demonstrates its usefulness for determining leg and trunk length when conducted under ideal conditions by a trained researcher. It is yet to be determined whether these results can be replicated in a busy practice setting where patients may not be disrobed and measurements are performed by a chiropractic assistant. Although many claims are made for the usefulness of the Metrecom in detecting spinal fixation, misalignments, and vertebral subluxations, little scientific evidence has been reported to validate such claims in clinical practice.—A.H. Adams, D.C.

Control and "Fibrositic" Tenderness: Comparison of Two Dolorimeters

Smythe HA, Buskila D, Urowitz S, Langevitz P (Univ of Toronto, Ont, Canada; Wellesley Hosp, Toronto, Ont, Canada)

J Rheumatol 19:768–771, 1992 2–9

Background.—Contrasting the tenderness of predefined "fibrositic" sites with a lack of tenderness at predefined "control" sites is central to objectively studying patients with chronic pain syndromes. Tenderness is measured in terms of the amount of force required to produce it. Because palpation detects tenderness only, dolorimeters have been developed to standardize measurements of tenderness. The usefulness of the Chatillon meter and the Fischer dolorimeter was compared.

Instruments.—The Chatillon meter uses a footplate with a diameter of approximately 1.4 cm. Tender sites will reach a threshold of pain with pressures of less than 4 kg, and sites with higher thresholds are rated as nontender. The Chatillon meter is satisfactory for measuring tenderness, but it is less satisfactory for quantifying lack of tenderness because its maximum scale is 9 kg. The Fischer dolorimeter has a scale maximum of 11 kg and a footplate approximately 1.1 cm in diameter. Both instruments provide about 1.1 cm scale length per kg increase in applied force.

Method.—Pain thresholds in 6 sites on 8 subjects were measured, using 2 observers and the Chatillon and Fischer dolorimeters.

Findings.—The Chatillon dolorimeter yielded 17 of 96 readings off its scale of 9 kg compared with 8 of 96 readings off the 11-kg upper limit of the scale of the Fischer instrument. Because of the smaller footplate of the Fischer instrument, the results using the 2 dolorimeters were not parallel. The median values for the 2 instruments were similar at 5.1 kg, but the Fischer instrument gave lower readings at tender sites and higher values at nontender sites. The control sites were much less tender than the fibrositic sites, but the pain thresholds at the fibrositic and control sites were significantly correlated within the same subject.

Conclusion.—In a comparison of the Chatillon meter and the Fischer dolorimeter, the Chatillon instrument had twice as many measurements off the upper limit of its scale. The Fischer dolorimeter had advantages of more tender points, less tender control points, and fewer observations off its 11-kg maximum scale. As in other studies, gender, steroid therapy, or associated diseases affected tenderness; however, there was significant correlation in the thresholds of both the control and fibrositic sites in the same subject.

▶ Dolorimetry holds great potential for quantifying tenderness in fibromyalgia, soft tissue dysfunction, and other pain syndromes. This study suggests that the Fischer instrument more accurately distinguished nontender from tender sites, and also is more sensitive sites.—A.H. Adams, D.C.

Evaluation of Pericranial Myofascial Nociception by Pressure Algometry: Reproducibility and Factors of Variation

Petersen KL, Brennum J, Olesen J (Gentofte Hosp, Hellerup, Denmark)

Cephalalgia 12:33–37, 1992 2–10

Introduction.—The detection of pressure pain is influenced by nociception from both skin and subcutis; the contribution of myofascia is unknown. This is of special interest in tension-type headache and fibromyalgia, in which nociception is believed to originate mainly from the myofascial tissues. Pressure algometry was used in neighboring locations with and without interposed myofascial tissues to study the effect of myofascial nociception on pressure pain detection and tolerance.

Subjects and Methods.—The study sample comprised 40 healthy volunteers who were equally distributed as to sex and handedness. The thresholds for both detection and tolerance of pressure pain were determined by pressure algometry in 2 neighboring temporal locations with and without interposed myofascial tissue—the temporalis muscle—and on the dorsum of the second finger.

Results.—The pressure pain thresholds were lower in the area over the temporalis muscle than in the area without interposed myofascial tissue. Within subjects, pressure pain tolerance was more reproducible; between subjects, tolerance differed more than detection did. Higher pain thresholds were noted in the fingers compared with the temples and in men compared with women. In right-handers but not in left-handers the pressure pain thresholds were lateralized.

Conclusion.—Nociception from myofascial tissue appears to contribute to pressure pain threshold as measured with pressure algometry. These thresholds are probably determined by the sum of nociception from all tissues. Future research should consider both pressure pain detection and tolerance thresholds.

▶ The pressure algometer, developed by Fischer (1), has shown promise as a tool to investigate somatic responses to pain. The contribution of myofascial structures to nociception is poorly understood, especially in regard to headache. This study demonstrates that the myofascial tissues do play a role in pressure pain threshold, but it also raises as many questions as it answers. (Why do right-handed people lateralize this pain whereas left-handed people don't?) The use of the algometer in clinical practice is only now beginning to grow, and research such as this helps point the way toward greater clinical use.—D.J. Lawrence, D.C.

Reference

1. Fischer A: *Pain* 30:115, 1987.

Electrophysiologic Evidence of Piriformis Syndrome

Fishman LM, Zybert PA (Flushing Hosp Med Ctr, NY; Columbia Univ, New York)

Arch Phys Med Rehabil 73:359–364, 1992 2–11

Introduction.—The symptoms of piriformis syndrome (PS) develop when 1 or both divisions of the sciatic nerve are entrapped as they emerge from the pelvis. The H-reflex is an electrically induced version of the Achilles reflex, which crosses the piriformis muscle in afferent and efferent orthodromic conductions. The H-reflex was used to diagnose PS in patients referred for low back pain and/or sciatica.

Methods.—The criteria for PS included a positive Lasegue sign at 45 degrees, tenderness at the sciatic notch, and increased sciatic pain in the AIF (flexion) position. The H-reflexes were recorded from 39 extremities of 34 patients, 21 of whom had normal conduction velocity and electromyography findings.

Findings.—The mean delay in the H-reflex when the PS-affected extremity was internally rotated in an adducted, flexed position was 2.66 msec compared with .36 msec for contralateral extremities and normal subjects. No differences in the H-reflex itself were observed in the different groups. Eleven of 12 patients having attempts at reducing mechanical impingement had substantial relief. Treatment included myofascial release maneuvers, McKenzie exercises, and stretching of the external rotators of the thigh.

Conclusion.—Recording the H-reflex is a simple, noninvasive means of distinguishing PS from clinically similar states.

▶ The H-reflex is basically an electrically stimulated verson of the Achilles reflex. It has been used to monitor a variety of low-back responses, and it is used in this study to examine the piriformis muscle. Piriformis syndrome results from compression of the sciatic nerve by the piriformis muscle, in some cases creating the so-called "hip pocket sciatica," a diagnosis that remains somewhat controversial. This study suggests that PS is indeed a mechanical impingement; it is, therefore, quite amenable to chiropractic intervention.—D.J. Lawrence, D.C.

Imaging Modalities

Plain Film

Plain Film Radiology in Chiropractic

Phillips RB (Los Angeles College of Chiropractic, Whittier, Calif)

J Manipulative Physiol Ther 15:47–50, 1992 2–12

Background.—The use of radiographs to evaluate patients with back pain must be justified by chiropractic physicians. Plain film radiography in the early stages of acute low back pain has been challenged. Both the high frequency of back pain and the possibility of misuse of radiographs when the caregiver owns the imaging equipment pose potential problems.

Indications.—Radiographs are used by chiropractic physicians to rule out pathology in patients seen with low back pain, as well as for biomechanical evaluation. Other reasons given are to protect against medicolegal action and to make money. The literature fails to support the use of x-ray films for any of these reasons.

Suggested Guidelines.—Deyo and Diehl proposed several indications for using x-ray films in diagnosis. They include age older than 50 years, significant injury, neuromotor deficit, unexplained weight loss, and drug or alcohol abuse. Other indications are suspected ankylosing spondylitis, a history of cancer, steroid therapy, and elevated body temperature. Radiographs also may be obtained in a patient who has not improved after a recent visit for the same problem, and for patients who seek compensation for back pain.

▶ Perhaps it is unfair to render a commentary on my own work. My objective in writing this paper was to draw attention to an issue in need of a solution—in health care generally and in chiropractic specifically. The time of accountability is at hand and we, as a profession, need to provide evidence of efficacy for what we do in practice. Radiographs expose patients to harmful radiation and are a large cost-driver in health care. Thus, this procedure becomes an early target for accountability. This article attempts to address the reasons why chiropractors use radiography. The evidence provided tends to fall short of providing the support necessary to justify our actions.

The clarion call to the profession remains to be answered. We must provide documented evidence to support what we do and then explain why we do it. The challenge remains, but if it is not soon removed, our opportunity to use this diagnostic procedure may well be curtailed.—R.B. Phillips, D.C., Ph.D.

An Analysis of Errors in Kinematic Parameters Associated With *in Vivo* Functional Radiographs

Panjabi M, Chang D, Dvořák J (Yale Univ, New Haven, Conn; Klinik Wilhelm Schulthess, Zürich, Switzerland)

Spine 17:200–205, 1992 2–13

Objective.—An attempt was made to quantify error in a computer analysis method based on functional lateral radiographic views of the lumbar spine, taken in passive flexion and extension. Sets of "normal," "good," and "poor" radiographs were selected from studies of 41 healthy subjects. The radiographs, imaging the entire lumbar spine, spanned the range of radiographic quality expected in the usual clinical setting.

Results.—Graphic construction and computer-assisted methods are used to analyze a pair of functional radiographs taken at each end of the range of motion. When the same pair of radiographs was redigitized several times, there were significant differences in errors resulting from the 2 digitizers. Only minimal differences, however, were seen when the radiographs were remarked and digitized. The ranges of error were ± 1.25 degrees for rotation ± .86 degrees for translation of the inferior posterior vertebral body corner, and ± 4.3 mm for the coordinates of the center rotation. The magnitude of errors was a function of both spinal level and radiographic quality.

Clinical Application.—If functional radiographs are used to monitor the outcome of treatment, measured change must exceed the error. The findings do not include the "biological" variability incurred when a functional test is repeated on the same patient at different times. These estimates are the lower limits of error associated with kinematic parameters.

▶ Functional radiographs have been advocated as a means for determining the effectiveness of treatment. The authors have demonstrated both the effectiveness of treatment and the limitation of this procedure, which results from the errors encountered when a set of radiographs are digitized and measured by different examiners. Even with the use of computerized sophistication, errors of 1.25 degrees or 4.3 mm are still present. The authors quite clearly point out that if functional radiographs are to be used to monitor the effects of treatment, then the effects must be greater than the potential measurement errors.

Other issues related to pre/post–x-ray evaluations include position errors, unnecessary radiation, escalating costs, and the clinical significance of the radiographic changes. Post-treatment x-ray evaluation as an outcome measure for the effectiveness of care is not a desirable procedure.—R.B. Phillips, D.C., Ph.D.

Lumbar Motion Trends and Correlation With Low Back Pain: Part I. A Roentgenological Evaluation of Coupled Lumbar Motion in Lateral Bending

Haas M, Nyiendo J, Peterson C, Thiel H, Sellers T, Mas ED, Kirton C, Cassidy D (Western States Chiropractic College, Portland, Ore)

J Manipulative Physiol Ther 15:145–158, 1992 2–14

Objective.—To relate coupled lumbar motion on lateral bending with the presence of low back pain, a prospective radiographic study was undertaken in 249 patients. The series included 114 individuals with low back pain; 106 asymptomatic subjects with a history of such pain; and 29 with no such history.

Methods.—Patients were categorized clinically using the Western States Questionnaire. Coupled motion was classified in 4 categories: (I)

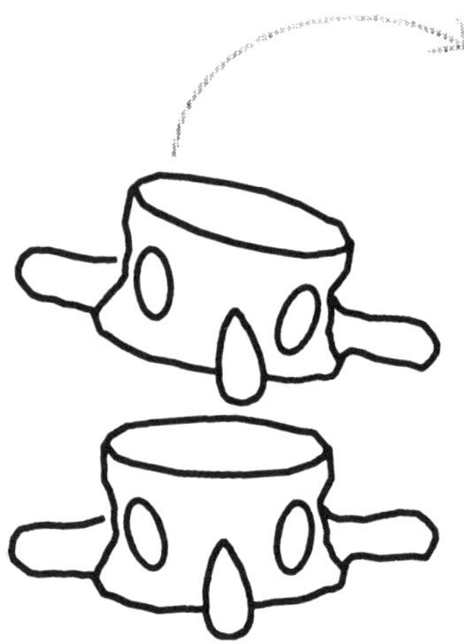

Fig 2–3.—Type I: ipsilateral tilt with contralateral rotation (right lateral bending). (Courtesy of Haas M, Nyiendo J, Peterson C, et al: *J Manipulative Physiol Ther* 15:145–158, 1992.)

ipsilateral tilt with contralateral rotation (Fig 2–3); (II) ipsilateral tilt with ipsilateral rotation; (III) contralateral tilt with contralateral rotation; and (IV) contralateral tilt with ipsilateral rotation.

Findings.—Correlation between low back pain and coupled motion was negligible at all lumbar spine levels. Correlation between pain and uniform sequential motion was poor. The average coupled motion frequencies did not differ significantly between different clinical groups of patients. The largest proportion of subjects had type I motion at L1–L5.

Implications.—Low back pain apparently does not predict qualitative segmental or global coupled lumbar motion on lateral bending. Pain is not an indication to use lateral bending radiographs to discover abnormal motion.

▶ The authors failed to support the belief that the presence of back pain is justification for taking lateral bending radiographs. It is generally believed that back pain is associated with abnormal spinal motion, either excessive or restricted. In this study, patients with low back pain, asymptomatic patients with a history of back pain, and a small group of individuals with no history of back pain were compared. Radiographic evidence of differences in spinal motion between the groups was not demonstrated.

Advocates of videofluoroscopy may argue that the end-range of motion demonstrated by static plain-film radiographs may fail to adequately demonstrate abnormal spinal motion and, thereby, may represent a flaw in this study. Such an argument awaits documented support. The authors' conclusions are consistent with those of other studies. The routine use of lateral bending studies on patients with low back pain is not supported by this work.—R.B. Phillips, D.C., Ph.D.

Evaluation of Quality of Lateral Full Spine Radiographs: A Statistical Study

Greko PJ, Thayer JD (Palmer College of Chiropractic, Davenport, Iowa; Andrews Univ, Berrien Springs, Mich)

J Manipulative Physiol Ther 15:217–223, 1992 2–15

Introduction.—The use of postural full-spine radiology by the chiropractic profession has led to some controversy. Matters of concern include radiation exposure levels, radiographic distortion effects, diagnostic quality, and radiographic quality control problems. To develop protocols optimizing radiographic quality, the effects of filtration on x-ray film quality were examined in full-spine radiographs of human subjects.

Methods.—Three chiropractic clinics provided 287 full spine lateral x-ray studies. One hundred eighty films were representative of a nonfiltration procedure; the remaining 107 films were obtained with a filtration procedure. Observers from various clinical backgrounds classified each film as adequate in quality or as over- or underexposed in each of the cervical, thoracic, lumbar, and sacral spinal regions. The effect of the subjects' sex and age on film quality was also examined.

Results.—In each of the 4 spinal areas, there were significant differences in the quality of film exposure between filtration and nonfiltration groups. The filtration group had significantly more films of adquate quality in all spinal regions except the cervical area. Regardless of filtration use, film quality decreased with increasing age in all spinal regions. Films of females had better quality in the upper spinal regions, whereas films of males were better in lower regions.

Conclusion.—Filtration procedures generally gave better results. Additional filtration over the cervical region should minimize the overexposure problem observed in these films. The practitioner should also take into account the sex and age of the patient when deciding on exposure factors and the use of sectional views.

▶ This interesting study calls into question the clinical efficacy of lateral full-spine radiographs for anything other than a postural screening. It was not designed to address the issue of radiographs and postural screening. Rather, the authors addressed the issue of filtration vs. nonfiltration for the lateral full-spine radiograph. They strongly recommended using appropriate filtration to obtain a radiograph of adequate diagnostic study.

There is a need for further study in this area. Are lateral full-spine radiographs necessary, even for postural screening? Can sectional views provide adequate information in place of the lateral full-spine radiograph? If filtration is to be used, what is the best method? What is recommended in terms of film-screen combinations and appropriate KVp techniques? The authors have done a good job of addressing a portion of a greater issue in chiropractic radiology.—R.B. Phillips, D.C., Ph.D.

The Ring of C2 and Evaluation of the Cross-Table Lateral View of the Cervical Spine

Van Hare RS, Yaron M (Overlake Hosp, Bellevue, Wash; Univ of Colorado, Denver)

Ann Emerg Med 21:733–735, 1992 2–16

Introduction.—The cross-table lateral view of the cervical spine is an essential part of the initial workup in a trauma patient with suspected cervical spinal injury. The criteria for clearing the cervical spine cross-table lateral view have previously been defined. Some physicians have proposed that identification of the radiographic ring of C2 on this view be added to the criteria for clearing the cervical spine cross-table lateral view of a trauma patient.

Discussion.—The ring of C2 is a composite shadow comprising several anatomical surfaces of the C2 vertebrae. Disruption of this ring represents a fracture of the body of C2 at the base of the dens or a type III odontoid fracture. Because identification of fractures of the second cervical vertebrae, particularly of type III odontoid fractures, may be subtle and difficult, a disruption of the ring of C2 may be the only direct sign of such a fracture on the cross-table lateral view.

▶ This article places needed emphasis on the use of a cross-table lateral view of the cervical spine in patients who have experienced significant trauma. This kind of patient usually is seen in the emergency room of a hospital, but chiropractors need to be aware of the potential of undetected cervical fractures in trauma patients who may arrive at their office, even after they have been cleared by a hospital. The use of cervical flexion and extension studies in accident victims, a common occurrence in chiropractic practice, should involve the use of a neutral lateral screening view to rule out the presence of a fracture before placing a patient in the flexed or extended position.—R.B. Phillips, D.C., Ph.D.

Lumbar Motion Trends and Correlation With Low Back Pain: Part II. A Roentgenological Evaluation of Quantitative Segmental Motion in Lateral Bending

Haas M, Nyiendo J (Western States Chiropractic College, Portland, Ore)

J Manipulative Physiol Ther 15:224–234, 1992 2–17

Background.—Some chiropractors have used lateral bending procedures as a quantitative technique for assessing patients with low back pain. The underlying premise, that specific spinal motion aberrations are related directly to symptoms, is still not validated. The relationship between the magnitude of coupled lumbar motion in lateral bending and the presence of low back pain was investigated.

Methods.—Two hundred forty-nine subjects were studied. One hundred fourteen had low back pain. Twenty-nine were asymptomatic and had no history of low back pain, and 106 were asymptomatic with a history of low back pain. One hundred ninety-four subjects were freshman volunteers. Fifty-five were new patients. The main outcome measures were net lumbar segmental tilt and rotation in lateral bending, corrected and uncorrected for segmental malposition with the patient standing upright in the neutral position.

Findings.—There was no statistically significant relationship between coupled lumbar motion and low back pain. On average, the presence of type II motion accounted for less than a 5% loss of segmental tilt in the lumbar spine. Asymmetries between left- and right-side motion averaged 45% to 100% of unilateral range of motion.

Conclusion.—Back pain is probably not an indication for the routine use of lateral bending films for the purpose of identifying changes in the magnitude of lumbar segmental motion in lateral bending. Furthermore, type II motion cannot be excluded as a normal variant. Segemental tilt or coupled rotation asymmetry probably should not, in itself, be considered an indication for spinal manipulation.

▶ This paper is a continuation of the report from the same study reported earlier. Further data analysis has demonstrated that type II motion (ipsilateral tilt with ipsilateral rotation) could not be ruled out as a normal variant. The difficulty of relating abnormal spinal motion to the presence of back pain and the need for additional radiographic studies using bending studies are underscored by the work of Haas et al. This is an area in which there is widespread use of a radiographic procedure with minimal evidence to support its usefulness. More research is needed to justify the indiscriminate use of stress radiographs to document the presence of abnormal spinal motion as a cause for low back pain.—R.B. Phillips, D.C., Ph.D.

The Value of Preemployment Roentgenographs for Predicting Acute Back Injury Claims and Chronic Back Pain Disability

Bigos SJ, Hansson T, Castillo RN, Beecher PJ, Wortley MD (Univ of Washington, Seattle; Sahlgren Hosp, Göteborg, Sweden)

Clin Orthop 283:124–129, 1992 2–18

Purpose.—Although industry has long used preemployment radiographs for screening purposes, little progress has been made toward curbing the cost of back problems. The usefulness of preemployment radiographs in predicting (1) back injuries in longshoremen and (2) back problems leading to disability lasting longer than 6 months was assessed.

Methods.—Two orthopedic surgeons evaluated 615 randomly selected sets of radiographs of longshoremen. Of these, 208 were preemployment screening radiographs, 207 were taken at the time of an acute back injury in workers whose employers did not use screening radiographs, and 200 were of patients who had been disabled with back problems for more than 6 months. The films were evaluated for spina bifida occulta, spondylolysis, spondylolisthesis, transitional vertebrae, the presence of more or less than 5 lumbar vertebrae, signs of Scheuermann's disease, changes of aging, retrolisthesis, and facet tropism.

Findings.—In all 3 groups, two thirds of the films showed no detectable abnormalities. Patients in the chronic group, who had a high incidence of spinal surgery, had a low incidence of spina bifida occulta; otherwise, there was no difference in the incidence of any of the radiographic abnormalities among the 3 groups. The groups had no significant difference in the absence of a detectable abnormality or multiple abnormalities.

Conclusion.—Lumbosacral radiographs do not appear to be useful in predicting which workers are likely to make a back injury claim or will have long-term disability. Because they have such limited association with back disorders, radiographs may discriminate against potential employees without reasonable cause. The radiation exposure in making these films is, therefore, not justified, particularly in young workers who generally have preemployment screening radiographs.

▶ This study adds to the prevailing evidence that preemployment screening radiographs of the low back are of little value in determining who is at risk for injury and/or back pain. By comparing the radiographs of 3 different populations (workers screening preemployment radiographs, (2) those workers with acute low back injuries, and (3) those who were disabled from back pain), no difference was found in the frequency of radiographic findings usually thought to put individuals at risk for back pain. This is a strong statement regarding the absence of a proven relationship between such radiographic findings as spina bifida occulta, spondylolysis, spondylolisthesis, transitional vertebrae, Scheuermann's disease, changes of aging, retrolisthesis, facet tropism, and low back pain.—R.B. Phillips, D.C., Ph.D.

Diagnostic Imaging of the Spine in Chiropractic Practice: Recommendations for Utilisation

Schultz G, Phillips RB, Cooley J, Hall T, Hoyt T, Gendreau D, Knudsen JT, Mitchel R, Taylor JAM (Los Angeles College of Chiropractic, Whittier, Calif; Univ of California, San Diego)

Chiroprac J Aust 22:141–152, 1992 2–19

Background.—Diagnostic imaging is frequently used in the evaluation of chiropractic patients. However, there is considerable lack of agreement between clinicians as to what constitutes proper x-ray use. The various types of radiographic imaging were discussed, and rationales for their use were represented.

Discussion.—The plain film is considered the mainstay in assessing chiropractic patients. It is an adequate first step in the evaluation of neoplasm, infection, fracture, and inflammatory joint disease. Traditionally, it has been used to diagnose occupational back pain, but this use has generated rigorous criticism because of the low diagnostic yield. In routine series radiographs, frontal and lateral views are generally considered to be the legal minimum. However, the inclusion of other views within this series continues to be controversial.

Full spine radiography has been used since 1924, and it remains an important diagnostic tool. New technical developments have increased its value as a safe and effective procedure. It is particularly useful for evaluating scoliosis, upper spine complaints, and complex biomechanical or postural disorders. However, it should never be used in routine screening or evaluations.

Spinal stress films are used to rule out degenerative, traumatic, inflammatory, or late postoperative instability, failed surgical fusion, osseous failure, high-risk ligamentous laxity, and scoliosis in growing skeletons. They provide little diagnostic information regarding hypomobility, aberrant biomechanics, or abnormal muscular activity. Cineradiography emerged in 1921 and is used to study the musculoskeletal system. Most reports of this method have focused on the cervical spine, although recent attention has also been given to the lumbar spine.

Computed tomography scanning is a very important tool for imaging various body systems, including the neuromusculoskeletal system and the abdomen. However, it should not be used in screening but, rather, in conjunction with plain film. Magnetic resonance imaging (MRI) is especially suited for stable, cooperative patients. It is less expensive than plain film, myelography, and CT, and it is as sensitive as other modes in diagnosing spinal compression and bony changes. However, as with many radiographic procedures, there are disadvantages and contraindications associated with the use of MRI. Conventional myelography is used only on a limited basis to evaluate radiculopathy of the cervical spine when CT or MRI findings are ambiguous. Scintigraphy, or nuclear medicine scanning, is a highly effective tool in the assessment of structure and function of many organ systems. It is based on biochemistry and is commonly used to stage and evaluate bone metastasis, as well as for screening the entire skeleton.

Conclusion.—Maintenance of reasonable boundaries and careful selection of appropriate populations are the keys to the future of diagnostic imaging. These strategies will help to hold down escalating costs while providing the positive diagnostic benefits of the technology.

▶ The chiropractic profession has received criticism for the what many view as overuse or inappropriate use of diagnostic imaging procedures. In this study, the authors provide a comprehensive list of criteria for the selection of x-ray and other imaging modalities. These recommendations ought to form the basis for the decision-making process regarding chiropractic use of diagnostic imaging. There is absolutely nothing in this paper with which I do not agree. We must at some point delineate standards for the use of these techniques, based on more than just opinion and past patterns of use. This has not yet happened to the degree necessary to allow us the best protection for our patients while still obtaining useful diagnostic information. There will still be those who order routine full-spine films and make measurements that have not been adequately tested. This must stop.—D.J. Lawrence, D.C.

Evaluation of Frontal Radiographs of Scoliotic Spines: Part I Measurement of Position and Orientation of Vertebrae and Assessment of Clinical Shape Parameters

Drerup B, Hierholzer E (Universität Münster, Germany)

J Biomech 25:1357–1362, 1992 2–20

Background.—The types of spinal deformities observed in patients with scoliosis usually include translations and rotations of the vertebrae. The position parameters describing these deformities may be obtained through calibrated stereoradiography or CT. Although both of these measurements provide a wealth of data, they are very expensive. It was demonstrated that limited positional information may be obtained from standard frontal radiographs by following the proposed data analysis.

Methods.—Four parameters, including lateral (x), and longitudinal (y) positions of the vertebra center, as well as lateral tilt (α) and vertebral rotation (ρ) angles were measured from 478 frontal radiographs of 113 patients. Smoothing of the data points was obtained by fitting the data to a first- or second-order harmonic equation using the basic harmonic function $H = A \sin (2\pi/ + \theta)$. In this equation, A represents the sine wave amplitude, λ is the wavelength, and θ is the phase with respect to the apex and the neutral vertebrae. These values were determined using least-squares approximations.

Results.—When using the harmonic approximations, a direct interpretation of functionally important clinical parameters was permitted. If lateral position, lateral tilt, and axial rotation were plotted as a function of longitudinal distance, a simple harmonic equation was seen to correlate well with the first 2 independent variables (Fig 2–4). However, to provide a better correlation with the data for axial rotation, a higher harmnonic is needed. Regression analysis demonstrated good agreement between conventional clinical parameters and those generated by the harmonic function. When compared with standard Cobb angle measurements, the measurements obtained with the harmonic approximation were shown to be more reproducible.

Conclusion.—Treatment of the data with sinusoidal functions resulted in less data scatter, and, therefore, improved reproducibility. This method of data treatment appears to be appropriate for the investigation of those spinal deformaties associated with scoliosis.

▶ Some of the best methods to assess scoliosis involve imaging procedures that are rather expensive to use. Therefore, some efforts have been put into

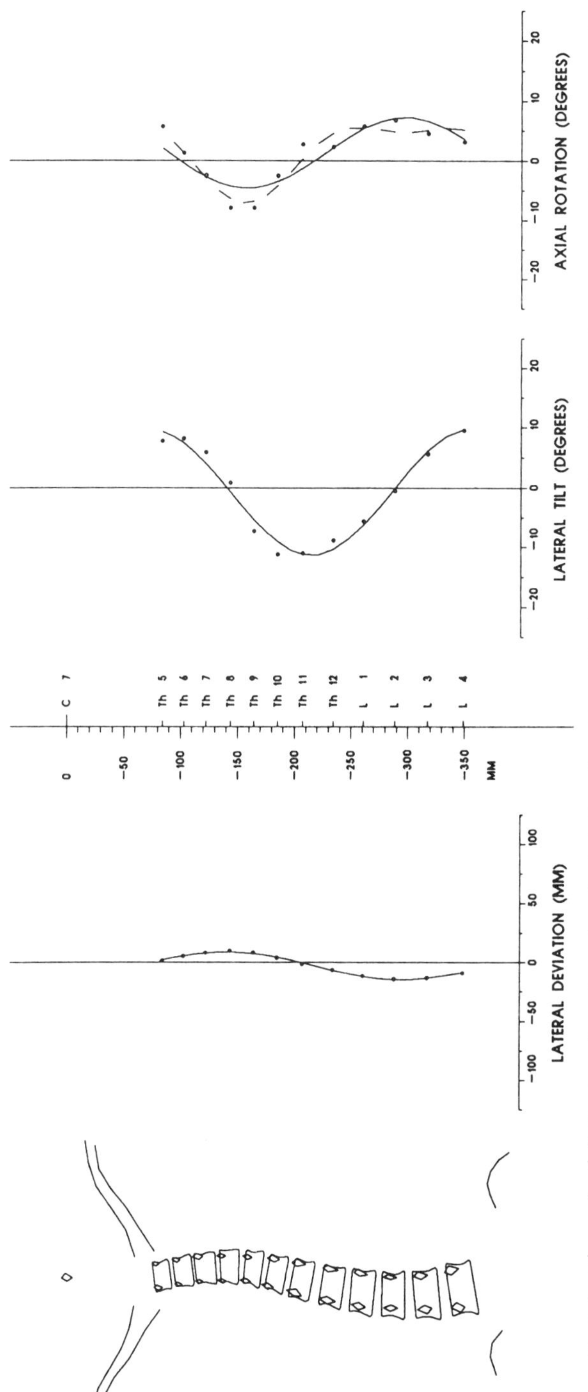

Fig 2–4.—The result of digitization of a radiograph and calculation of position and orientation of vertebrae. (Courtesy of Drerup B, Hierholzer E: *J Biomech* 25:1357–1362, 1992.)

refining standard radiographic analysis. The methods offered by Drs. Drerup and Hierholzer are complex and are probably outside the purview of the average busy practitioner. However, these methods do help to smooth reliability in the standard Cobb measurement.—D.J. Lawrence, D.C.

Macrodystrophia Lipomatosa: Radiographic Observations

Gupta SK, Sharma OP, Sharma SV, Sood B, Gupta S (Banaras Hindu Univ, Varanasi, India; Sanjay Gandhi Post-Graduate Inst of Med Sciences, Lucknow, India)

Br J Radiol 65:769–773, 1992 2–21

Background.—Macrodystrophia lipomatosa (MDL), also known as macrodactyly, megalodactyly, congenital localized gigantism, dactylomegaly, gigantomegaly, or partial acromegaly, is identified at birth or during the neonatal period and comprises a rare form of localized gigantism of 1 or more fingers or toes. As the child grows, this anomaly can disrupt joint function, vascular supply, or innervation. A wide range of MDL radiographic findings was described, with an emphasis on less frequently reported associated findings, including polydactyly, brachydactyly, early maturation of epiphyseal centers of ossification, metacarpal or metatarsal thinning, and symphalangism.

Patients.—A total of 23 cases of MDL were reviewed for clinical and radiographic findings. The patients were 16 males and 7 females, ranging from 2 to 24 years of age.

Results.—Single limb involvement was noted in 20 cases, whereas the remaining 3 patients demonstrated bilateral involvement. Five patients had upper limb and 18 had lower limb involvement. In a few cases, hypertrophy also affected the forearm and leg. The digits involved included 1 in 2 patients, 2 in 10 patients, 3 in 5 patients, 4 in 5 patients, and 5 in 2 patients. The palm of the hand and the sole of the foot were also affected, with or without metacarpal or metatarsal involvement, in 14 patients. The most frequently seen combination of digit involvement included the second and third digits. No evidence of symmetrical involvement was noted in bilateral cases. An increase in length and width was seen in affected bones, although the trabecular pattern was maintained. In some cases, the distal phalanx was surrounded by a fatty tissue ring. Lucent fatty tissue zones were also detected on some radiographs. The great toe phalanges and the first metatarsal were smaller than expected in 2 patients. In addition, early bone maturation, as demonstrated by the larger size of epiphyseal centers of ossification of phalanges and metatarsals, was also noted in several patients. In 1 patient, the metatarsals were elongated yet thinned. The articular surfaces of the phalanges were frequently slanted. Polydactyly was seen in 2 cases, syndactyly in 3, brachydactyly in 2, and symphalangism. Angiography revealed that the distal vessels were proportionately enlarged.

Conclusion.—Overgrowth of the mesodermal tissues is a common finding in MDL. However, the associated findings of syndactyly, polydactyly, brachydactyly, and even underdevelopment in a significant number of patients have demonstrated that the interaction of many different factors, including genetic factors, can result in a wide spectrum of anomalies in this disorder.

▶ Chiropractors need to at least be aware of the rarer conditions that may be seen in their offices. Few cases of macrodystrophia lipomatosa have been reported in the past, and this particular paper offers the single largest series ever published and the only reports of this disease seen in the little toes. The radiographic findings to be mindful of include overgrowth of the tissues of the digits, elongation of the digits and enlargement of their diameter, and lucent zones of fatty tissue. The authors provide some beautiful radiographs demonstrating these changes.—D.J. Lawrence, D.C.

Suggested Reading

Tiel-van Buul MMC, van Beek EJR, Broekhuizen AH, et al: Diagnosing Scaphoid Fractures: Radiographs Cannot Be Used as a Gold Standard! *Injury* 23:77–79, 1992

▶ It might surprise the reader to know that the most standard of diagnostic procedures carry with them interrater differences. If we were to have 10 doctors interpret blood pressure readings, there would be differences in measurement. That there can be these same differences in interpreting radiographs should come as no surprise, but it should also make us realize that "gold standards" may not be realistic. This simply points out that clinical uncertainty is part and parcel of medical and chiropractic practice. We may want to consider increasing the use of chiropractic specialists (such as diplomates in radiology) to decrease the level of misinterpretation; this merits further investigation within a chiropractic setting.—D.J. Lawrence, D.C.

Computed Tomography

Diagnosis of Lumbar Spinal Stenosis in Adults: A Metaanalysis of the Accuracy of CT, MR, and Myelography

Kent DL, Haynor DR, Larson EB, Deyo RA (VA Med Ctr, Seattle; Univ of Washington, Seattle)

AJR 158:1135–1144, 1992 2–22

Introduction.—The disabling chronic illness of lumbar spinal stenosis (LSS) arises from developmental anomalies or degeneration of the lumbar spine. Computed tomography (CT), MRI, and myelography are accurate techniques for the evaluation of the lumbar spine, but questions remain about the clinical relevance of differences in their technical capa-

Distribution of Quality Ratings in Each Assessment Category

Category	Number of Studies*			Quality Rating	Rating Criteria
	MR	CT	Myelography		
Index test Technical quality (by test)	1	1	3	High	Best state-of-art techniques (see text).
	3	7	3	Intermediate	Average techniques found in usual practice.
	1	3	0	Low	Obsolete, technically flawed, or not described.
Reference test quality (by study)		6		High	Surgical findings or overall impression after technical imaging and follow up; explicit criteria for surgical or clinical final diagnosis.
		8		Intermediate	Surgical or clinical follow up without explicit criteria.
		0		Low	Unacceptable or unspecified reference test.
Application of reference test		12		High	Single reference test applied to all analyzed cases.
		2		Intermediate	Mixed reference tests, all cases analyzed.
		0		Low	Acceptable reference test not applied to all cases.
Independence of interpretations		3		High	Study protocol prevented both test review and diagnosis review biases.
		7		Intermediate	One of two biases present or cannot be excluded.
		4		Low	Both biases present, or no information to assure independence of test results and reference standard determinations.

bilities. Therefore a meta-analysis of CT, MRI, and myelography studies was undertaken to evaluate the use of these imaging techniques in the evaluation of LSS.

Methods.—From a review of the literature, 116 articles were found concerning LSS in adult patients without prior surgery. Of these, 14 used some reference standard other than the technique of interest. Nine studies used CT only, 6 used myelography, 3 used both CT and MRI, and 2 used MRI only. Diagnostic accuracy was estimated by the quality of the research methods, which were assigned rating categories, A being highest and D lowest (table).

Clinical description	5	High	Description includes demographics (age, sex), duration of symptoms, and percent of cases with usual symptoms and physical findings.
	5	Intermediate	Incomplete demographic or clinical description.
	4	Low	No description other than "low back pain" or "radiculopathy."
Cohort assembly	0	High	Wide spectrum of clinical severity, enrolled prospectively from typical clinical practice sources.
	8	Intermediate	Retrospective case finding; limited spectrum of types or severity, referral filtering due to enrollments after tests ordered from specialized center.
	6	Low	Workup bias present or procedure for assembling study cohort not described.
Sample size	0	High	≥35 diseased and ≥35 nondiseased.
	11	Intermediate	≥35 diseased and <35 nondiseased or reverse.
	3	Low	<35 diseased and <35 nondiseased.

*Of The 14 studies, 5 reported on MRI, 11 on CT, and 6 on myelography.
(Courtesy of Kent DL, Haynor DR, Larson EB, et al: *AJR* 158:1135–1144, 1992.)

Results.—Of the 14 studies reviewed, all received a rating of C or D; common problems included failure to include a representative cohort, small sample size, and failure to be independent between image readings and reference standards. The reported sensitivities were .81 to .97 for MRI, .70 to 1 for CT, and .67 to .78 for myelography; pooled estimates were impossible because of the wide range of cases, test definitions and disease categories, and geographic locations. As many as 28% of asymptomatic patients showed abnormal CT or MRI findings; this was more common in the elderly.

Conclusion.—Meta-analysis of studies of CT and MRI for the evaluation of LSS does not permit strong conclusions about the relative accuracy of these techniques because of their lack of methodologic rigor. Until better studies appear, the decision to use one technique over the other will depend on cost, reimbursement, access, radiologic skill, and patient safety. Future studies need to use larger sample sizes, direct more attention to methodologic bias, and assess contribution to clinical outcome.

▶ Kent et al. have hit the nail on the head with their article assessing the quality of the literature reporting the accuracies of various imaging modalities with respect to spinal stenosis. There are many radiologists who do research, but too few researchers do radiology research. All too frequently, the hypothesis set forth by the investigating radiology department is a non-hypothesis. Also too frequently, the premise for a study assessing radiologic procedures is to "prove" or "disprove" a notion or belief. Inconsistencies in terminology, condition definition, and interpreter training, as well as bias, render many radiologic studies dangerous to draw conclusions from.

Spinal stenosis is a serious condition that is encountered in chiropractic practice. Accurate diagnosis is predicted largely on the basis of clinical parameters. The determination of where to—or what to—apply therapeutically is best *confirmed* by imaging and is not primarily *determined* by imaging. This statement is never more true than when studies such as this objectify the quality of the literature upon which we are basing our decisions.

To a large degree, interpreter experience is going to play an important role in the accuracy of any imaging interpretation. It is safest at this point to consider the options, consult with a radiologist, and then acquire imaging based on that consultation. It probably is not in the patient's best interest to undergo MRI when the interpreter is much more confident about making a diagnosis with CT. In addition to the accuracy issues, it is important to consider the cost-benefit and risk-benefit issues, especially in this era of cost-containment.—G. Schultz, D.C., D.A.C.B.R.

The Reliability of Imaging (Computed Tomography, Magnetic Resonance Imaging, Myelography) in Documenting the Cause of Spinal Pain

Wiesel S (Georgetown Univ Hosp, Washington, DC)

J Manipulative Physiol Ther 15:51–53, 1992 2–23

Background.—Computed tomography (CT), MRI, and myelography have been used in diagnosing low back pain. Each modality has different strengths and weaknesses.

The Reliability of CT, MRI, and Myelography.—Until recently, myelography has been reserved for preoperative assurance to confirm the location of the damaged disk or to determine whether there are any congenitally anomalous nerve roots, tumors, or double disks. Most studies report that CT and meylography are comparably accurate. However, a recent carefully controlled study found that myelography was more accurate than CT. However, it is unable to diagnose foraminal pathology and has been associated with complications, which make it a second choice in centers with CT and MRI. Myelography still has a role in confirming the diagnosis of arachnoiditis and in imaging the spine postoperatively when metal hardware would distort or prevent CT or MRI. Myelography is also useful in patients with multiple levels of degenerative disease with spinal stenotic symptoms when it must be decided which levels are to be decompressed. Comparisons of myelography and CT have shown that CT is just as sensitive and specific in diagnosing herniated disks. When used appropriately to confirm clinical findings, CT is very valuable. The most recent evidence suggests that MRI is more accurate than myelography in detecting degenerative disk disease. Magnetic resonance imaging is at least as accurate as CT in the diagnosis of spinal stenosis, sequestered lumbar intervertebral disk, and far lateral disk herniation.

Conclusion.—Myelography, CT, and MRI are very useful in diagnosing spinal problems. Each technique has its own role. Each should be used to confirm clinical impressions based on history and physical examination. These tests alone should not be relied upon in making a decision about surgery, because the clinical false positive rate is too high.

▶ Wiesel has pointed out the controversies surrounding the use of imaging to determine the location or need for surgery in patients with spinal pain. His article points out that clinical parameters should remain the foundation of therapeutic planning, with imaging providing necessary anatomical correlates. It is interesting to see the perceptions of a nonradiologist with respect to imaging. Thankfully, Dr. Wiesel has not been swayed by the "technocratic revolution," which has consumed so many specialists. He recognizes the advantages that new technologies bring, but is quick to point out that clinical parameters should always be the basis of therapeutic decision-making.—G. Schultz, D.C., D.A.C.B.R.

A Comparative Study of Computed Tomographic and Plain Radiographic Methods to Measure Vertebral Rotation in Adolescent Idiopathic Scoliosis

Ho EKW, Upadhyay SS, Ferris L, Chan FL, Bacon-Shone J, Hsu LCS, Leong JCY (Duchess of Kent Children's Hosp, Hong Kong; Univ of Hong Kong; Queen Mary Hosp, Hong Kong)

Spine 17:771–774, 1992 2–24

Background.—Vertebral rotation is a most important aspect of scoliosis. Initially, rotation was measured by displacement of the spinous process from the midline, but Nash and Moe found this method to be unreliable because of acquired asymmetry of the spinous processes of the scoliotic spine. Instead, they proposed that displacement of the convex-side pedicle toward the midline is directly proportional to the degree of rotation.

Objective.—The current Nash-Moe method was compared with a modified CT method of measuring vertebral rotation in 17 girls aged 12.5 to 14.5 years who had idiopathic scholisis. Cobb angles ranged from 25 to 68 degrees, with a mean of 46 degrees.

Methods.—Computed tomography scans of supine subjects were done using a low-mAS technique (120 kV, 40 mamp, 2 sec) to image the entire spinal curvature. A total of 173 vertebrae located in scoliotic curves were measured for rotation. Nash-Moe measurements were made on magnified supine anteroposterior (AP) scout films obtained during CT scanning, which were then graded by 2 observers using the pedicle shift method.

Results.—Vertebrae graded 0 by the Nash-Moe method had as much as 11 degrees of rotation by CT assessment. In Nash-Moe grade 1 and 2 vertebrae, CT showed significantly greater rotation for lumbar than for thoracic vertebrae. The mean difference between CT measurements and rotation, as predicted by the Nash-Moe grade, was not significant for either thoracic or lumbar vertebrae.

Implications.—The Nash-Moe grade 0 is not, in fact, a neutrally rotated vertebra. Nash-Moe grades may readily be converted into angles of vertebral rotation, as measured by CT, for the thoracic and lumbar vertebrae.

▶ The most commonly used procedure for measuring vertebral rotation in children with scoliosis is measurement of pedicle rotation. Developments in imaging technique have made it possible for these measurements to be made from CT. These new procedures show greater precision and reliability than those of the original. Because it is not cost-effective to obtain the serial CT scans of children necessary to make this measurement, the authors supply a simple formula that allows you to convert the old measurement into the new angle of rotation. This should be instituted into chiropractic practice.—D.J. Lawrence, D.C.

MRI

MRI and Discography of Annular Tears and Intervertebral Disc Degeneration: A Prospective Clinical Comparison

Osti OL, Fraser RD (Royal Adelaide Hosp, South Australia)

J Bone Joint Surg (Br) 74-B:431–435, 1992 2–25

Introduction.—Diskography has been used extensively to identify annular tears, a main feature of intervertebral disk degeneration. Recent studies have suggested that MRI might also be used to reveal such tears.

Patients and Methods.—Researchers evaluated 114 lumbar intervertebral disks in 33 patients with low back pain. The T2-weighted spin-echo sagittal images of 5-mm thickness were obtained with MRI. According to the signal intensity from the central zone, the disk images were classified as normal, reduced, or absent. Diskography was performed after MRI with a posterolateral approach and a 2-needle technique with stilettes. Four patterns were identified at diskography, based on the outline of the nucleus and the presence and extent of annular tears. The pain reproduced and the pressure accepted were also recorded.

Results.—All disks identified as abnormal by MRI also showed abnormal diskography patterns. However, 6 disks with normal MRI findings were found to exhibit marked degenerative changes at diskography. All symptomatic disks had degenerative contrast patterns at diskography; 27 of 39 disks that caused typical pain on diskography had normal signals on MRI.

Conclusion.—These findings indicate that MRI, using current techniques, fails to demonstrate some of the structural changes in the annulus that would be evident on diskography. Thus, patients with a normal MRI and continuing pain should undergo diskography.

▶ The study presents some interesting concepts for the evaluation of patients with low back pain. In many instances, the need for imaging beyond plain films is limited to complicated or therapy-resistant patients. There is a population of patients who demonstrate few or no findings on any imaging typically used to evaluate low back pain. This population may need a more functional study to determine their pathology. Diskography has been used to evaluate diskogenic spinal pain for many years, but it has fallen out of favor because of the invasive nature of examination and the advent of less invasive, quicker forms of imaging.

There remains a population of patients who possess abnormalities that are not visualized by the less invasive means. These patients probably need the more invasive, more sensitive studies, such as diskography, for accurate diagnosis and therapy planning. This study confirms that there are instances where diskography is uniquely diagnostic and is of therapeutic importance, even when compared with MRI, which has excellent sensitivity for the evaluation of degenerative disk disease and its complications.

Diskography has a role in the evaluation of complicated or therapy-resistent diskogenic symptomatology, where less invasive studies have failed to demonstrate the pathologic lesion. In addition to the anatomical advantages of injection of contrast directly into the nuclear space of the disk, there are provocative and palliative tests that can be performed during the procedure, as well as dynamic disk assessment that can be done under fluoroscopic observation. This study confirms the superior sensitivity of diskography as well as the role of diskography as a unique modality in certain circumstances.—G. Schultz, D.C., D.A.C.B.R.

Degeneration of the Posterior Columns of the Spinal Cord: Postmortem MRI and Histopathology

Okumura R, Asato R, Shimada T, Kusaka H, Mizutani T, Miki Y, Konishi J (Kyoto Univ, Japan; Kitano Hosp, Osaka, Japan)

J Comput Assist Tomogr 16:865–867, 1992 2–26

Introduction.—A wide range of pathologic conditions involve diffuse degenerative changes in the spinal white matter. Postmortem MR images were examined in 2 patients with spinal ataxia and 1 without neurologic abnormality. Axial spin echo images were acquired using a surface coil.

Case 1.—Man, 33, was seen with paresthesia of the legs and lumbar pain. There was progressive neurologic deterioration, as well as a disturbance in gait and urinary incontinence over 1 year. Polyneuropathy, systemic edema, 1gA gammopathy, and dermal pigmentation were found upon examination, and Crow-Fukase disease was diagnosed. The patient succumbed to lung edema 3 years after onset.

Case 2.—Man, 48, was seen with paresthesias of the extremities. A lung tumor was found on routine chest radiography, and a small cell carcinoma was seen on bronchoscopic biopsy. The patient died 3 years after the onset of symptoms, after experiencing progressive ataxia and severe vibratory sense loss.

Findings.—The 2 patients with severe posterior column syndrome and losses of vibratory and position sensation exhibited posterior column degeneration of the spinal cord. Pain and temperature sensation was relatively preserved in these cases. The MR images demonstrated high sig-

Conditions Causing Spinal Cord Degeneration (Other Than Multiple Sclerosis)

- Gracile funiculus
  - Peripheral neuropathy
  - Subacute combined degeneration of spinal cord
  - Carcinomatous radiculopathy
  - Tabes dorsalis
  - Toxins
    - Organophosphorus
    - Clioquinol (SMON)
    - Vincristine
    - Thallium
- Cuneate funiculus
  - Ascending, from lower spinal trauma or tumor
  - Friedreich's ataxia
  - Joseph disease and other system degenerations

Abbreviation: SMON, subacute myeloopticoneuropathy.

(From Okumura R, Asato R, Shimada T, et al: *J Comput Assist Tomogr* 16:865–867, 1992. Modified from Erisi MM, Oppenheimer DR: *Diagnostic Neuropathy.* London, Blackwell Scientific Publications, 1989.)

nal intensity and loss of volume, resembling what is seen in amyotrophic lateral sclerosis and Wallerian degeneration.

Discussion.—Secondary degenerative changes in the posterior columns of the spinal cord are found in many disorders other than multiple sclerosis, including peripheral neuropathy and diseases of the dorsal ganglia and/or root (table). Factors contributing to column degeneration may include Wallerian degeneration, axonal degeneration, and secondary demyelination.

MRI.—Degenerative changes in white matter are better demonstrated on spin-density-weighted images than on T2-weighted images. Image contrast is unsatisfactory in T1-weighted images. However, the fixation process may influence postmortem MR images.

► Spin-density-weighted imaging was shown to be more precise than T2-weighted images in studying degeneration in the posterior columns of the spinal cords of 2 recently deceased patients. One of the most common causes of cord degeneration is multiple sclerosis; another is diabetic neuropathy. With further refinement, MRI should soon identify the presence of these processes in an intact, live spinal cord.—D.J. Lawrence, D.C.

ULTRASOUND

Duplex Ultrasonography of Vertebral Arteries: Examination, Technique, Normal Values, and Clinical Applications

Bartels E, Fuchs H-H, Flügel KA (Städtisches Krankenhaus Bogenhausen, München, Germany)

Angiology 43:169–180, 1992 2–27

Background.—Duplex scanning is now widely accepted as a noninvasive method for detecting carotid artery disease. However, few studies have focused on duplex scanning of vertebral arteries. One possible reason for this is the anatomical position of these vessels and the consequent technical problems in imaging them. A practical method for investigating the vertebral arteries was described, and the pathologic findings diagnosed using this method were demonstrated.

Methods.—Fifty-four patients aged 22–75 years were included. None had a history of cerebrovascular disease. A duplex scanner with a 7.5- or a 10-MHz transducer was used because of its advantage of the simultaneous registration of the B-mode image and Doppler signal, during which the pulsed Doppler sample volume can be placed in any desired location in the artery. The patients were examined in the supine position, with the head in the middle position, in contrast to the carotid artery examination position, in which the head is turned away from the examined side. The vertebral artery was distinguished from the vertebral vein by its pulsatility and evidence of the typical Doppler signal in the vessel. The vertebral artery in the lower neck was examined first to locate its origin from the subclavian artery. The thyrocervical trunk can

Results in 54 Patients		
Visualization of the vertebral artery:		
in the intertransverse segment	C4-C5	100%
	C5-C6	100%
Visualization of the vertebral origin		
on the right side in 43 cases		81%
on the left side in 35 cases		65%
Maximal systolic velocity in the segment	C5-C6	
on the right side	43.0 ± 8.9 cm/s	
on the left side	43.3 ± 9.6 cm/s	
Diameter in the segment C5-C6:		
on the right side	3.81 ± 0.46 mm	
on the left side	3.88 ± 0.47 mm	
Side asymmetries in 18 cases:		33%

(Courtesy of Bartels E, Fuchs H-H, Flügel KA: *Angiology* 43:169–180, 1992.)

usually be visualized lateral from the vertebral artery, which is easily detectable by its high resistance flow characteristics. The course of the vertebral artery was then scanned longitudinally in its pretransverse and intertransverse C6–C5, C5–C4, and C4–C3 segments in the anteroposterior and lateral level, to look for plaques and flow characteristics.

Findings.—The vertebral artery was distinguished in the pretransverse and intertransverse segment C5–C6 in all of the patients. The mean diameters were 3.81 mm on the right and 3.88 on the left. The average maximal systolic velocity on the right and the left sides were 43 and 43.3 cm/second, respectively. In 81%, the vertebral origin was located on the right; in 65%, it was located on the left. The depth of the structure examined greatly influenced the technical quality of visualization, especially of the vertebral origin (table).

Conclusion.—The vertebral arteries have an important role in supplying blood to the brain. Duplex scanning, as a noninvasive method complementing continuous-wave Doppler assessment, provides more accurate hemodynamic and morphologic data on the vertebrobasilar system. It is hoped that the development of new instrumentation will eventually improve the accuracy of the examinations done.

▶ This article presents an interesting and promising technological development in the noninvasive imaging of the vertebral arteries. In the past, this area of vasculature has been difficult to image because of the complex anatomy of the region and the amount of bony overlap of the spine with the arteries. Although it is clear that the results are, at best, preliminary, this study by Bartels et al. presents evidence that this area can be effectively imaged without the use of ionizing radiation or injected contrast material. Both of these items carry an inherent morbidity with their application and, as such, should be avoided if at all possible. One of the advantages of diagnostic ultrasound is that the vascular structures can be imaged in real time. This would presumably allow the blood-flow characteristics of any segment to be evaluated during spinal motions and at certain positions.

The exciting potential for this work is that the craniovertebral junction could be noninvasively imaged, allowing a great deal more to be learned about vertebral artery insult during chiropractic manipulation. No effective, safe, inexpensive method of prospectively evaluating the complex vasculature of this area currently exists. Computed tomography, MRI angiography, and conventional angiography are the studies currently available clinically to evaluate the vertebral arteries, and they all involve considerable risk or expense. It is hoped that additional work in this area will be done to refine the technology and to increase the knowledge of this area using noninvasive means.—G. Schultz, D.C., D.A.C.B.C.

General Diagnostics

Incidence of Cancer Among Patients With Rheumatoid Arthritis

Gridley G, McLaughlin JK, Ekbom A, Klareskog L, Adami H-O, Hacker DG, Hoover R, Fraumeni JF Jr (Natl Cancer Inst, Rockville, Md; Univ Hosp, Uppsala, Sweden; Information Management Services, Silver Spring, Md)
J Natl Cancer Inst 85:307–311, 1993 2–28

Background.—Because of the presence of altered immune function in rheumatoid arthritis (RA), a chronic, autoimmune disease, numerous studies have investigated the incidence of cancer in patients with RA. In most of those studies, no increase in total incidence of cancer was revealed, except for a reported increased risk of hematopoietic cancer, including lymphoma, multiple myeloma, and leukemia. Risk clarification could aid in a better understanding of the interplay between immune disorders and their treatment, and cancer risk. The relationship between RA and subsequent specific cancer development was investigated in a large population-based cohort.

Methods.—A total of 11,683 Swedish men and women, all with a diagnosis of RA, were included. Identification of the case patients occurred from 1965 through 1983. Patient follow-up continued through 1984 via computer linkage of the Swedish Hospital Inpatient Register to the National Swedish Cancer Registry and the Swedish Registry of Causes of Death. Standardized incidence ratios were used to estimate cancer risk for specific cancers.

Results.—The overall incidence of cancer within this group of patients with RA was 840, which was close to expectation in both genders (table). A reduced risk for colon, stomach, rectum, and liver cancers was found in both sexes. For other digestive tract cancers, including cancer

Standardized Incidence Ratios (SIRs) for Selected Cancers in Swedish Male and Female Patients With Rheumatoid Arthritis

	Men			Women			Total		
Cancer site (ICD7 code)	Observed	SIR	CI	Observed	SIR	CI	Observed	SIR	CI
All (140-209)	331	1.08	1.0-1.2	509	0.88	0.8-1.0	840	0.95	0.9-1.0
Buccal (140-148)	1	0.13	0.0-0.7	16	1.77	1.0-2.9	17	1.03	0.6-1.7
Digestive (150-159)	73	0.79	0.6-1.0	108	0.65	0.5-0.8	181	0.70	0.6-0.8
Esophagus (150)	7	1.81	0.7-3.7	4	0.90	0.2-2.3	11	1.32	0.7-2.4
Stomach (151)	17	0.62	0.4-1.0	22	0.64	0.4-1.0	39	0.63	0.5-0.9
Colon (153)	15	0.70	0.4-1.2	29	0.60	0.4-0.9	44	0.63	0.5-0.9
Rectum (154)	11	0.74	0.4-1.3	17	0.73	0.4-1.1	28	0.72	0.5-1.1
Liver (155.0)	2	0.45	0.1-1.6	2	0.29	0.0-1.0	4	0.35	0.1-0.9
Gallbladder (155.1)	5	1.28	0.4-3.0	10	0.52	0.3-1.0	15	0.65	0.4-1.1
Pancreas (157)	15	1.12	0.6-1.8	17	0.68	0.4-1.1	32	0.83	0.6-1.2
Lung (162, 163)	39	1.19	0.9-1.6	29	1.50	1.0-2.2	68	1.31	1.0-1.7
Breast (170)	0	—	—	106	0.79	0.6-1.0	106	0.79	0.6-1.0
Cervix (171)	0	—	—	17	0.90	0.5-1.4	17	0.90	0.5-1.4
Uterine corpus (172)	0	—	—	27	0.86	0.6-1.1	27	0.86	0.6-1.3

Ovary (175)	0	—	—	30	0.96	0.7-1.4	30	0.96	0.6-1.4
Prostate (177)	90	1.16	0.9-1.4	0	—	—	90	1.16	0.9-1.4
Kidney (180)	16	1.25	0.7-2.0	26	1.38	0.9-2.0	42	1.33	1.0-1.8
Renal cell (180.0)	14	1.27	0.7-2.1	22	1.31	0.8-2.0	36	1.29	0.9-1.8
Pelvis (180.1)	2	1.62	0.2-5.9	2	1.74	0.2-6.3	4	1.68	0.5-4.3
Bladder (181)	14	0.73	0.4-1.2	10	0.74	0.4-1.4	24	0.74	0.5-1.1
Melanoma (190)	1	0.25	0.0-1.4	11	1.23	0.6-2.2	12	0.93	0.5-1.6
Other skin (191)	13	1.26	0.7-2.2	14	1.09	0.6-1.8	27	1.17	0.8-1.7
Brain and central nervous system (193)	8	1.20	0.5-2.4	22	1.46	0.9-2.2	30	1.38	0.9-2.0
Hematopoietic (200-209)	47	2.06	1.5-2.7	43*	1.18	0.9-1.6	90	1.52	1.2-1.9
Lymphoma (200-202, 205)	22	2.38	1.5-3.6	26	1.73	1.1-2.5	48	1.98	1.5-2.6
Hodgkins (201)	9	4.61	2.1-8.8	3	0.95	0.2-2.8	12	2.34	1.2-4.1
Non-Hodgkins (200, 202)	13	1.78	1.0-3.0	23	1.94	1.2-2.9	36	1.88	1.3-2.6
Multiple myeloma (203)	9	1.83	0.8-3.5	7	0.80	0.3-1.6	16	1.17	0.7-1.9
Leukemia (204-207)	15	1.86	1.0-3.1	9	0.79	0.4-1.5	24	1.23	0.8-1.8
CLL (204.0, 204.1)	9	2.34	1.1-4.4	2	0.52	0.1-1.9	11	1.43	0.7-2.6
Other†	30	1.13	0.8-1.8	57	0.90	0.7-1.2	87	1.02	0.8-1.3

*This number includes 1 case with 1CD7 code 208, polycythemia vera.

†Includes 3 small intestine, 5 secondary liver, 3 nose or middle ear, 4 larynx, 2 uterus (not otherwise specified), 3 vaginal and/or vulvar, 1 testis, 1 penis, 2 eye, 6 thyroid, 20 other endocrine, 3 bone, 6 connective tissue, and 28 other and/or not otherwise specified.

(Courtesy of Gridley G, McLaughlin JK, Ekbom A, et al: *J Natl Cancer Inst* 85:307–311, 1993.)

of the gallbladder and pancreas, decreased risks were found only in women. Men were at increased risk for lymphoma, multiple myeloma, and leukemia, whereas women were prone to non-Hodgkin's lymphoma only. The risks for Hodgkin's disease, multiple myeloma, and leukemia were slightly below the expected levels in women. Among men, the leukemia excess consisted primarily of chronic lymphocytic leukemia.

Conclusion.—The reduced colorectal cancer risk was consistent with that found in previous investigations of patients with RA, and with that found in reports which have indicated that nonsteroidal anti-inflammatory drugs may aid in protecting against the development of large bowel cancer. The excess of lymphomas also correlates with several studies of patients with RA.

► There are few studies that examine the incidence of cancer in patients with rheumatoid arthritis, and those that do are biased because few patients are included in the study. It is difficult to assess the risk of cancer in such patients because of their use of therapeutic pharmaceuticals. Nonsteroidal anti-inflammatory drugs are increasingly being used within medical and chiropractic settings, and these drugs have a mitigating effect on the development of certain cancers, including those of the stomach, rectum, and colon. However, the incidence of lymphoma in patients with RA is higher than that in the general population, a finding that is not explained by drug therapy and certainly worthy of note to chriropractic diagnosticians.—D.J. Lawrence, D.C.

Thermographic Imaging of Myofascial Trigger Points: A Follow-Up Study

Kruse RA Jr, Christiansen JA (Natl College of Chiropractic, Lombard, Ill)

Arch Phys Med Rehabil 73:819–823, 1992 2–29

Background.—Myofascial trigger points (TrPs) are hyperirritable spots usually found within a band of skeletal muscle or in the muscle fascia. They cause pain when compressed and may give rise to referred pain and autonomic phenomena. Examination of the affected muscle will identify a taut or palpable band. The pressure threshold for examining TrPs is the minimal force that induces pain.

Objective and Methods.—Thermographic studies were done in 11 adult subjects with myofascial TrPs and in 11 asymptomatic control subjects. Infrared thermography was used to obtain images with which to compare the sensory referral areas of myofascial TrPs with their thermal referral patterns. The images were taken at and distal to the sensory referral area of each TrP during its compression, and dynamic temperature changes were monitored.

Results.—Compression of the TrP led to an average decrease of .6°C in mean temperature at several thermal referral areas, including the lat-

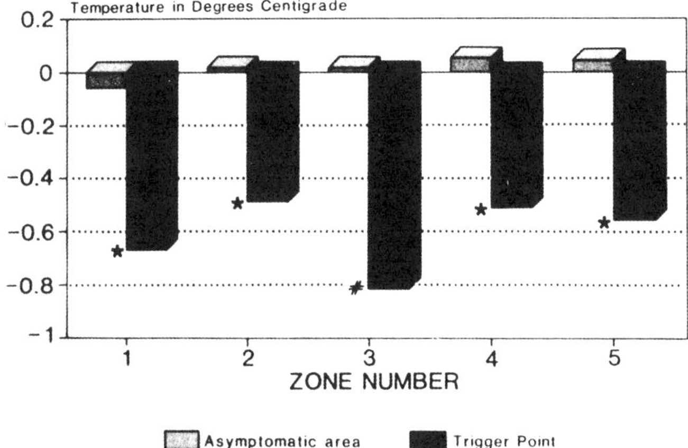

Fig 2–5.—Thermal responses of trigger point referral zones after compression of the trigger point or asymptomatic muscle areas. $n = 11$; *star*, $P < .01$; *pound sign*, $P < .05$. (Courtesy of Kruse RA Jr, Christiansen JA: *Arch Phys Med Rehabil* 73:819–823, 1992.)

eral aspects of the deltoid, arm, and forearm, the dorsum of the wrist, and the dorsum of the hand. Compression of the same areas in control subjects was associated with a mean temperature increase of .02°C. The forearm (zone 3) exhibited the greatest decrease in temperature when TrPs were compressed (Fig 2–5). The pressure thresholds for TrPs were significantly lower than those for control areas.

Discussion.—Direct compression of a specific region of somatic tissue is a consistent means of identifying TrPs. Myofascial TrPs are more sensitive than either contralateral TrP-free muscle areas or surrounding healthy tissues. The TrPs in myofascial pain syndrome probably have a peripheral autonomic component and increased sensitivity both locally and distally, in contrast to TrPs in primary fibromyalgia syndrome. Thermography may help distinguish between these syndromes.

▶ Thermography shows increasing promise as a diagnostic tool, and, in the past, it has been used to demonstrate the presence of TrPs. Diagnostic standards are being established through work such as this.—D.J. Lawrence, D.C.

Persistent Antinuclear Antibodies in Children Without Identifiable Inflammatory Rheumatic or Autoimmune Disease

Cabral DA, Petty RE, Fung M, Malleson PN (Univ of British Columbia, Vancouver, Canada)

Pediatrics 89:441–444, 1992 2–30

Background.—General pediatricians often do an antinuclear antibody (ANA) test in the evaluation of children with musculoskeletal complaints. The presence of ANAs in such cases is thought to strongly suggest significant underlying disease. The clinical and laboratory course of a group of children with musculoskeletal pain (MSP) and a positive ANA test, but with no readily identifiable rheumatic disease, was reported.

Methods.—A group of 108 children with MSP believed not to be caused by an autoimmune of inflammatory disease underwent ANA testing. Of these children, 24 were ANA positive on HEp-2 cell substrate at a 1:20 screening serum dilution.

Outcomes.—During a mean of 38 months, a positive result persisted in 21 children. None of the sera from any child at initial assessment had anti-DNA antibodies by radioimmunoassay or direct immunofluorescence on *Crithidia luciliae.* One child recently had increased anti-DNA antibodies but still had a negative assay on C. *luciliae.* Four children had antibodies to core histones according to immunoblotting. None of the children had an overt inflammatory or autoimmune disease develop during a mean 61-month follow-up.

Conclusion.—Because ANAs have been found to occur frequently in normal children, children with nonrheumatic diseases, and children with MSP, it is suggested that in the absence of clinical signs, demonstrating ANAs is unhelpful in screening for rheumatic diseases. Testing should be done only in those children with physical evidence suggesting an inflammatory rheumatic disease or a history of symptoms that strongly suggest systemic lupus erythematosus.

► Positive ANA tests generally are seen as indication of the presence of an autoimmune or rheumatic disorder. These authors found that the incidence of positive ANA tests in children without the presence of these serious underlying diseases was surprisingly high (21 of 24 patients with musculoskelatal pain). The ANA titers may be normal in children; conversely, they may be caused by viral conditions in the recent past. In the absence of clinical signs, the ANA titer may be a helpful test for screening rheumatic diseases.—D.J. Lawrence, D.C.

Human Immunodeficiency Virus Testing: Update

Hook WC, Fernandes JJ (Philadelphia College of Osteopathic Medicine)

J Am Osteopath Assoc 92:485–498, 1992 2–31

Introduction.—The acquired immunodeficiency syndrome is associated with HIV types 1 and 2. These infections are detected by screening serum samples for the presence of antibodies to HIV proteins; a confirmatory test is needed for serum samples with a positive screening test. The available screening and confirmation tests were described.

Screening Tests.—Currently used screening tests are basically enzyme linked immunosorbent assays (ELISAs), which use a mixture of HIV antigens as an immunoreactant. Most have a specificity greater than 99.8%. However, if used to screen populations at low risk for HIV infection,

Criteria for Interpretation of Western Blot Assays

	Interpretive criteria		
Organization	**Positive**	**Negative**	**Indeterminate**
American Red Cross	Minimum of 3 bands: 1 each of *env*, *gag*, *pol*	No bands	Failure to meet positive test criteria
Centers for Disease Control	Minimum of 2 of the p24, gp41, or gp160/120	No bands	Failure to meet positive test criteria
Food and Drug Administration	p24, p31, and gp41 and/or gp120/160	No bands	Failure to meet positive test criteria
Consortium for Retrovirus Serology Standardization	p24 or p31 and gp41 or gp160/120	No bands	Failure to meet positive test criteria

(*Adapted from CDC: *MMWR* 33:1–7, 1989. Courtesy of Hook WC, Fernandes JJ: *J Am Osteopath Assoc* 92:485–498, 1992.)

their positive predictive value may be 10% or less. A positive ELISA test does not prove that HIV is present, nor does a negative test rule out exposure. The physician must be aware of the patient's anxieties and present both pretest and post-test counseling, and a positive result should be not be reported until confirmation has been obtained.

Confirmatory Tests.—The most widely used confirmatory test is the Western blot technique. With this method, after HIV is grown and purified, the virus is lysed and the lysate is separated by electrophoresis. The proteins, as bands, are then transferred to nitrocellulose, from which they can be cut and used to detect the presence of antibodies to HIV proteins. Similar, but not identical, criteria for interpretation of Western blotting have been proposed by 4 major organizations (table). Although these criteria concur that the absence of bands denotes a negative result, there is considerable disagreement as to which bands must be present for a positive result. In one study, interpretation with each set of criteria gave variable numbers of positive, negative, and indeterminate findings.

Conclusion.—Although many advances have been made in the detection of HIV infection, there is no inexpensive, simple test with 100% predictive value. For now, the practice of screening with subsequent confirmatory testing for the diagnosis of HIV infection will continue. The results must be interpreted carefully, because with HIV, even a negative test result cannot be considered to indicate accurately that the subject is not infected.

▶ Although ELISA tests may be in common use, their effectiveness in screening nonrisk populations may be less than 10%. The most frequently used confirmatory test is the Western blot, but even it is not 100% effective in any population. When the screening and confirmatory tests are coupled, the effectiveness increases, but it still is not perfect. Caution is indicated when interpreting these tests with patients, because both false positive and false negative results can and do occur.—D.J. Lawrence, D.C.

Discriminating Ability of Plasma Viscosity and Erythrocyte Sedimentation Rate; A Prospective Study at the Rheumatology Outpatient Department

Dinant GJ, Habets GPA, van der Tempel H, Knottnerus JA (Univ of Limburg, Maastricht, The Netherlands; De Wever Hosp, Heerlen, The Netherlands)
Scand J Rheumatol 21:186–189, 1992 2–32

Background.—Measures of plasma viscosity (PV) and the erythrocyte sedimentation rate (ESR) are important as general parameters of inflammatory disease activity. They are thought to reflect the complex of acute-phase reactants in inflammations. The PV and ESR tests were prospectively studied at a rheumatology outpatient department to determine their ability to discriminate between inflammatory and noninflammatory rheumatic diseases in new patients.

Methods and Findings.—Two hundred thirty-five patients were included. Plasma viscosity was measured using the Coulter Viscometer II, and ESR was measured using the Westergren method. The receiver operating characteristic curve was slightly better for PV than for ESR. However, using the higher cutoff points of more than 1.81 miliPascal × seconds for PV and more than 25 mm/L/hour for ESR, ESR had more favorable sensitivities, specificities, predictive values, and odds ratios.

Conclusion.—The erythrocyte sedimentation rate, at the higher cutoff points, is superior to PV in sensitivities, specificities, predictive values, and odds ratios. In addition, measurement of PV is considerably more expensive than measurement of ESR. Thus, there is no reason to implement PV in the daily routine of the rheumatologist at the outpatient department. The possible methodologic flaws in this research were discussed.

▶ The ESR has been viewed as a useful tool in evaluating inflammatory diseases. In the case of an inflammatory process, the ESR measures combined acute-phase protein concentration. The same is true for the measurement of plasma viscosity. Studies comparing the 2 procedures have shown mixed responses. Therefore, the authors studied the 2 procedures in a group of selected, prospectively collected patients; they found that, based on their results coupled with cost-containment issues, the use of ESR should remain routine. They do not recommend adding PV as a routine screen for rheumatic disease. Chiropractors should note that ESR remains a standard screen for rheumatic and inflammatory disease.—D.J. Lawrence, D.C.

Prevalence of Vitamin B_{12} Deficiency Among Geriatric Outpatients

Yao Y, Yao S-L, Yao S-S, Yao G, Lou W (New York Med College, Kingston, NY; Dartmouth Univ, Hanover, NH; Boston Univ, Mass; Yale Univ, New Haven, Conn)

J Fam Pract 35:524–528, 1992 2–33

Introduction.—Low levels of vitamin B_{12}, or cobalamin (Cbl), can be seen in healthy subjects with no signs or symptoms of Cbl deficiency. Early detection is vital, and radioimmunoassays have improved the accuracy of Cbl determinations. Nevertheless, there is a wide variation in studies of Cbl deficiency because of the differing study populations. The prevalence of Cbl deficiency was evaluated in 100 elderly outpatients in a primary care setting.

Methods.—The patients (mean age, 77 years) had their serum Cbl levels tested during visits to a private office practice during an 11-day period. Almost all were white, and most were in the upper-middle socioeconomic class. Those with a Cbl level of 299 pg/mL or lower had testing of the serum intrinsic factor and parietal cell antibodies, serum gastrin, part 1 schilling test, serum methylmalonic acid, and total homocysteine, if possible, for the diagnosis of type A gastritis and intracellular Cbl deficiency.

Results.—The serum Cbl levels were 200 pg/mL or less in 16% of subjects. In this group, there were 2 patients with macrocytic anemia, 3 with peripheral neuropathy, and 8 with type A gastritis. In the 21% of patients with Cbl levels between 201 and 299 pg/mL, there were no cases of macrocytic anemia, 2 of peripheral neuropathy, and 9 with type A gastritis. The methylmalonic acid and total homocysteine levels were high in 80% of the patients with Cbl levels of 200 pg/mL or less and in 33% of those with Cbl levels of 201 to 299 pg/mL.

Conclusion.—A 37% prevalence rate of Cbl deficiency was found in geriatric outpatients, which is a higher rate than in any recent report. It is suggested that all patients aged 65 years or older have serum Cbl screening, and that the lower limit of normal be increased to 300 pg/mL. Below this level, serum methylmalonic acid and total homocysteine levels should be tested, especially in patients with unexplained hematologic and neuropsychiatric disorders. These tests should also be done in patients with signs of Cbl deficiency, even if their screening results are normal.

▶ There is a single lesson to be learned from this study: geriatric patients are at much higher risk of having nonsymptomatic vitamin B_{12} deficiency. Because this study examined only geriatric outpatients, it is not possible to determine the extent of deficiency within the general population of healthy individuals; however, screening should be considered for geriatric patients. The authors do suggest that further metabolic testing (for levels of methylmalonic acid and total homocysteine) should be checked in those individuals with low levels of cobalamine, but cost makes this prohibitive (the average cost of these procedures is more than $273). For patients with low levels of B_{12}, this testing may, however, reduce any risk of neuropsychiatric disorder.—D.J. Lawrence, D.C.

Dynamic Muscular Endurance in Primary Fibromyalgia Compared With Chronic Myofascial Pain Syndrome

Jacobsen S, Danneskiold-Samsøe B (Frederiksberg Hosp, Denmark)

Arch Phys Med Rehabil 73:170–173, 1992 2–34

Introduction.—Patients with primary fibromyalgia (PF) have chronic widespread muscle pain and easy muscle fatigability. They also often have functional disability and decreased work capacity. In the current study, subjective reports of easy fatigability in PF were quantified by determining the voluntary dynamic muscular endurance (DME).

Methods and Results.—The study included consecutive outpatients referred to a rheumatology clinic specializing in PF. Thirty-six patients with PF and 18 with chronic myofascial pain (CMP) syndrome were investigated. The 2 groups were matched for sex, age, height, weight, peak torque, and contractional work. Dynamic muscular endurance was defined as the number of repeated knee extensions needed for contractional work in 2 successive knee extensions to be equal or less than 70% of the initial value measured with an isokinetic dynamometer. The group with PF had a significantly lower DME than the CMP group—11 and 18, respectively.

Conclusion.—Compared with patients with CMP, those with PF have a low voluntary muscular endurance. The reduced capacity for muscle work in patients with PF most likely has both central and peripheral origins.

▶ Fibromyalgia is a perplexing clinical problem composed of muscular weakness, tender points at specific locations, and certain various organic and other symptoms. By comparing the muscle weakness in fibromyalgia to that of chronic myofascial pain, the authors hoped to demonstrate a greater amount of muscle weakness in the fibromyalgia group. They did so. By using strength dynamometry, it may be possible to clinically differentiate between these 2 similar conditions.—D.J. Lawrence, D.C.

Complications/Contraindications

Quadriplegia After Chiropractic Manipulation in an Infant With Congenital Torticollis Caused by a Spinal Cord Astrocytoma

Shafrir Y, Kaufman BA (St Louis Children's Hosp, Mo; Washington Univ, St Louis, Mo)

J Pediatr 120:266–269, 1992 2–35

Background.—An infant with congenital torticolls secondary to a holocord astrocytoma had respiratory insufficiency develop and became quadriplegic within a few hours of chiropractic manipulation.

Case Report.—Boy, 4 months, had a fluctuating but persistent head tilt and underwent manipulation that included flexion, extension, and axial loading/unloading. The infant was hard to arouse the next day but underwent another manipulation and immediately began moaning and grunting. A fever of 39.3°C was present a few hours later, as well as tachypnea and tachycardia and mild, diffuse hypotonia. A seizure occured the next day, followed by gasping respirations and cyanosis necessitating tracheal intubation. Hyponatremia was treated with 3% saline.

The infant was comatose when admitted to the intensive care unit and had repeated hypotensive/bradycardic episodes. Erythema waxed and waned in various parts of the body. An asymmetrical midcervical sensory level was identified. The infant was areflexic and retained urine. The spinal canal was enlarged from C3 through T8 and MRI demonstrated a mass within the spinal cord, extending into the medulla and into the lower thoracic region.

The cervical and lower thoracic parts of the tumor were easily removed from normal-appearing cord tissue, but normal cord was evident in the midthoracic region. Most of the tissue was acutely necrotic, but areas of low-grade astrocytoma were seen. Motor and sensory function returned to the T4 level and, after 18 months, the child had full use of his arms and senory function at about T9. There also was some nonfunctional motion of the right leg.

Discussion.—It seems likely that the extensive acute necrosis in this tumor resulted from neck manipulation. The blood supply to the tumor and spinal cord probably was compromised by the mass itself, and further impaired by manipulation. Any child with torticollis should have radiographic and neurologic evaluation before receiving physical treatment.

▶ Relatively few case reports of the complications resulting from spinal manipulation in patients with torticollis are available. Therefore, from this report, a great deal can be learned to develop clinical strategies for the prevention of such accidents involving manipulation of the cervical spine. It is important to note that more than half of all children with a cervical intramedulallary astrocytoma have torticollis as a presenting symptom (1). Children who are seen with torticollis should have an appropriate physical examination and plain-film radiographs of the cervical spine before cervical manipulation is performed. Magnetic resonance imaging may also be useful in the evaluation of children with torticollis, where the pretest probability is sufficiently high enough to consider cervical spine anomalies and tumors as diagnostic possibilities.—H. Adams, D.C.

Reference

1. Epstein F: *Adv Techn Stand Neurosurg* 13:135, 1986.

Complications From Manipulation of the Low Back

Terrett AGJ, Kleynhans AM (Royal Melbourne Inst of Technology, Bundoora, Victoria, Australia)

Chiroprac J Aust 22:129–140, 1992 2–36

Overview.—Complications of spinal manipulative therapy (SMT) of the lower back may be categorized as (1) accidents; (2) incidents that are particularly serious or long-lasting; (3) slight, short-lived reactions; or (4) indirect complications when SMT delays diagnosis and appropriate treatment.

Complications.—By far, the most common complication with low-back SMT is disk pathology or injury. Diagnostic errors and vascular insults are the next most frequent causes. Lumbar disk-related complications predominate in males, with the most common serious complication of low-back SMT being the cauda equina syndrome. Diagnostic errors occur when spinal pain is ascribed to a manipulable lesion, whereas serious underlying pathology goes undetected or is ignored. The vascular complications of SMT include hematoma formation, aortic occlusion, and thrombosis. Infrequently reported complications include excessive SMT, rib fracture, and inguinal and abdominal hernias.

Causes.—Only minor complications have resulted from a lack of technical knowledge or skill, unless a diagnostic error has occurred. Adequate patient instruction and preparation are required to make patients tolerant of SMT. Psychological intolerance and an excessive pain response may dispose patients to complications.

Clinical Decision-Making.—Patients who feel an improvement after treatment may continue to be treated until they are free of symptoms or until the treatment goal is reached. Treatment may also continue if symptoms become worse hourse after treatment but improve on the next day. If symptoms worsen immediately after treatment, the diagnosis should be reviewed and the patient treated with gentle traction, ice massage, or physiologic therapeutics. Progressive worsening of symptoms calls for a change in treatment or appropriate referral of the patient. Referral is also necessary if new signs and/or symptoms develop.

▶ In studying an 80-year database of the medical literature, the authors were able to locate a total of 86 cases of complications resulting from manipulation of the lower back. Of those cases, less than half could be attributed to chiropractic intervention. The complications identified included disk pathology, diagnostic error, vascular insult, hernia, rib fracture, etc. The authors identify the potential causes of complications, including a lack of historical data, inadequate patient assessment, excessive manipulation, and diagnostic error. They also provide a list of absolute and relative contraindications to low back manipulation. Not everyone will agree with these recommendations, but they do provide a framework to ensure that the already low incidence of such complications is made even lower. Even one complication in all of chiropractic history is too many, and some of these complications might have been avoided had a more rigorous standard of care been followed.—D.J. Lawrence, D.C.

Cryotherapy-Induced Nerve Injury

Bassett FH III, Kirkpatrick JS, Engelhardt DL, Malone TR (Duke Univ, Durham, NC)

Am J Sports Med 20:516–518, 1992 2–37

Background.—Cryotherapy is commonly used for a wide range of acute athletic injuries. However, disabling neuropathies after prolonged ice application have been reported.

Patients.—Six male athletes, aged 20–24 years, who received cryotherapy after sustaining acute sports-related injuries had peripheral nerve in-

Cryotherapy-Induced Neuropathy

Case	Nerve affected	Duration of ice (min)	Disability duration	EMG	Motor deficit	Sensory deficit
1	Peroneal	30–45	6 Months	Pos.*	Yes	Yes
2	Peroneal	20–30	1 Hour	None	Yes	Yes
3	Peroneal	60	3–4 Months	None	Yes	Yes
4	Lat. femoral condyle	60	3–4 Months	None	No	No
5	Lat. femoral condyle	15–20	96 Hours	None	No	Yes
6	Supraclavicular	15–20	3 Weeks	None	No	Yes

*Axonotmesis.
(Courtesy of Bassett FH III, Kirkpatrick JS, Engelhardt DL, et al: *Am J Sports Med* 20:516–518, 1992.)

juries (table). Three peroneal nerves, 2 lateral femoral cutaneous nerves, and 1 supraclavicular nerve were involved. The duration of cryotherapy ranged from 15–20 minutes to 2 hours, and the peripheral nerve injuries lasted from 1 hour to 6 months. Three nerves had motor deficits, and all nerves had sensory deficits. Electromyography was performed in 1 patient with a peroneal nerve injury, and the findings were consistent with axonotmesis.

Recommendations.—Peripheral nerve injury can be avoided by limiting ice applications to, at most, 20 minutes. Caution must be used when applying ice to areas overlying subcutaneous fat. Cold whirlpools or chemical cold packs may be safer than plastic ice bags because their temperatures do not drop below 10°C. Compression of the injured region must be avoided at all times when applying ice.

▶ A simple warning: excessive cryotherapy carries risk just as the overuse of hot packs do. The danger here is not of a burn (although that too can occur), but of nerve damage. In particular, the more body fat a patient has, the less likely the incidence of this injury. The authors recommend quite prudent guidelines: keep temperatures above 10°C, don't compress, use massage rather than continuous application, and keep the time of contact to less than 20 minutes.—D.J. Lawrence, D.C.

Post-Laminectomy Pseudomeningocele: An Unusual Cause of Bone Erosion

Lau KK, Stebnyckyj M, McKenzie A (Repatriation Gen Hosp, Victoria, Australia)

Australas Radiol 36:262–264, 1992 2–38

Introduction.—Pseudomeningocele is a rare complication of laminectomy that occurs secondary to a dural tear. Recurrent back pain has been a consistent feature. Complications include infection with chronic meningitis and lumbar nerve root entrapment.

Case Report.—Man, 64, had had low back pain radiating down the left leg for several years. Lumbar myelography showed spinal canal stenosis. A decompressive laminectomy was done at L5–S1. The patient recovered well but had increasing right leg pain 3 weeks later; the left leg pain recurred after 9 months. An x-ray examination showed scalloping of the posterior aspects of L3 and L4, as well as recent destruction of the inferior parts of the inferior articular processes of these vertebrae and the left L4 lamina. Myelography then demonstrated a large pseudomeningocele posterior to the spinal theca at L4 and a slight narrowing of the lumbar spinal theca adjacent to L4–5. A postmyelographic CT scan suggested mild arachnoiditis.

Mechanisms.—The postlaminectomy pseudomeningocele results from a dural or arachnoid tear during spinal surgery. It probably forms mechanically, its size being dependent on the extent of the defect, the spinal fluid pressure, and the resistance of the soft tissues. Outflowing spinal fluid keeps the defect open, and the lesion tends to enlarge over time.

Diagnosis.—A pseudomeningocele may be missed on lumbar myelography if the communication with the subarachnoid space closes. Hydrosoluble contrast medium, which readily diffuses in the CSF, may be helpful in defining the sac. Postmyelographic CT will show whether the pseudomeningocele fills with contrast, and it will clearly demonstrate such sequelae as bone erosion and vertebral body scalloping.

▶ Postsurgical patients are increasingly common in chiropractic offices. We should be aware of the complications that may occur in these patients. A pseudomeningocele occurs when there is a dural or arachnoid tear during surgery. It fills with CSF and will grow over time. Although it is, in itself, rare, in this case it was accompanied by an even rarer finding: it eroded parts of the third and fourth lumbar vertebrae. Computed tomography is believed to be the best procedure with which to identify this complication.—D.J. Lawrence, D.C.

3 Basic Sciences

Biomechanics and Functional Anatomy

Effect of Pelvic Position and Stretching Method on Hamstring Muscle Flexibility

Sullivan MK, Dejulia JJ, Worrell TW (Univ of Indianapolis, Ind)

Med Sci Sports Exerc 24:1383–1389, 1992 3–1

Background.—Hamstring muscle strain can develop in athletes for a variety of reasons, including strength imbalance, inadequate flexibility, poor warm-up, and muscle fatigue. Hamstring stretching reportedly is effective, but the role of pelvic position during stretching has not been adequately recognized in the literature. Many athletes compensate by flexing the spine in bringing the chin to the knee of the stretched leg.

Objective.—Static stretching and the proprioceptive neuromuscular facilitation (PNF) technique were compared in 20 subjects who had hamstring flexibility of less than 70 degrees bilaterally, as measured by the active knee extension test (AKET). Stretching was done with the pelvis maintained in an anterior or a posterior tilt.

Stretching.—Eight 5-minute treatment sessions were held on a daily basis, 4 days per week, for 2 weeks. Static hamstring stretching was done in the posterior pelvic tilt position by assuming a trunk-forward/flexed position, touching the chin to the chest, and then leaning forward to touch the head to the knee. The PNF stretching used the contract-relax-contract method.

Results.—Comparison of pre- and post-test AKET values showed the anterior pelvic tilt position to be significantly more effective than the posterior pelvic tilt position in enhancing hamstring muscle length. The method of stretching was not a significant factor, nor was there any apparent interaction between pelvic position and the stretching method used.

Conclusion.—Hamstring muscle length is optimally increased by performing stretching exercises in the anterior pelvic tilt position, regardless of the particular stretching technique used.

▶ One of the more common athletic injuries is hamstring muscle strain, and one of the chief causes of hamstring strain is lack of hamstring flexibility. Increasing flexibility is a desirable means of preventing these injuries, but there are a number of questions as to the best method of accomplishing that stretching. One factor affecting a stretching exercise is body position; another is the type of stretching technique. Of these 2 factors, body position is more important, and a position of anterior pelvic tilt while stretching is most important. The technique is much less important.—D.J. Lawrence, D.C.

Cross Talk in Surface Electromyograms of Human Hamstring Muscles

Koh TJ, Grabiner MD (Cleveland Clinic Found, Ohio)
J Orthop Res 10:701–709, 1992 3–2

Introduction.—Surface electromyograms (EMGs) are clinically used to assess muscle activation and also to estimate muscle forces during various movements. Signals deriving from muscles other than those studied may, through volume conduction, "contaminate" the tracing and distort its interpretation. This "cross talk" is especially a problem when recording from inactive or relatively inactive muscles close to highly active muscles.

Objective.—Cross talk was quantified in the human hamstring muscles by electrically stimulating the quadriceps femoris via the femoral nerve, and by recording EMGs from the vastus lateralis and the medial and lateral hamstring muscle groups. Six healthy men with a mean age of 30 years participated in the study.

Methods.—Silver/silver chloride surface electrodes that were 8 mm in diameter were used. The amplitude of the EMG response of the vastus lateralis to electric stimulation was adjusted to match that of its maximum voluntary effort (MVE) under isometric conditions. Power density spectrum analysis showed that the median frequencies of the signals generated electrically and by MVE did not differ significantly.

Findings.—In conventional bipolar recordings, cross talk in lateral hamstring EMGs averaged 17% of MVE and, in medial hamstring tracings, 11%. The double differential technique of data analysis significantly reduced cross talk to 8% and 4%, respectively.

Conclusion.—The double differential approach is a relatively selective means of recording the EMG from muscles having active neighbors. A software version is available for use when the number of amplifiers is limited.

▶ Surface electromyography is a diagnostic tool that is increasingly being used within the chiropractic profession. Interpretation of the signal readings requires intensive training and can easily be confounded by "cross talk", i.e., the presence of signals generated from muscles others than those of interest. Procedures that limit or eliminate signal confounders need to be developed, and these procedures will need to be site-specific for each individual muscle. With respect to the quadriceps femoris, the double differential technique is more effective at eliminating "cross talk" than is the more common bipolar technique.—D.J. Lawrence, D.C.

Forces and Moments on the Human Leg in the Frontal Plane During Static Bipedal Stance

Carmines DV, MacMahon EB (Georgetown Univ, Washington, DC; Catholic Univ of America, Washington, DC)

J Orthop Res 10:917–925, 1992 3–3

Background.—External loading of the foot has an important role in the research on and clinical evaluation of lower extremity abnormalities. An experimental apparatus was designed to allow measurement of the vertical and lateral ground reaction forces as the hip is abducted, resulting in foot separation of .25 to 71 cm with the knee in 0 degrees of flexion.

Methods.—Eight men and 4 women volunteered for the study. The hip joint was located by using the center of rotation measurements on each volunteer's legs. Knee joint locations were determined by using anatomical measurements.

Observations.—Even when the subjects' feet were placed together, the mediolateral force was nonzero and directed toward the body midline. The population mean mediolateral force was 3% of body weight, with the feet positioned at shoulder width. Simplifying assumptions based on zero lateral force or zero hip moment produced errors, compared with measured values, over various ranges of foot separation, with the zero hip moment assumption providing accuracy over a broader range.

Conclusion.—These measurements provide a means of modeling the lateral forces on the foot of healthy persons when performing research or clinical analyses. In contrast to the simplified assumptions commonly used, the lateral ground reaction force in static bipedal stance is almost always a nonzero quantity directed toward the body midline.

▶ The measurement of ground reaction forces and external loads on the foot has important implications in chiropractic research and clinical assessment. Past studies have examined the changes in ground reaction forces after chiropractic adjustment of patients with specific low back conditions. Foot loading is categorized 3 ways: static one-legged stance (which allows for simplified analysis); dynamic loading (gait analysis, which is probably best studied by chiropractors); and static bipedal stance (a compromise between the first two, used for analysis and modeling). Static bipedal stance provides a means with which to model the lateral forces on the foot as well as a method for computing the zero shear angle of the tibial plateau in the knee. The ultimate potential may be to provide new and novel methods for diagnosis of knee pathologies.—D.J. Lawrence, D.C.

Reliability of Measuring Forward Head Posture in a Clinical Setting

Garrett TR, Youdas JW, Madson TJ (Mayo Clinic and Found, Rochester, Minn)

J Orthop Sports Phys Ther 17:155–160, 1993 3–4

Background.—Faulty posture of the shoulders, neck, and head may produce and perpetuate cervical pain dysfunction syndrome. In many vocations, workers sit in ways that exaggerate forward head posture and put stress on specific regions of the musculoskeletal system by increasing flexion of the lower cervical spine and extension of the upper cervical spine. An assessment of posture is important in the physical examination of patients because it affects the treatment plan.

Methods.—Because of the need for a practical method of determining objective measurement of forward head posture, within-tester and between-tester reliabilities for clinical measurements of static, sitting, forward head posture were determined by using the cervical range of motion (CROM) instrument. Repeated measurements were obtained from 40 patients seated in a standardized position. A standardized protocol was used. Seven testers, with 1–8 years of clinical experience, participated in the study.

Findings.—Measures of forward head position performed by the same physical therapist were highly reliable. When different physical therapists measured the forward head posture of the same patient, reliability was good.

Conclusion.—Forward head posture measurements obtained by physical therapists trained in using the CROM instrument were found to be reliable. The CROM instrument will help clinicians objectively assess and reassess patients who demonstrate forward head posture.

▶ Poor posture is one of the most common yet significant factors that contributes to cervical pain syndromes. The postural components of cervical pain are endemic in chiropractic practice. Many methods have been devised to assess posture, ranging from visual assessment to radiographic mensuration. These methods have reliabilities that range from good to untested. The CROM instrument is a recently developed device designed to measure cervical range of motion, as well as forward and backward head motion. The device generates highly repeatable results; therefore, its use in assessment and evaluation is promising.—D.J. Lawrence, D.C.

The Influence of Dance Training and Foot Position on Landing Mechanics

McNitt-Gray JL, Koff SR, Hall BL (Univ of Southern California, Los Angeles; Pennsylvania State Univ, State College)

Med Probl Perform Art 7:87–91, 1992 3–5

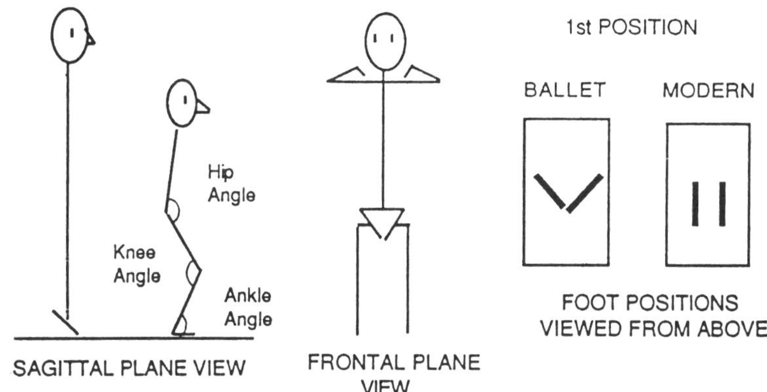

Fig 3–1.—Geometric arrangement of body segments during landings performed in first-position ballet and first-position modern from 3 perspectives. (Courtesy of McNitt-Gray JL, Koff SR, Hall BL: *Med Probl Perform Art* 7:87–91, 1992.)

Background.—Dancers experience many musculoskeletal injuries to the lower extremities. To identify ways of effectively attenuating forces during landing, the relationship between landing techniques that dancers prefer and the internal and external forces occurring during landings needs to be studied. The influence of dance training and foot position on landing mechanics was examined.

Methods.—The landings from jumps in modern dance and ballet performed by dancers, dance students, and nondancers were compared (Fig 3–1). The dancers had an average of 13 years of semiprofessional dance experience, and the dance students had completed 15 weeks of training. Ankle, knee, and hip kinematics, and vertical impulse characteristics of straight body jumps done in first-position parallel and first-position ballet were quantified.

Findings.—There were significant differences in minimum knee and hip angular positions among groups. However, there were no significant differences in minimum ankle dorsiflexion (table). The dancers had significantly greater knee angular velocities than did the students or control subjects. Peak vertical reaction forces did not differ among the groups or foot positions.

Conclusion.—Dance training apparently influences landing mechanics. Differences in the temporal characteristics and joint kinematics between subjects with and without dance training tended to be more marked for experienced dancers compared with dance students. Dance training may modify muscle activation patterns and joint kinetics before and during landings.

▶ Musculoskeletal injuries in dancers are quite common and often are caused by the ground reaction forces resulting from repeated landing from the many jumps a dancer makes. Dancers are trained in landing technique to

Mean (Standard Deviation) Kinematic Characteristics of First-Position Modern Dance Landings

	Ankle		*Knee*		*Hip*	
	Minimum Angle (°)	Maximum Angular Velocity (°/s)	Minimum Angle (°)*†‡	Maximum Angular Velocity (°/s)*†	Minimum Angle (°)*†‡	Maximum Angular Velocity (°/s)
Dancer (n = 6)	74 (3)	567 (32)	117 (4)	371 (31)	143 (8)	190 (37)
Student (n = 6)	77 (5)	502 (48)	123 (9)	329 (78)	142 (14)	162 (57)
Control (n = 6)	80 (9)	490 (99)	136 (11)	271 (70)	158 (11)	122 (54)

*Statistically significant difference exists between groups ($P < .05$).
†Follow-up pairwise comparisons indicate statistically significant difference exists between dancers and controls ($P < .05$).
‡Follow-up pairwise comparisons indicate statistically significant difference exists between students and controls ($P < .05$).
(Courtesy of McNitt-Gray JL, Koff SR, Hall BL: *Med Probl Perform Art* 7:87–91, 1992.)

minimize these injuries. They also modify their knee and hip angular positions more so than the general population to mitigate landing forces. Examination of mechanics can help decrease incidence of injury in professional dancers.—D.J. Lawrence, D.C.

Effects of Cervical Collars on Standing Balance

Burl MM, Williams JG, Nayak USL (Royal Orthopaedic Hosp, Birmingham, England; Univ of Liverpool, England; Univ of Birmingham, England)

Arch Phys Med Rehabil 73:1181–1185, 1992 3–6

Background.—Wearing of a cervical collar is often prescribed to relieve symptoms of pain and muscle spasm or to limit neck movement. Physiotherapists generally believe that wearing the collar can be detrimental to balance, especially when vision is decreased, such as in the dark. However, studies on whether the wearing of a cervical collar alone significantly affects balance have yielded conflicting evidence.

Methods.—The effects of cervical collars on standing balance were examined in 20 healthy women aged 60–78 years, and in 20 healthy women aged 18–29 years. The subjects stood on a Kistler force platform with and without a cervical collar. Total, lateral, and anteroposterior sway velocity were determined with the subjects in each of 3 positions: long-base stance with eyes open, wide-base stance with eyes open, and wide-base stance with eyes closed.

Findings.—The analysis of variance showed no significant difference between the collar and no-collar conditions for any of the standing balance measures. The older women had significantly more sway velocity than the younger women with and without the collar during long-base standing. In addition, they had significantly more sway velocity in the total and anteroposterior (AP) directions of wide-base standing. No significant differences in lateral sway velocity were noted. In the wide-base position, sway velocity was greater in both age groups, both with and without the collar, when subjects had their eyes closed. There were significant differences in sway velocity between AP and total and lateral conditions in the wide-base stance.

Conclusion.—A cervical collar does not significantly affect standing balance in able-bodied women. In standing balance, minimizing the role of the neck proprioceptors by limiting neck motion did not adversely affect balance in normal individuals.

▶ Cervical collars are used to help decrease pain and limit motion in the neck. The interruption of flow from mechanoreceptors in the neck may disturb postural reflexes and alter balance. Balance is a complex function involving muscular, vestibular, and neurologic components. Although physiotherapists have postulated that the use of the collar may disturb balance by affecting mechanoreceptor impulse flow, the results of this study indicate that this does not happen. Cervical collars do not affect postural sway or balance, at least in the 2 age ranges tested.—D.J. Lawrence, D.C.

Intersegmental Sagittal Motion in the Lower Cervical Spine and Discogenic Spondylosis: A Preliminary Study

Good CJ, Mikkelsen GB (Anglo-European College of Chiropractic, Bournemouth, England)

J Manipulative Physiol Ther 15:556–564, 1992 3–7

Background.—Radiographs are routinely obtained in the evaluation of patients with spinal conditions. When radiographs are being reviewed, the presence and severity of diskogenic spondylosis should be noted. Correlation between diskogenic spondylosis and the type of motion found in the sagittal plane of the intervertebral motion units of the lower cervical spine was examined in a case-control study.

Methods.—The records of 100 patients aged 15–73 years were reviewed. All had cervical spine-related symptoms. The cases were selected randomly from a cohort attending the clinic from 1987 to 1990 who had normal radiographic anatomy and for whom cervical spine neutral, flexion, and extension lateral radiographs had been made. A method of measuring interspinous angles is shown in Figure 3–2, and visual assessment of the motion of an intervertebral motion unit is diagramed in Figure 3–3.

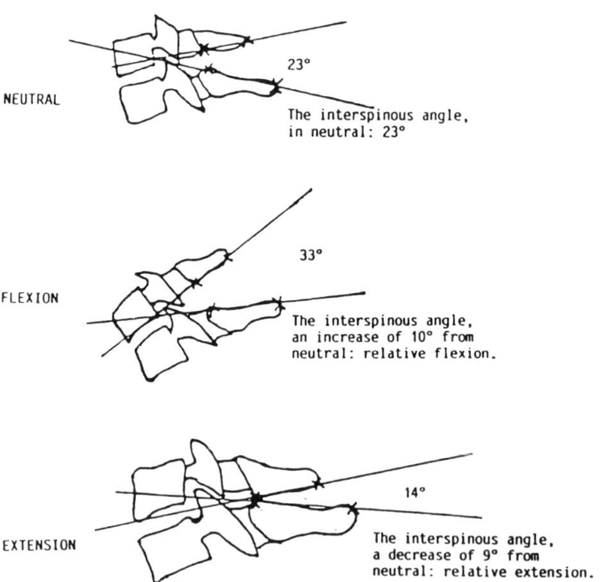

Fig 3–2.—illustration of interspinous angle measurements. (Courtesy of Good CJ, Mikkelsen GB: *J Manipulative Physiol Ther* 15:556–564, 1992.)

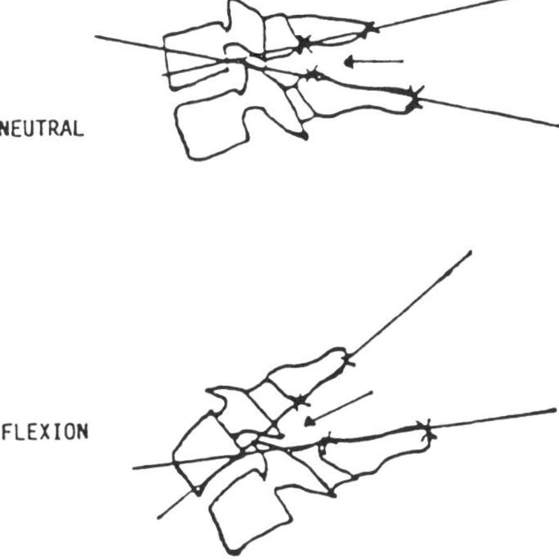

Fig 3–3.—Visual assessment of motion of intervertebral motion unit. This is easily done by observing change in gap at intersection of adjacent spinout processes. (Courtesy of Good CJ, Mikkelsen GB: *J Manipulative Physiol Ther* 15:556–564, 1992.)

Findings.—Flexion and extension films suggested that intervertebral motion units with and without varying severities of diskogenic spondylosis differed in type of motion. Intervertebral motion units with diskogenic spondylosis were more likely to exhibit motion abnormalities, and all types of motion apparently depended on its severity. In general, normal motion occurred approximately 60% of the time when diskogenic spondylosis was absent or mild, and it declined precipitously as moderate and severe amounts of diskogenic spondylosis appeared. In global cervical flexion, intersegmental hypermobility predominated when there was little or no diskogenic spondylosis and abnormal motion. Hypomobility predominated overall with moderate and severe diskogenic spondylosis. Intersegmental hypomobility was predominant in global cervical extension for all severities of diskogenic spondylosis when there was abnormal motion. Paradoxical motion occurred in 11% of the intervertebral motion units without diskogenic spondylosis.

Conclusion.—Trends occur with differing amounts of diskogenic spondylosis when considering intersegmental cervical sagittal motion. Further research is needed to corroborate these findings and to determine their clinical significance.

▶ Kirkaldy-Willis has shown a progression in degenerative changes in the spine, which moves from an initial hypomobility in early spondylosis to a hypermobility that accompanies moderate degenerative changes and, finally, back to a hypomobility with severe degeneration. Assessment of vertebral motion is one of the chief diagnostic indicators that chiropractors use in diagnosis and treatment. The radiographic procedures used in this study show that patients with diskogenic spondylosis do show differences in motion from those without. However, the findings in this case seem to contradict the model advanced by Kirkaldy-Willis, although the authors do point out potential biases that may explain or impact their findings.—D.J. Lawrence, D.C.

Evaluation of the Metrecom and Its Use in Quantifying Skeletal Landmark Locations

Smidt GL, McQuade KJ, Wei S-H (Univ of Iowa, Iowa City)

J Orthop Sports Phys Ther 16:182–188, 1992 3–8

Background.—Assessment of the posture and joint motion is the key to evaluating physical function for a variety of abnormalities. The value of the Metrecom Skeletal Analysis System (Metrecom method) and its use in quantifying skeletal landmark locations were investigated.

Methods.—The accuracy, repeatability, and linearity of the Metrecom System and the reliability of bony landmark identification with a technique using the Metrecom System to obtain coordinates for human skeletal landmarks were studied. A calibration control object with 20 known 3-dimensional coordinates in a rectangular field served as the standard in the first part of the study. The Metrecom method was assessed by using a test-retest approach for 10 bony landmarks on each of 10 healthy individuals studied by 2 different examiners.

Findings.—The hysteresis of the Metrecom System was minimal, and the linearity was excellent. The differences between the true and measured distances for 20 known points were not statistically significant. Within the field of measurement, the variability for any point was homogeneous. The Metrecom System had an accuracy of 2.7 mm. The repeatability reflected by deviations along the X, Y, and Z axes was .22, .57, and .31 mm, respectively. When the Metrecom method was used, the intraexaminer and interexaminer differences were not statistically significant. The ICC reliability values for identifying coordinates for 10 bony landmarks were .95 for 1 examiner and .96 for the other. The mean interrater ICC was .87.

Conclusion.—The Metrecom system appears to be valid and reliable, and the Metrecom method appears to be reliable. A common Metrecom linkage position should be used for each skeletal landmark location. Human factors seem to influence the Metrecom method; thus, examiner training, competence in identifying bony landmarks, and familiarity with the use of the instrument are important.

► Any new procedure, however exciting it initially appears to be, must undergo testing to determine both its reliability and validity. The Metrecom is a new device that analyzes motion by using an electrogoniometric data-acquisition system and sophisticated computer programs. Metrecom analysis is becoming more prevalent in chiropractic practice. The mechanical system used by the device is reliable and valid in determining cartesian (*x*-, *y*-, and *z*-axis) coordinates in space. The authors do note, however, that human factors *do* influence the methods used by the system. Therefore, training and competency in determining bony landmarks is necessary to achieve the most effective use of the system.—D.J. Lawrence, D.C.

Effect of Backrest Inclination on the Transmission of Vertical Vibrations Through the Lumbar Spine

Magnusson M, Pope M, Rostedt M, Hansson T (Sahlgren Hosp, Göteborg, Sweden; Univ of Vermont, Burlington)

Clin Biomech 8:5–12, 1993 3–9

Background.—Increasing evidence suggests that driving is associated with low back pain, emphasizing the need for ways to attenuate vibrations on the spine. The inclination of a backrest was assessed.

Methods.—Three young women who were free of low back pain and other health problems were studied. The impact device consisted of a suspended seat platform, a frame, and a pendulum. Various postures were evaluated.

Findings.—The subjects showed a marked transmissibility peak at the L4 vertebra at 4 to 8 Hz, and a transmissibility valley at 8 to 10 Hz. There was no trend of either frequency or gain at the transmissibility peak, with the inclination angle for the supported postures at 110–112 degrees. The data were similar between subjects and were repeatable within subjects. Almost complete attenuation was found for the horizontal response of unsupported subjects. For most of the frequency range, attenuation was noted. For supported postures, phase-angle plots demonstrated no shift of phase with frequency up to 4 Hz. In the unsupported postures, the phase declined with increasing frequency. Attenuation occurred throughout the range for the *x*-axis gain, indicating that the *x*-axis response is not problematic for the lumbar spine under vertical vibration input.

Conclusion.—The backrest had only a minor effect on the attenuation of vibrations in this study. The backrest resulted in a slight decrease in resonant frequency and in the peak gain.

▶ Dr. Pope was instrumental in demonstrating the effects of vibration on the spine. His work supported that of previous researchers who had shown that there was an increased risk of low back pain in individuals who either sit or drive when working. One way in which to help decrease the effect of vibration on the back is to design seating systems that limit these effects, but few such studies examining this option exist. In this study, the authors show that the inclination of the backrest has little, if any, effect on vibration attenuation; seating ergonomics will need to examine other factors in limiting the effects of vibration on those who are subject to its effects.—D.J. Lawrence, D.C.

Reliability of Hindfoot Goniometry When Using a Flexible Electrogoniometer

Ball P, Johnson GR (Durham School of Podiatric Medicine, England; Univ of Newcastle upon Tyne, England)

Clin Biomech 8:13–19, 1993 3–10

Background.—Clinically assessing subtalar motion is an essential part of examining pathologic conditions in the foot. Establishment of the subtalar neutral position is required for producing many foot orthoses. The use of an electrogoniometer for obtaining the relevant measurements and the important aspects of the clinical procedure were examined.

Methods.—Three methods were used for measuring passive motion. In the first, the subtalar joint was removed by grasping the calcaneus to invert and evert the hindfoot maximally relative to the lower leg, which was stabilized by firmly holding it with 1 hand. In method 2, the subtalar joint was moved by grasping the forefoot instead of the calcaneus (Fig 3–4). Lower leg stabilization was achieved as in method 1. Method 3 involved active inversion and eversion. Twenty-five subjects with a mean age of 25 years were included in the study of intersubject variability. For intrasubject variability, 15 consecutive measures were sufficient.

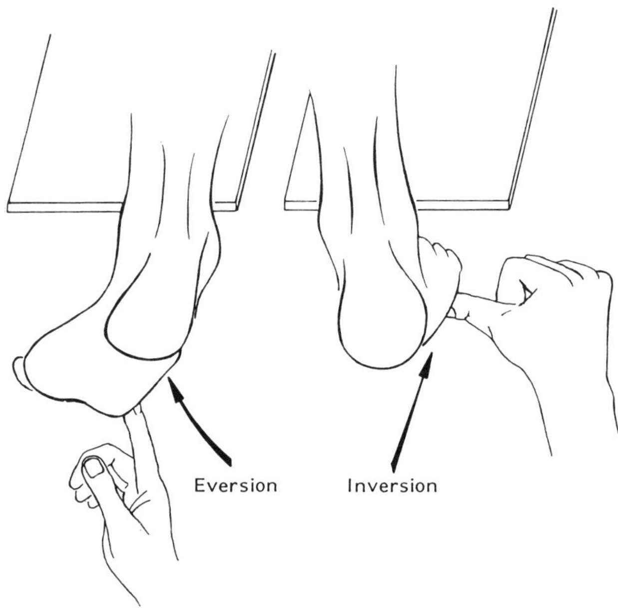

Fig 3–4.—Application of force to forefoot while measuring subtalar joint movement. (Courtesy of Ball P, Johnson GR: *Clin Biomech* 8:13–19, 1993.)

Effect of Active or Passive Motion on Range of Motion

	Passive			*Active*		
	Inv	*Ev*	*RoM*	*Inv*	*Ev*	*RoM*
(a) Inter-subject study						
Mean	31.5	5.8	37.3	22.2	4.8	27.0
SD	5.2	2.4	5.4	6.2	3.2	6.1
Min	23.0	1.0	28.0	12.0	0.0	15.0
Max	44.0	11.0	48.0	35.0	11.0	42.0
(b) Intra-subject study						
Mean	24.8	6.6	31.4	14.9	5.3	20.2
SD	1.5	1.5	2.2	2.3	3.3	2.1
Min	23.0	5.0	30.0	10.0	0.0	18.0
Max	28.0	10.0	38.0	19.0	14.0	24.0

Abbreviations: Inv, inversion; *Ev,* eversion; RoM, range of motion.
(Courtesy of Ball P, Johnson GR: *Clin Biomech* 8:13–19, 1993.)

Results.—In all cases, there were significant differences between the results obtained by using the different subject positions. The passive ranges of motion were always greater than the active ranges of motion (table). However, the differences could be attributed almost entirely to changes in inversion. The changes in measured eversion were not significant. The study of symmetry relative to the palpated subtalar neutral position demonstrated that although the overall range between the 2 sides did not differ, the difference between measured inversion was significant. The right side tended to be more inverted than the left. Measurements of symmetry using a resting zero position revealed no significant differences between the 2 sides.

Conclusion.—There were large variations, up to 7 degrees, between the neutral positions determined by different observers. Although the electrogoniometer is a reliable instrument, the methods currently used for assessing neutral position and, therefore, inversion and eversion of the hindfoot, are unreliable.

▶ The motions of inversion and eversion of the foot primarily occur at the subtalar joint, whose function is critical to the overall function of the foot. Chiropractors often assess motion in this joint as part of a motion palpation procedure; however, there are great variations in the methods used to do this in practice. Assessing joint play is based in part on the assumption of a neutral position for the subtalar joint, yet no clear understanding of that neutral position exists. In the past, traditional goniometers have been used in attempts to understand this position, but have been found inadequate. The electrogoniometric procedure used here, although more sophisticated than standard goniometry, had poor reliability in the determining ranges of inversion and eversion based on a neutral position. One implication involves the preparation of custom foot orthotics, many of which are based on the establishment of neutral subtalar position, something that is exceedingly difficult to accomplish.—D.J. Lawrence, D.C.

The Effects of Armrests and High Seat Heights on Lower-Limb Joint Load and Muscular Activity During Sitting and Rising

Arborelius UP, Wretenberg P, Lindberg F (Karolinska Inst, Stockholm)

Ergonomics 35:1377–1391, 1992 3–11

Background.—Seat heights that are higher than normal may be better for performing certain jobs, especially those that involve standing and sitting. High seats may also be of benefit to individuals with disabilities of the lower extremities that make it difficult to rise from a seat of standard height.

Methods.—The loading moment of force on the hip, knee, and ankle joints of 9 healthy men rising from 4 different stool types was studied. The levels of myoelectric activity in 4 leg muscles were also investigated. Two types of stools, called stand stools, had higher-than-normal seats. The other 2 were of standard height; 1 had armrests.

Findings.—The mean maximum knee moment was more than 60% lower when subjects rose from the high stool. In addition, the difference between the high and low stand stools was significant. Using the high stool or help with the arms decreased the mean maximum hip moment by about 50%. Different stools only marginally affected the mean maximum ankle moment. Seat height influenced knee moment more than hip moment. Vastus lateralis activity was significantly greater when subjects rose from seats of standard height than when they rose from high or low stand stools. The rectus femoris muscle was minimally activated. The semitendinosus muscle was activated sooner when subjects rose from higher seats. All subjects believed that the effort of rising from the higher stand stool was less than that from rising from the lower stand stool or from the seat of standard height without armrests.

Conclusion.—The largest decrease in muscular activity and maximum moments occurred when subjects rose from a high stand stool. Stand stools are good alternatives for workers who frequently change from sitting and standing positions.

► Office ergonomics is receiving greater scrutiny as industrialized nations attempt to come to grips with the increase in job-related spinal and extremity pain. Seat design is one major factor being examined. We often pay little attention to seat designs when selecting office furniture, yet if we were to do so, it might help to decrease the incidence of pain and lost days at work. The authors of this study examined a number of different parameters with 4 different seating designs, including electromyography and loading forces. A higher than normal seat height may help to decrease load forces and should be recommended for chiropractic patients who combine tasks that require both sitting and standing.—D.J. Lawrence, D.C.

Apophyses of the Sacro-Iliac Joints on CT

Funke VM, Götz W, Fischer G, Grabbe E, Herken R (Klinikum der Georg-August-Universität Göttingen)

Rofo Fortschr Geb Rontgenstr Neuen Bildgeb Verfahr
157:43–46, 1992 3–12

Introduction.—Computed tomography (CT) is extremely useful for studying the sacroiliac (SI) joint. During the imaging of young patients, opacities in the area of the SI joint that had not previously been described in the CT literature were seen. However, similar structures have been described as apophyseal elements in the anatomical and radiographic literature. Correlation of the anatomical, radiographic, and CT appearances of these bony structures was investigated.

Materials.—Twelve macerated pelvic preparations from young individuals aged 12–20 years at the time of death were obtained from the anatomical research institute. The SI joints from 2 young men aged 15 and 17 years were harvested at autopsy and prepared for conventional radiographic and CT examinations. The CT scans from 29 patients younger than 30 years of age who underwent CT scanning of the pelvic area during the past 6 months were also examined.

Results.—No apophyseal structures were found in any of the macerated preparations. Conventional radiography of the 2 autopsied joints showed round, sharply delineated, bony structures (2–5 cm in length) located at the ventral aspect of the SI joint. Histopathologic examination confirmed that those ossicles had a spongiosa structure. The CT findings agreed with the radiographic findings. The CT scans of 7 patients aged 15–19 years also showed the narrow, round, or bandlike opacities on the ventral aspect of the SI joint. The bony structures were not associated with any pathologic changes of the SI joints. None of the CT scans of adult patients showed similar bony structures near the SI joint.

Conclusion.—The bony structures sometimes seen within the SI joint of young individuals are considered normal. These structures are apophyseal elements that later fuse with the sacrum.

▶ Dr. J. David Cassidy and his colleague Dr. Bowen were among the first to demonstrate age-related changes in the SI joint. In Cassidy's original work, the ages studied ranged over several decades. The authors of this study demonstrate the presence of apophyseal structures within the SI joints during adolescence and the teenage years. There are clinical implications to these structures, because they appear radiographically and on CT images. Because they are normal findings, they should not be confused with any pathologic process.—D.J. Lawrence, D.C.

Comparisons Between Active vs. Passive End-Range Assessments in Subjects Exhibiting Cervical Range of Motion Asymmetries

Wong A, Nansel DD (Palmer College of Chiropractic-West, Sunnyvale, Calif)

J Manipulative Physiol Ther 15:159–163, 1992 3–13

Objective.—Cervical range of motion was compared in a double-blind, within-subject study after active and passive (practitioner-aided) movement of the head to end range.

Subjects and Methods.—Chiropractice college students (age, 22–38 years) who lacked neck pain participated in the study. A goniometric device, the inclinometer, was used for cervical end-range determinations. Active studies were followed immediately by passive assessments.

Findings.—The extent of end-range asymmetry apparent after active assessment was only about half of that seen on passive assessment. Active end-range values were about 5 degrees less than passive values on the more restricted side of passive motion, and they were about 10 degrees less on the less restricted side.

Implications.—Cortical influences on active motion apparently limit active head motion on the side of the greatest potential passive end range. The effect is to preserve symmetry at the expense of the overall range of motion. Range of active motion may be much harder to assess accurately.

▶ Nonpractitioner goniometric assessment using an inclinometer provides results lower than when the assessment is done passively (practitioner-assisted). It is unknown whether there is any clinical significance to this, and the authors speculate that the answer may depend on several factors, such as magnitude of range of motion restriction or whether end-range capability is a significant consideration. Cortical control may mediate active movement and be intolerant of asymmetry, yet this has to be confirmed experimentally. Nevertheless, this has implications for how manipulation may be used in returning normal symmetric motion to restricted vertebral levels.—D.J. Lawrence, D.C.

Reproducibility and Accuracy of Angle Measurements Obtained Under Static Conditions With the Motion Analysis Video System

Vander Linden DW, Carlson SJ, Hubbard RL (Univ of Florida, Gainesville)

Phys Ther 72:300–305, 1992 3–14

Introduction.—Newer, increasingly automated systems are thought to have increased the accuracy of kinematic analysis of human motion.

Many such systems are currently used by physical therapists, yet the accuracy and reproducibility of computerized and semi-automated motion analysis systems have not been reported. These qualities were evaluated in the Motion Analysis video system.

Methods.—The Motion Analysis™ Expert Video system, designed for 3-dimensional motion tracking and analysis, was evaluated under static conditions using a standard goniometer. The reflective markers placed on a goniometer were recorded by 2 video cameras at 17 angles, from 20 to 180 degrees, in increments of 10 degrees. The recordings were made at 3 locations within the cameras' field of view. Separate intraclass correlation coefficients (ICC) were calculated for each of the 3 locations.

Results.—The system was consistent in calculating angles from the reflective markers, regardless of the location of the goniometer in the calibration field; under static conditions, the ICC exceeded .99 for each of the 3 locations. At all locations, the average within-trial variability was less than .4 degrees. The slopes of the linear-regression equations comparing the mean system-calculated angles and reference angles were near 1; the intercepts were not statistically different from zero. A preliminary assessment of the system was made under dynamic conditions. The results revealed that distances were somewhat underestimated, regardless of where the movement occurred within the calibration cube.

Conclusion.—These findings suggest that the system evaluated has acceptable error in calculating angles from reflective markers. Clinicians and researchers should be aware that other sources of error, such as placement of markers on a subject on multiple days, might jeopardize the reliability of computerized systems.

▶ Video kinematic analysis is a new procedure that uses an optoelectric system to analyze human motion via a digitizing algorithm. Because it is new, the reproducibility and reliability of the procedure is unknown. The Motion Analysis system was found to be highly reproducible for measuring angles, with low error measurements. The application of the analysis system to clinical situations is only in its infancy and awaits testing. Video analysis will likely become an important diagnostic tool as the clinical issues are resolved and the price of the system decreases.—D.J. Lawrence, D.C.

Postural Control in Young and Elderly Adults When Stance Is Perturbed: Kinematics

Alexander NB, Shepard N, Gu MJ, Schultz A (Univ of Michigan, Ann Arbor; Ann Arbor VA Med Ctr, Mich)

J Gerontol 47:79M–87M, 1992 3–15

Introduction.—Increased postural sway and falling, which are associated with aging, are probably related to difficulties with postural control in elderly individuals. It was hypothesized that healthy elderly individuals would respond differently to 4 postural control tasks compared with young adults. The tasks compared a full vs. reduced support surface and a quiet vs. perturbed stance.

Subjects and Methods.—Twenty-four healthy young adults and 15 elderly adults, aged a mean of 26 and 72 years, respectively, were studied. The motions of individual body segments were assessed in response to standing with the feet flat on an anteriorly accelerating platform, or Flat Translation; standing on a narrow beam support that was stationary, or Beam Standing; standing on a narrow beam support that was accelerating anteriorly, or Beam Translation; and standing on a rotatable but otherwise stationary springboard, or Springboard Standing. The rotations of body segments, especially maximum excursions, time to first rotation response, direction of initial rotation, and time to first rotation reversal were measured with an optoelectronic camera system.

Results.—Larger rotation excursions were generally noted in the elderly individuals rather than in the younger persons, particularly in the Beam Standing and Beam Translation tasks. However, the magnitude of rotation difference was small. All rotation magnitudes were well within the available ranges of body joint motions. The elderly showed greater variability than the young in excursion magnitudes and directions of initial rotation. In the Beam Translation task, the elderly tended to rotate their upper body segments more than in the Flat Translation task when compared with the young adults.

Conclusion.—Healthy elderly adults with no apparent musculoskeletal or neurologic impairment appear to have small but consistent differences in postural control kinematics, especially in more challenging circumstances. These findings provide the basis for biomechanical analyses of joint torques and other dynamic requirements of such responses.

▶ Falls in the elderly are common, debilitating, and even life-threatening. Loss of postural control in the elderly accounts for the increased number of falls that are seen. This study used a sophisticated optoelectric system to study 4 different stance activities, finding differences of body segment movement in the elderly when compared with the young.—D.J. Lawrence, D.C.

Laterally Transposed Pelvis: A New and Proper Name for an Old Problem

Patriquin DA (Ohio Univ, Athens)

J Am Osteopath Assoc 92:472–476, 1992 3–16

Introduction.—Efforts to standardize the terminology describing osteopathic findings are ongoing, including terminology relating to postural examination. In the diagnosis of postural imbalance, particularly minor

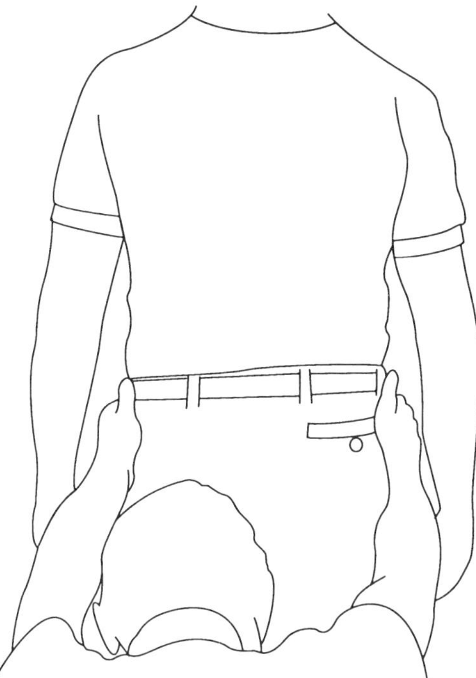

Fig 3–5.—The examiner crouches behind the patient, eyes at the level of the iliac crests, both arms fully extended with the palms against the most lateral portion of the trochanteric area. The examining physician compares the distances from his/her palms to the vertically extended midheel line. When the distances are unequal, laterally transposed pelvis exists. (Courtesy of Patriquin DA: *J Am Osteopath Assoc* 92:472–476, 1992.)

forms, a static test for laterally transposed pelvis may be critical. Some term is needed to refer to this clinical finding and nothing else. The terminology of this aspect of the postural examination is discussed, and the term laterally transposed pelvis is recommended.

Terminology.—Previously used terms for laterally transposed pelvis have included lateral shift or displacement of the pelvis, lateral shift of the sacrum, hip shift, and pelvic sideshift. Each has many definitions; none is universally used to describe the static finding of pelvis-sacral position in the coronal place in relation to the vertically extended midheel line. The literature reveals no conventions related to the meaning of these varied terms except for the usage in this article.

Recommendation.—The word shift was favored to describe this motion, but it carries the idea of change or motion. Therefore, the use of the term laterally transposed pelvis is recommended to indicate this finding. It is identified by the examiner crouching behind the patient, who is standing straight. The examiner places the palms against the most projecting areas of the lateral hip; he or she then visually extends a reference line of place vertically from between the patient's heels up through the pelvic-sacral area and compares the distance from the palm of each hand to the vertical midheel line. If the distances from each hand to the midheel line appear unequal, then a laterally transposed pelvis is present (Fig 3–5). In less obvious cases, other visual cues help in the identification and quantification of this condition.

Conclusion.—The term laterally transposed pelvis should be the standard for this aspect of the static postural examination. If this term were applied universally, it would avoid the semantic problem noted in the literature and in discussions.

▶ This author is essentially describing a lateral pelvic subluxation in this study, and he fails to investigate the chiropractic literature regarding its effect on postural biomechanics. Interdisciplinary consultation may help to describe such pelvic patterns, which the chiropractic profession has long studied and incorporated into clinical practice.—D.J. Lawrence, D.C.

Sensory Innervation of Human Thoracolumbar Fascia: An Immunohistochemical Study

Yahia L, Rhalmi S, Newman N, Isler M (Ecole Polytechnique, Montreal; Hôtel-Dieu Hospital, Montreal)

Acta Orthop Scand 63:195–197, 1992 3–17

Introduction.—The thoracolumbar fascia appears to play a significant role in the biomechanics of the lumbar spine. In addition, the thoracolumbar fascia might have a sensory function in the flexion-relaxation phenomenon. Immunohistochemical techniques were applied to an examination of the sensory innervation of the human thoracolumbar fascia, an area that has thus far received little attention.

Methods.—Seven patients who were undergoing various surgical procedures provided thoracolumbar fascia specimens. These specimens were studied with light microscopy; antiserum against neurofilament protein (NFP) and S-100 protein were used to identify sensory nerve fibers and their endings.

Results.—The thoracolumbar fascia was found to be well innervated. Stained sections showed nerve-bundle NFP immunoreactivity. Two encapsulated mechanoreceptors, namely Ruffini's and Vater-Pacini corpuscles, were observed with S-100 protein antiserum. The Ruffini receptor was characterized by its single axon and a dense arborization of nerve tissue within the collagen bundles.

Conclusion.—A neurosensory role for the thoracolumbar fascia in the lumbar spine mechanism is supported. The finding of Pacinian and Ruffini's receptors confirms that neural elements are present in the thoracolumbar fascia.

▶ The thoracolumbar fascia acts with the posterior lumbar ligaments to support the flexed vertebral column. This might be considered its mechanical role. It may also have a neurosensory role, where it may initiate postural reflexes and muscular activity. This study does indicate such a role, and it suggests that it may be mediated in part by Ruffini endings and Vater-Pacinian corpuscles. These same nerve receptors play roles in the afferent dorsal horn cell bombardment from a spinal fixation; therefore, there may be an unknown role for the fascia to play in the creation of spinal dysfunction.—D.J. Lawrence, D.C.

Skeletal Muscle Tone and the Misunderstood Stretch Reflex

Davidoff RA (Univ of Miami, Fla; VA Med Ctr, Miami, Fla)

Neurology 42:951–963, 1992 3–18

Introduction.—Because it is defined so differently by neurologists and neurophysiologists, the term muscle tone has been used imprecisely in the neurologic literature. A revision of long-accepted tenets about the genesis of muscle tone in humans was presented.

Discussion.—Muscle tone in humans has been compared to the reflex tone described by Sherrington in decerebrate animals. In this tradition, muscle tone is presumed to be fully determined by the monosynaptic stretch reflex, tonic fusimotor activity is thought to be necessary for its production in normal humans, and tonic muscle tone in antigravity leg muscle is believed to be responsible for posture maintenance. The data reviewed indicate that nonreflex, mechanical mechanisms are involved in the maintenance of resting muscle tone. In addition, spinal cord reflex responses are not stereotyped responses but, rather, depend on the ongoing activity in interneurons, on which inputs from various peripheral sensory receptors and descending fiber systems converge. Long-latency transcortical responses are elicited when a muscle is stretched, and these responses effectively address large displacements. Also, inertial components and viscoelastic muscle forces can counterbalance small amounts of body sway during quiet standing.

Conclusion.—Modern approaches to muscle tone have made obsolete the traditional view that the resistance to stretch could be attributed solely to the monosynaptic reflex actions from the activation of primary muscle spindle endings receiving tonic background fusimotor innervation. The response to muscle stretch is not fixed and inflexible; it can be adjusted according to the demands of the moment.

▶ This paper reviews the literature discussing the concept of muscle tone. It suggests that muscle tone results from a variety of interacting mechanisms from spinal, supraspinal, and peripheral levels.—D.J. Lawrence, D.C.

The Effects of Compression on the Physiology of Nerve Roots

Rydevik BL (Univ of Goteborg, Sweden)
J Manipulative Physiol Ther 1:62–66, 1992 3–19

Introduction.—The spinal nerve roots are located in narrowly confined spaces where they pass through the spinal column; consequently, they are vulnerable to mechanical compressive forces from such states as herniated disk, spinal stenosis, and spinal trauma. Relatively low levels of compression probably cause damage by impairing the blood supply to neural tissue, whereas higher forces can have direct mechanical effects on nerve tissue.

Experimental.—By altering the permeability of the endoneurial capillaries, compression can produce intraneural edema, which may in turn increase endoneurial fluid pressure and further impede capillary flow. Such edema may also lead to intraneural fibrosis. The substances released by degenerated disk tissue or facet joints may contribute to symptoms in various spinal pain syndromes; glycoprotein is a possible example. If a nerve root is irritated, as by a herniated disk, even minimal mechanical deformation can produce radiating pain. Experiments with whole body vibration suggest that the dorsal root ganglion is mechanosensitive and probably has a critical role as a mediator of pain in the lumbar spine.

Summary.—The mechanisms of clinical nerve root compression are quite complex, especially in chronic disorders.

▶ This paper discusses the pathophysiologic mechanisms that cause nerve root compression. The standard model begins with venous compression and congestion and then cascades to pressure buildup, capillary congestion, capillary wall damage, protein leakage, and endoneural edema; fibrosis of the nerve root is not reversed. There may also be axoplasmic blockages as well. Such compressions may be the result of osteoarthritic spur formation, tumor, pressure, or even subluxation.—D.J. Lawrence, D.C.

Line of Gravity Relative to Upright Vertebral Posture

Pearsall DJ, Reid JG (Queen's Univ, Kingston, Ont, Canada)
Clin Biomech 7:80–86, 1992 3–20

Introduction.—The mechanisms of the vertebral column have been studied extensively. However, knowledge of its physical arrangement in the line of gravity is conflicting. The sagittal thoracolumbar spine posture, as represented by the vertebral centroids, was investigated, and the position of these centroids relative to the line of gravity of the whole body was determined.

Subjects and Methods.—Twenty-eight boys and 15 girls, aged 14 and 15 years, were assessed noninvasively. The thoracolumbar centroid curve within the sagittal plane was calculated from back skin profiles.

Results.—The vertebral centroid postures were varied. The girls' curve was significantly more posterior of the line of gravity than the boys' curve. In addition, the degree of kyphotic curvature was significantly greater in boys. As indicated by the kyphotic and lordotic curvatures, the posture assumed by the spine was significantly correlated with the cumulative centroid displacement of the line of gravity and with gender. It was also correlated with height, mass, and spine depth.

Conclusion.—The findings from the comprehensive noninvasive analysis of spine posture relative to the line of gravity of the whole body differ from previous hypotheses on the relationship of the spine to the line of gravity of the body within the sagittal plane. Postural differences between adolescent girls and boys were also demonstrated.

▶ This paper may have critical ramifications for the chiropractic profession because it demonstrates differences in posture between boys and girls, and also throws into question our understanding of the spine's relation to the gravity plumbline. If this is indeed so, then our entire assessment procedure using postural analysis may have to be reexamined, and those x-ray films marking systems that depend upon postural radiography may have to be reassessed. Further study is obviously needed.—D.J. Lawrence, D.C.

A Comprehensive Evaluation of Trunk Response to Asymmetric Trunk Motion

Marras WS, Mirka GA (Ohio State Univ, Columbus)
Spine 17:318–326, 1992 3–21

Introduction.—In a review of workplace lifting conditions, almost all situations involving manual materials handling (MMH) were found to involve asymmetric lifts with significant trunk motion. Most lifting guides, however, assume that the trunk is in a sagittally symmetric position, and biomechanical analyses are based on static investigations of the spine. The reaction of the trunk muscles and intra-abdominal pressure to components of trunk loading commonly seen in the workplace during MMH was determined.

Methods.—The components studied (using electromyography) included angular trunk velocity, trunk position in 3-dimensional space, and trunk torque exertion level. Forty-four subjects participated in the study. They produced constant trunk exertion torque around the lumbosacral junction while moving the trunk under constant angular velocity conditions.

Results.—There were significant reactions to trunk angular velocity, trunk torque level, and unique combinations of trunk position and velocity in all trunk muscles. The other components selectively affected the muscles according to function. The only significant intra-abdominal pressure reaction was to trunk angle and some unique trunk angle-symmetry positions.

Conclusion.—These findings can facilitate our understanding of spine loading during MMH movements. Most of the reactions of the trunk muscles and intra-abdominal pressure to trunk motion, trunk asymmetric position, exertion level, and combinations of these factors resulted in an increased coactivation between muscle groups. The added trunk muscle force associated with trunk concentric and eccentric motions primarily occurs in muscles other than those in the erector spinae group. Intra-abdominal pressure activity declined as trunk asymmetry increased and was unaffected by velocity or load level.

▶ This study examines what happens to trunk muscles when a load similar to that experienced at work is applied. It provides a more detailed understanding of both muscle function and the action of isolated muscles in the process of loading weight. Some asymmetrical responses appear to be common, although it is not known whether these are normal.—D.J. Lawrence, D.C.

Studies on the Biomechanical Effect of a Spinal Adjustment

Triano JJ (Natl College of Chiropractic, Lombard, Ill)

J Manipulative Physiol Ther 15:71–75, 1992 3–22

Introduction.—Although manual treatment is perhaps the most carefully studied treatment for spine-related disorders, too little is known

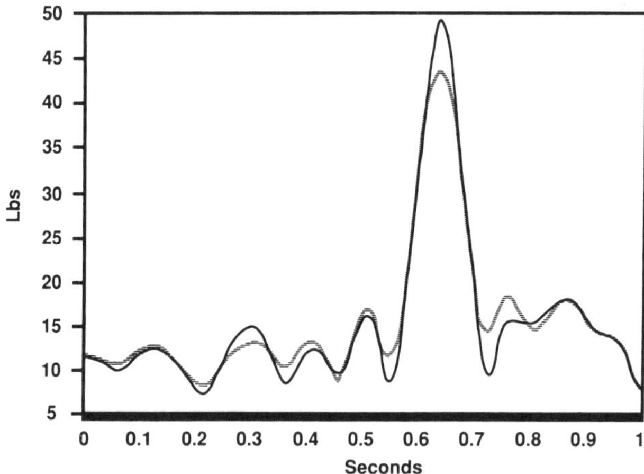

Fig 3–6.—Amplitude of axial forces on the cervical spine during a manipulation at C2. The *solid line* represents applied forces; the *shaded line* indicates the forces transmitted to the spine. (Courtesy of Triano JJ: *J Manipulative Physiol Ther* 15:71-75, 1992.)

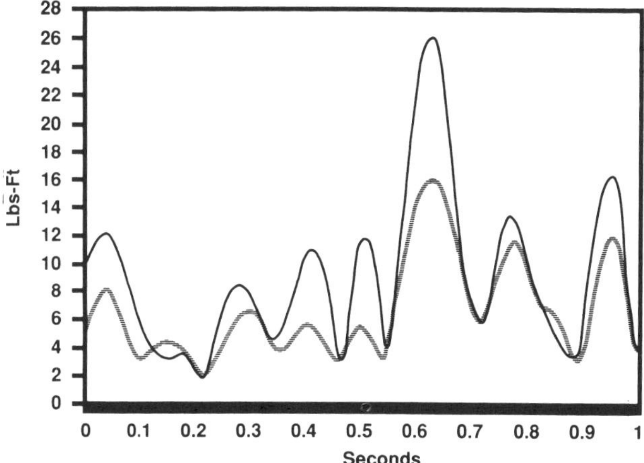

Fig 3–7.—Amplitude of moments (torques) acting on the cervical spine during a manipulation at C2. The *solid line* represents applied moments; the *shaded line* indicates the moments transmitted to the spine. *Author's Note:* "These first efforts to model transmitted moments may be high in their estimation and remain to be validated." (Courtesy of Triano JJ: *J Manipulative Physiol Ther* 15:71–75, 1992.)

scientifically about these methods. What manual methods have in common is the application of an external load to the spine and surrounding tissues.

Lesions.—The functional spinal lesion is a biological biomechanical concept that may be a component of diverse clinical conditions. Views of subluxation mechanics still primarily rely on blocked motion. Recent biomechanical work has revealed a previously unrecognized phenome-

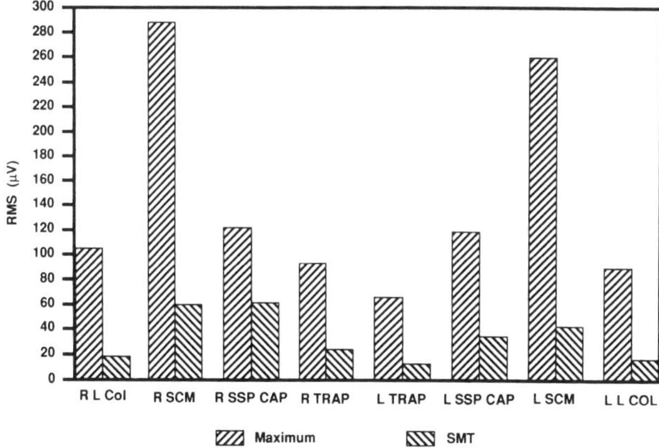

Fig 3–8.—Relative muscle activity as a proportion of maximum voluntary contraction for neck muscles in response to a C2 manipulation. *Abbreviations:* *L*, left; *R*, right; *L Col*, longus colli; *SCM*, sternomastoid; *SSP Cap*, semispinalis capitis; *Trap*, trapezius. (Courtesy of Triano JJ: *J Manipulative Physiol Ther* 15:71–75, 1992.)

non, motion-segment buckling, which occurs when a structure undergoes large deformation with a relatively small increase in load.

Loads and Effects.—Modern biomechanical research is able to quantify the loads associated with manipulation, as illustrated in Figure 3–6. Initial efforts to model transmitted moments (Fig 3–7) may yield high estimates, and they remain to be validated. A comparison of muscular activity in voluntary neck motion and the reaction to manipulation is shown in Figure 3–8. The patient's muscular response can modify the mechanical effect of an applied manipulative load, and different patients probably recruit different muscles to varying degrees. Severe muscular reaction might explain some complications of manipulation.

Discussion.—Manipulation is, biomechanically, a very complex event. Much remains to be done in quantifying the changes in biomechanical function after manipulation in different areas of the spine.

▶ This paper by Dr. Triano develops a new approach to the chiropractic lesion. Dr. Triano views the functional spinal lesion (FSL) in terms of the information we can learn from it and about it. He asks (1) how the FSL behaves in contrast to healthy motion segments; (2) what loads are applied during a manipulation; (3) what loads pass through the spine; (4) how the behavior of the FSL is changed by manipulation; etc. These questions reflect his training as a biomechanist, and this is essentially a mechanical model. These questions have allowed Dr. Triano to substantially add to the chiropractic profession's understanding of the effects of manipulation and to model in new ways (such as with finite element analysis) how the lesion leads to biomechanical dysfunction.—D.J. Lawrence, D.C.

Cervical Spine Motion in the Sagittal Plane II: Position of Segmental Averaged Instantaneous Centers of Rotation: A Cineradiographic Study

van Mameren H, Sanches H, Beursgens J, Drukker J (Univ of Limburg, Maastricht, The Netherlands)

Spine 17:467–474, 1992 3–23

Introduction.—An instantaneous center of rotation (ICR) reflects the quality of motion—both rotary and translatory—between adjacent vertebrae. It remains uncertain to what extent ICRs in an individual are identical at consecutive measurement sessions, or to what degree they differ in asymptomatic persons.

A Proposal.—Segmental ICRs based on only extreme cervical spine positions on 2 static radiographs may involve considerable random measurement error. When using cineradiographic films of sagittal-plane motion, many more positions per segmental bony structure are available. "Averaged" ICRs are the mean of a cluster of ICRs, each deduced from

Moving?

I'd like to receive my ***Year Book of Chiropractic*** without interruption.
Please not the following change of address, effective:

Name: ______________________________

New Address: ______________________________

____

City: ______________________ State: __________ Zip: __________

Old Address: ______________________________

____

City: ______________________ State: __________ Zip: __________

Reservation Card

Yes, I would like my own copy of ***Year Book of Chiropractic.*** Please begin my subscription with the current edition according to the terms described below.* I understand that I will have 30 days to examine each annual edition. If satisfied, I will pay just $64.95 plus sales tax, postage and handling (price subject to change without notice).

Name: ______________________________

Address: ______________________________

City: ______________________ State: __________ Zip: __________

Method of Payment
❍ Visa ❍ Mastercard ❍ AmEx ❍ Bill me ❍ Check (in US dollars, payable to Mosby, Inc.)

Card number: ______________________ Exp date: __________

Signature: ______________________________

LS-0908

*Your *Year Book* Service Guarantee:

When you subscribe to the *Year Book*, we'll send you an advance notice of future volumes about two months before they publish. This automatic notice system is designed to take up as little of your time as possible. If you do not want the *Year Book*, the advance notice makes it quick and easy for you to let us know your decision, and you will always have at least 20 days to decide. If we don't hear from you, we'll send you the new volume as soon as it's available. And, of course, the *Year Book* is yours to examine free of charge for 30 days (postage, handling and applicable sales tax are added to each shipment.).

BUSINESS REPLY MAIL

FIRST CLASS MAIL PERMIT No. 762 CHICAGO, IL

POSTAGE WILL BE PAID BY ADDRESSEE

Chris Hughes
Mosby-Year Book, Inc.
200 N. LaSalle Street
Suite 2600
Chicago, IL 60601-9981

BUSINESS REPLY MAIL

FIRST CLASS MAIL PERMIT No. 762 CHICAGO, IL

POSTAGE WILL BE PAID BY ADDRESSEE

Chris Hughes
Mosby-Year Book, Inc.
200 N. LaSalle Street
Suite 2600
Chicago, IL 60601-9981

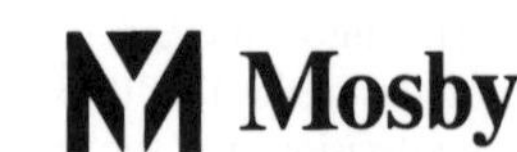

Dedicated to publishing excellence

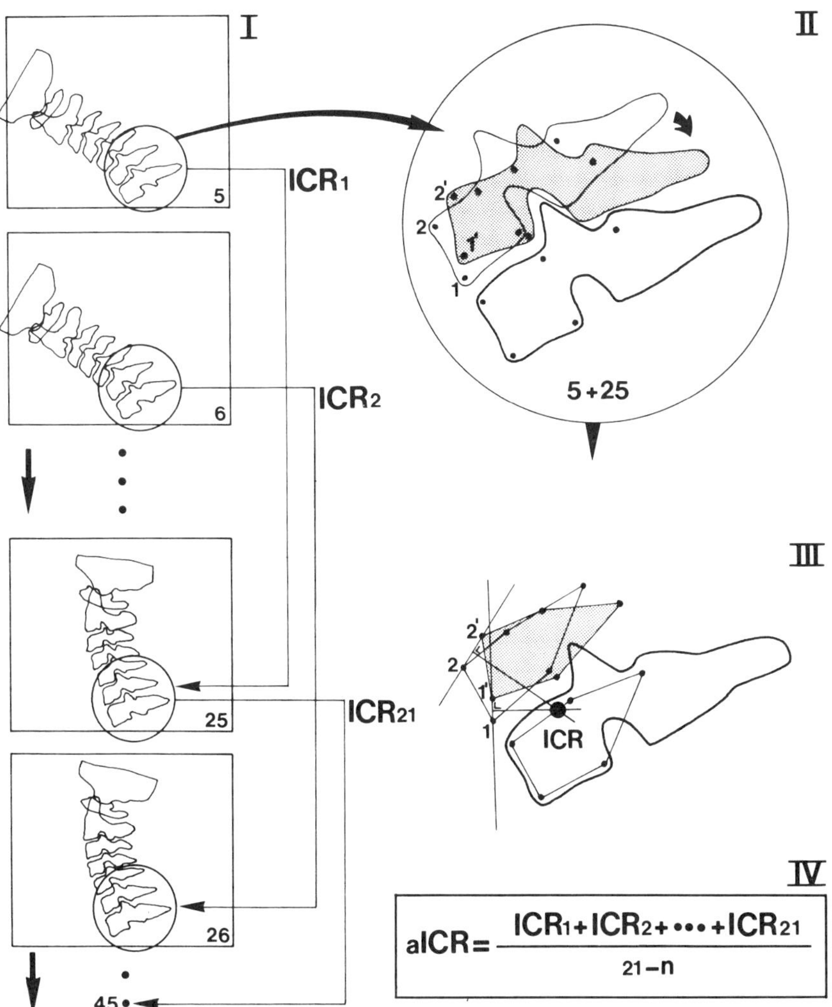

Fig 3–9.—Visualization (given for C6-C7) of the calculation of the aICR of a cineradiographic film with 1 = 20 frames and minimal angle (MA) = 7 degrees between frames 5 and 45. Starting from frame 5, the frames are subdivided into pairs of frames with I = 20. Thus, an arithmetic series of pairs, (5, 25), (6, 26), (7, 27), . . . , (25, 45), is created (I). The ICR is calculated for each pair of frames using corresponding positions of points 1 and 2 of the average pentagon of the cranial vertebra on both frames (1 and 1′, respectively 2 and 2′) (II and III). The average pentagon of the caudal vertebra is superimposed, fitting exactly. Thus, for each segment, 21 ICRs are calculated. The ICRs of the pairs for which holds true segmental rotation equal to or greater than 7 (MA = 7 degrees) are selected, resulting in a group of (21 − ⁻*n*) ICRs. The aICR, the average position of this group of selected ICRs, is computed (IV). (Courtesy of van Mameren H, Sanches H, Beursgens J, et al: *Spine* 17:467-474, 1992.)

the position of segmental structures on a pair of nonadjacent cineradiographic frames (Fig 3–9).

Study.—Ten healthy subjects aged 19–22 years participated in the study. Eight of them were filmed 2 and 10 weeks after initial evaluation. The images were recorded in maximum active anteflexion as well as retroflexion. Segmental averaged ICRs were calculated using the positions of ICRs estimated from pairs of frames between the 5th and 45th virtual frame of the film.

Findings.—In contrast to segmental range of motion, the position of the averaged ICRs exhibited low variability. Dispersion of averaged ICRs was less than that of standard ICRs in most clusters, particularly for C0-C1 and C1-C2. Within individuals, the averaged ICRs of each anteflexion and retroflexion registration were clustered close together (except for C0-C1).

Conclusion.—The position of averaged ICRs of the cervical spine may be used to diagnose abnormal mobility and to evaluate treatment.

▶ Cineradiography was used to determine the instantaneous axis of rotation for the cervical vertebrae. By developing these standards, we can begin to understand the full effects of spinal dysfunction in the human.—D.J. Lawrence, D.C.

Pathoanatomic Studies and Clinical Significance of Lumbosacral Zygapophyseal (Facet) Joints

Giles LGF (Griffith Univ, Queensland, Australia)

J Manipulative Physiol Ther 15:36–40, 1992 3–24

Introduction.—It has been proposed that the effects of joint dysfunction on soft tissue structures, including vascular stasis, neural ischemia, and soft tissue entrapment, may be one mechanism of back pain of mechanical origin. The soft tissue structures associated with the zygapophyseal joints were assessed histologically.

Methods.—The lumbosacral spine was removed from 16 cadavers (aged 50–92 years) and trimmed into blocks of osteoligamentous tissues including the paired zygapophyseal joints at the L4–L5 and L5–S1 levels. The soft tissue structures were examined by low-magnification light microscopy.

Fig 3–10.—A, 100-micron thick section cut in the horizontal plane from the lower one third of the lumbosacral joint of a 74-year-old male cadaver. The right (*R*) zygapophyseal joint shows a large highly vascular intra-articular synovial fold inclusion with a fibrotic tip, projecting between the osteoarthritic hyaline articular cartilage surfaces. This tip is probably fibrotic as a result of nipping of the synovial fold between the joint surfaces during life. C represents the fibrous capsule, some fibers of which have become attached to the surface of the hyaline articular cartilage (*H*) on the sacral facet (*diagonal arrow*) between the articulating surfaces. *D* represents the dural sac containing the cauda equina; *IVD*, a small midline bulge of the intervertebral disk; *L*, lamina; *L5*, inferior articular process of the fifth lumbar ver-

(continued)

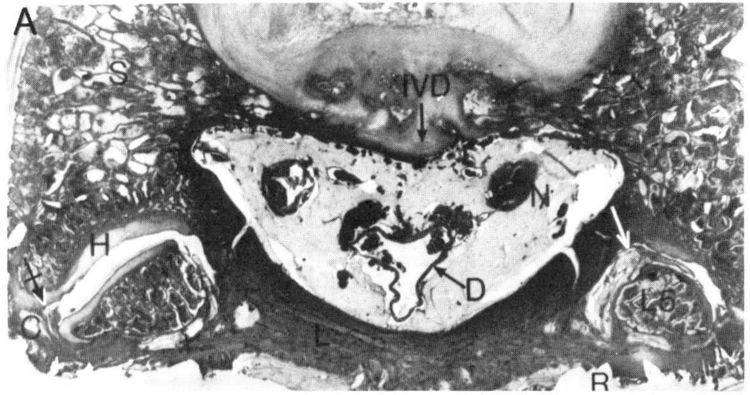

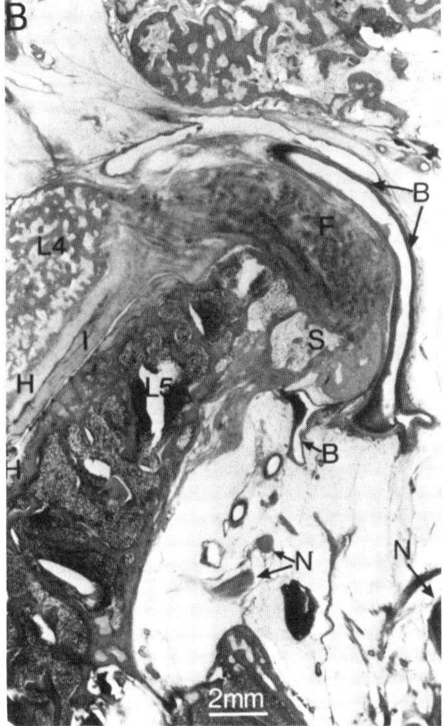

Fig 3–10 (cont).

tebra; *N*, nerve roots; *S*, sacral ala. **B,** parasagittal section of part of the left L4–L5 zygapophyseal joint and adjacent intervertebral canal from a 79-year-old man. Note how the blood vessels (*B*) can be deformed and tractioned by an osteophytic spur (*S*) projecting from the superior articular process of the L5 vertebra, and how the large blood vessel conforms to the contour of the osteoarthritic joint as it passes around the margin of the zygapophyseal joint and its capsule. *F* represents the fibrous joint capsule-ligamentum flavum junction; *H*, hyaline articular cartilage (osteoarthritic); *I*, intra-articular synovial-lined fold arising from the fibrous joint capsule-ligamentum flavum junction superiorly; *L4*, part of the inferior articular process of the L4 vertebra; *L5*, part of the superior articular process of the L5 vertebra; *N*, neural structures within the intervertebral canal. (Courtesy of Giles LGF, *J Manipulative Physiol Ther* 15:36-40, 1992.)

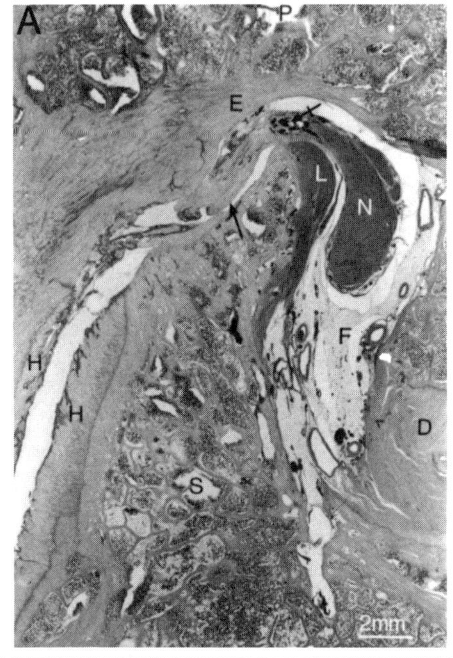

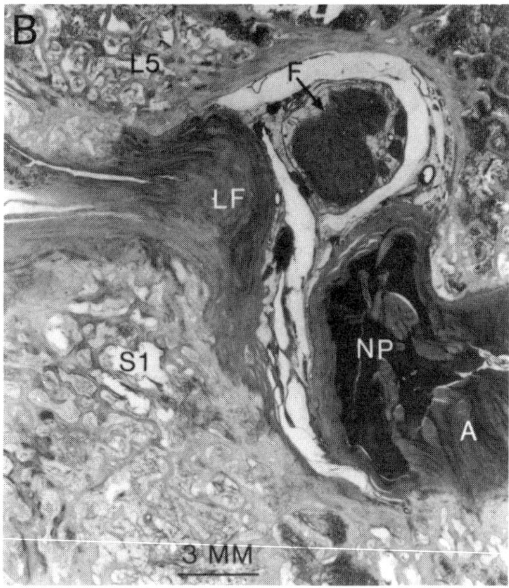

Fig 3–11.—A, parasagittal section of the left lumbosacral intervertebral canal from a woman, 82, showing how the neural complex (*N*) and a dense fibrous intraarticular synovial joint inclusion (*arrow*) have become attached to each other via a highly vascular connective tissue adhesion (*diagonal arrow*). *D* represents intervertebral disk; *E,* eburnation of the inferior aspect of the pedicle (*P*) of the L5 vertebra; *F,* intervertebral canal "foramen"; *H,* hyaline articular cartilage (osteoarthritic); *L,* ligamentum flavum,

(continued)

Findings.—Several soft tissue structures possibly involved in low back pain were identified. They included the large intra-articular synovial folds of the zygapophyseal joints (Fig 3–10A); the fiborus joint capsule tissues attached to hyaline articular cartilage; and the vessels within the intervertebral canal. Neural structures attached to the intra-articular synovial folds or altered by canal stenosis also were observed. These vessels can be deformed by osteophytic spurs projecting into the intervertebral canal (Fig 3–10B). Vascular connective tissue adhesions (Fig 3–11A) and canal stenosis (Fig 3–11B) are other possible cause of lumbar symptoms, as is focal epineural fibrosis.

Conclusion.—Soft tissue structures not visualized by common imaging procedures may contribute to zygapophyseal joint dysfunction and the low back facet syndrome. Spinal motion could produce low back pain when adhesions develop between the fibrous capsule and the surface of hyaline articular cartilage. Adhesions between zygapophyseal joint structures may compromise the neural complex and microvascular structures.

▶ Dr. Giles has developed some highly elegant staining techniques that allow him to examine anatomical structures in fine detail. In this study, he is able to locate several structures associated with the apophyseal joints that may contribute to low back pain. These include synovial folds, joint capsule tissue, and blood vessels. This significantly complicates our clinical picture of low back pain and makes isolating the involved tissues that much harder.—D.J. Lawrence, D.C.

Investigation of Evidence for Anticipatory Postural Adjustments in Seated Subjects Who Performed a Reaching Task

Moore S, Brunt D, Nesbitt ML, Juarez T (Univ of Oregon, Eugene; Univ of Florida, Gainesville; Texas Woman's Univ, Houston)

Phys Ther 72:335–343, 1992 3–25

Background.—The paradigm for studying anticipatory postural adjustments allows exploration of the coordination of postural and voluntary components of functional movement. Seated subjects were investigated under clinically relevant conditions to determine whether there were anticipatory postural adjustments for voluntary movement.

Fig 3–11 (cont).

S, superior articular process of the sacrum. **B,** the large posterolateral contained intervertebral disk herniation shown in this parasagittal section from the left intervertebral canal of a man 74, projects 5 mm into the lower half of the intervertebral canal, below the neural complex, causing advanced stenosis of the canal. *A* represents the anulus fibrosus; *LF,* ligamentum flavum; *L5,* fifth lumbar vertebra; *NP,* contained herniated nucleus pulposus; *S1,* sacral superior articular process. There appears to be some disruption and congestion of the blood vessels in the lower half of the intervertebral canal opposite the contained herniation. There is evidence of minor focal epineurial fibrosis (*F*) of the neural complex, particularly on the opposite side to that adjacent to the hernation. (Reproduced with permission from Giles and Kaveri. Courtesy of Giles LGF: *J Manipulative Physiol Ther* 15:36–40, 1992.)

Methods.—Eight neurologically normal volunteers, aged 23–38 years, participated in the study. The subjects performed a reaching task to a target placed at shoulder height 45 degrees to the right of the midline. The onsets and magnitudes of lateral and fore-aft reactive forces and of electromyographic (EMG) activity of the ipsilateral deltoid and external abdominal oblique and contralateral paraspinal muscles were monitored. Trunk support, reach speed, and distance reached conditions were manipulated.

Findings.—In 70% of all trials for seated subjects, the onsets of deltoid muscle EMG activity preceded the onsets of postural muscle EMG activity. This is in contrast to the findings of reports of EMG activity onset in the postural muscles before the prime mover in standing subjects performing a similar task. The role of trunk musculature and the significance of reactive forces before hand movement were not established.

Conclusion.—There was no clear evidence that anticipatory postural adjustments are needed in seated subjects reaching from an unsupported position. Further research is being done to clarify these findings and to determine the existence of anticipatory postural adjustments in seated individuals.

▶ Postural adjustments occur nearly all the time as we move about, yet we rarely think about them. The intent of this study was to examine one specific postural event: reaching forward when sitting. There were no anticipatory postural adjustments, so all involved movements must be considered voluntary.—D.J. Lawrence, D.C.

Leg Extensor Power and Functional Performance in Very Old Men and Women

Bassey EJ, Fiatarone MA, O'Neill EF, Kelly M, Evans WJ, Lipsitz LA (Univ of Nottingham, England; Tufts Univ, Boston; Hebrew Rehabilitation Centre for Aged, Boston)

Clin Sci 82:321–327, 1992 3–26

Background.—Leg extensor power is needed for many basic activities, such as walking. Various impairments in old age (which probably include lack of muscle power) threaten an individual's ability to do such basic activities. A rig that enables safe, convenient measurement of the power available in a single extension of 1 leg was developed. The extent to which power output measured in the rig predicted performance in older individuals was investigated.

Methods.—Leg extensor capability was assessed in 13 men and 13 women, aged a mean 88.5 and 86.5 years, respectively, who lived in a chronic care hospital and had many pathologies. The custom-built rig was used to assess maximal power output over less than 1 second in a single extension of 1 leg. Performance measures were obtained by timing chair rises, stair climbing, and walking.

Findings.—Leg extensor power was significantly correlated with all performance measures. However, the performance measures were unrelated to each other, except for chair rising and walking speed. Although women had significantly less extensor power than men, their power accounted for more of the variance in performance. No relationship could be found between age and any of the variables measured.

Conclusion.—Measuring leg extensor power in frail elderly individuals may be useful in determining effective rehabilitation programs. In this series, all subjects were able to undergo testing on the rig, despite their advanced age and frailty. All appeared to give a maximal effort.

▶ Rehabilitation of the elderly can be time consuming, frustrating, and difficult. Any information that would allow us to develop an appropriate plan would help to decrease the impact of these problems. From this work, one important factor for such a plan appears to be leg extensor power, and this should be built into rehabilitation plans for elderly patients.—D.J. Lawrence, D.C.

Influence of Body Segment Dynamics on Loads at the Lumbar Spine During Lifting

Tsuang YH, Schipplein OD, Trafimow JH, Andersson GBJ (Natl Taiwan Univ Hosp, Taipei; Rush-Presbyterian-St Luke's Med Ctr, Chicago)

Ergonomics 35:437–444, 1992 3–27

Introduction.—Lifting-induced back pain is common in the industrial setting. Dynamic models, which recently were introduced to assess the forces and moments associated with lifting, indicate that static models may underestimate these measurements. The moments at the L5/S1 level and the hip joint were compared by analyzing the same lifts with dynamic and static models.

Methods.—Ten healthy men (mean age, 27.9 years) with normal physical findings and no history of back problems took part in the study. Each was asked to lift a box from the floor to a shelf at knuckle height directly in front of them. Two different loads (50 N and 150 N) were lifted, and 2 different speeds (fast and normal) were used. The subjects were free to choose their own lifting technique. Two of the men were also asked to perform 3 static lifting tasks, holding the 150-N box at waist level, knee level, and just above the floor.

Results.—When holding weights in static postures, the moments predicted by the dynamic analysis and the static analysis were the same. When performing the lifts, differences in peak moments influenced by external load and by lifting speed occurred between the dynamic and static analyses. When the effect of the inertia of the load was taken into account in the static analysis, there was an increase in the moment magnitude. The predicted moment, however, was still much less than in the dynamic analysis. The differences between dynamic and static analyses were greatest when the 50-N box was lifted at fast-speed; when the pure static was replaced with a dynamic analysis, there was an 87% increase in L5/S1 moment and a 95% increase in hip moment.

Conclusion.—These findings appear to confirm the importance of using a dynamic analysis when studying spinal loading during lifting. A static evaluation greatly underestimates predicted moments and always ignores the speed factor.

The Anatomical Basis for Cervicogenic Headache

Bogduk N (Univ of Newcastle, New South Wales, Australia)

J Manipulative Physiol Ther 15:67–70, 1992 3–28

Introduction.—In patients with cervicogenic headache, pain perceived as arising in the head actually has its origin in the cervical spine. The neuroanatomical basis of cervicogenic headache, its sources, clinical features, and diagnosis were investigated.

Neuroanatomical Basis and Sources.—Convergence in the trigeminocervical nucleus between nociceptive afferents from the field of the trigeminal nerve and the receptive fields of the first 3 cervical nerves forms the neuroanatomical basis for cervicogenic headache. The possible sources of this headache are any structures innervated by the C1–C3 nerves. Structures experimentally shown to cause this headache include the dura matter of the posterior cranial fossa and the vertebral artery, the postvertebral muscles, and the C2–C3 zygapophyseal joint. Structures innervated by lower nerves can also cause referred pain, but this does not encompass the head.

Clinical Features.—Cervicogenic headache can be diagnosed only by exclusion of other causes of headache and confirmation of a cervical abnormality. The verified causes of headache are rheumatoid arthritis and trigger points in the muscles innervated by C1–C3. The current gold standard for diagnosis is injection techniques; plain radiographs are of limited value, as are CT and MRI.

Conclusion.—The prevalence of cervicogenic headache is uncertain, but many patients thought to have tension headaches may have cervicogenic headache. No methods of treatment, whether manipulation or injection, have been evaluated in a controlled trial.

▶ Cervicogenic headache arises from the trigeminocervical nucleus, where convergence of both trigeminal and cervical input occurs. This allows information concerning pain to be transmitted to the thalamus, where cervical pain ends up being interpreted as trigeminal pain, i.e., as a headache. It may be that the joint proprioceptor activity from adjustment helps to break this cycle and thus prevent the convergence from occurring. This awaits further study.—D.J. Lawrence, D.C.

Preparation of Dynamic Posture and Occurrence of Low Back Pain

Omino K, Hayashi Y (Keio Univ, Yokohama, Japan)

Ergonomics 35:693–707, 1992 3–29

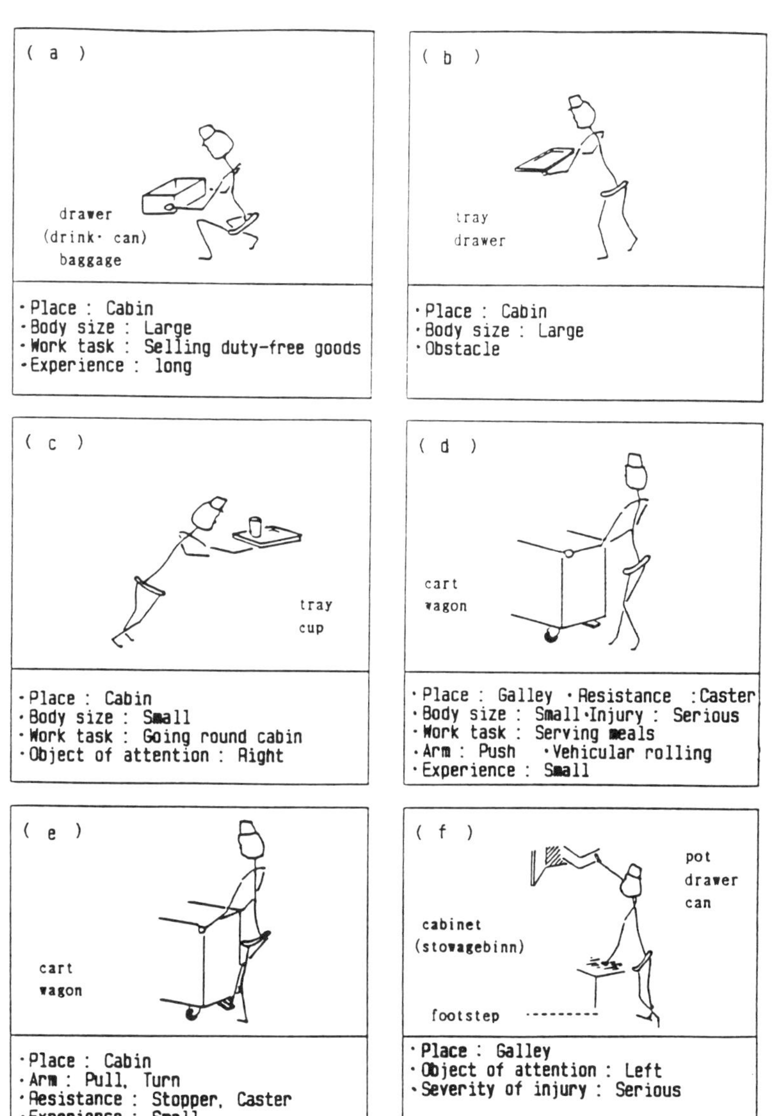

Fig 3–12.—Schematic illustration of 6 postural patterns associated with occurrence of low back pain. (Courtesy of Omino K, Hayashi Y: *Ergonomics* 35:693–707, 1992.)

Background.—Improper posture is thought to be 1 cause of low back pain. Low back pain occurring when individuals adopt a dynamic posture was studied.

Methods.—Low back pain was investigated in flight attendants, who provide a typical example of low back pain in a dynamic posture. Multidimensional quantification III was applied to survey results.

Findings.—Low back pain occurred in 6 postural patterns: bending knee posture, the posture of lifting and holding a light object, the posture of tilting the trunk, working posture to push a cart, the posture of turning or lifting a cart, and stretching. Low back pain often occurred when an unexpected load was imposed on the lumbar region. In experiments conducted to simulate the unexpected loading of this area, the results showed that lumbar muscular activity was not fast enough to cope with the load and resulted in an increased trunk swaying. This swaying was thought to induce a lumbar region load (Fig 3–12).

Conclusion.—Many low back pain occurrences observed in this group were probably the consequence of unexpected loading of the lumbar region. These findings support the notion that basic dynamic posture is important in preventing low back pain.

▶ That posture can lead to low back pain will come as a surprise to no one, but it is heartening to see other researchers note this fact in greater detail. The import of this study concerns therapy; restoration of normal dynamic posture becomes critical in restoring full function to the spine and allowing it to handle the loads that have been placed on it. Chiropractors are uniquely qualified to make this assessment, and they have done so for nearly their entire history.—D.J. Lawrence, D.C.

Parietal Bone Mobility in the Anesthetized Cat

Adams T, Heisey RS, Smith MC, Briner BJ (Michigan State Univ, East Lansing)

J Am Osteopath Assoc 92:599–622, 1992 3–30

Background.—Because of the paucity of direct quantitative data on cranial bone motion, it has traditionally been thought that the bones of the head are immobile and that the cranial vault is a rigid container. Direct quantitative evidence indicates that the parietal bones in the anesthetized cat move laterally and rotationally in reference to the medial sagittal suture that separates them on the dorsal surface of the skull.

Methods and Observations.—A newly developed instrument was attached to the surgically exposed skull of anesthetized adult cats. Lateral and rotational parietal bone movements around the fulcrum of the suture were differentiated. External forces applied to the skull and changes in intracranial pressure associated with induced hypercapnia, intravenous injections of norepinephrine, and controlled injections of artificial CSF into the lateral cerebral ventricle were used to produce bone movement. The cats' responses varied greatly. Lateral head compression generally caused sagittal suture closure, small inward rotation of the parietal bones, elevated intraventricular pressure, transient apnea, and unstable systemic arterial blood pressure. Graded intracranial volume increases produced stepped increases in pressure, lateral expansion at the sagittal suture, and outward rotation of the parietal bones. Variations among the cats were mostly attributed to differences in intracranial and suture compliance.

Conclusion.—Cranial compliance is defined at least in part by cranial suture mobility. Although the differences among animals were great, increases in intracranial pressure and inward lateral compressive forces on the temporal bones have a general effect, causing the parietal bones to change their relative positions.

▶ Practitioners of cranial therapy have long held that the bones of the skull move in the adult, but this has remained poorly studied and quite controversial. It has been claimed that this movement is involved in CSF flow, in respiration, and in cardiac function. This study demonstrates bone motion in a cat skull and then correlates that motion to changes in specific physiologic function (such as blood pressure and heart rate). This seems to lend credence to the claims of some osteopaths and chiropractors concerning the possibility of cranial motion; however, caution is indicated because the model was a cat. What happens in the human may be very different.—D.J. Lawrence, D.C.

The Role of the Rotator Interval Capsule in Passive Motion and Stability of the Shoulder

Harryman DT II, Sidles JA, Harris SL, Matsen FA III (Univ of Washington, Seattle)

J Bone Joint Surg (Am) 74-A:53–66, 1992 3–31

Background.—There has been much recent progress in defining the relationship of specific ligaments to glenohumeral motion and stability. However, the effects of operative modification of the interval capsule on glenohumeral motion or stability are not well understood. The role of the capsule in the interval between the supraspinatus and subscapularis tendons was characterized with respect to glenohumeral motion, translation, and stability.

Methods.—The glenohumeral rotations and translations resulting from applied loads in 8 cadaver shoulders were determined using a 6-degrees-of-freedom position sensor and a 6-degrees-of-freedom force and torque transducer. In each specimen, the range of motion was measured with the capsule in the rotator interval in a normal state, after the capsule had been sectioned, and after it had been imbricated.

Findings.—Surgical alteration of the capsular interval affected flexion, extension, external rotation, and adduction of the humerus with respect to the scapula. Modifying this part of the capsule also affected obligate anterior translation of the humeral head on the glenoid during flexion. Limitation of motion and obligate translation increased with operative imbrication and decreased with sectioning of the rotator interval capsule. Assessments of passive stability of the glenohumeral joint showed instability and occasional frank dislocation of the glenohumeral joint occurring inferiorly and posteriorly after section of the rotator interval capsule. Imbrication of this portion of the capsule raises resistance to inferior and posterior translation.

Conclusion.—The capsule in the rotator interval plays an important role in glenohumeral motion and stability. Release of this capsule portion may improve the range of motion of shoulders that have limited flexion and external rotation. Conversely, posterior and inferior instability may be controlled in part by imbrication of the rotator interval capsule.

▶ The rotator interval capsule functions to check a wide range of motions in the shoulder and, therefore, acts in concert with the ligamentous structures located there. Stretching it may be a necessary component of a shoulder rehabilitation program.—D.J. Lawrence, D.C.

A Universal Model of the Lumbar Back Muscles in the Upright Position

Bogduk N, Macintosh JE, Pearcy MJ (Univ of Newcastle, Australia; Univ of Durham, England)

Spine 17:897–913, 1992 3–32

Background.—Research into the biomechanics of the lumbar spine must rely on mathematical or computer modeling techniques. Construction of a comprehensive model of the back musculature relies on several data. These data have been largely unavailable until the recent appearance of detailed morphologic descriptions of the lumbar back muscles and the axes of rotation of the lumbar vertebrae. These data were used to construct a model representing the lumbar spine's action on every fascicle of the lumbar back muscles.

Methods.—The model was constructed using the 49 fascicles described in the anatomical descriptions of Macintosh and co-workers. The 3-dimensional orientation of the fascicles was determined by plotting each onto radiographs of 9 healthy volunteers in the upright position.

Findings.—Of the total extensor moment exerted on L4 and L5, the thoracic fibers of the lumbar erector spinae were found to contribute half. Approximately 20% was contributed by the multifidus, and the rest was exerted by the erector spinae lumbar fibers. Seventy percent to 86% of the total extensor moment in the upper lumbar levels was contributed by the thoracic fibers of the lumbar erector spinae. The net shear force of the lumbar back muscles on segments L1 to L4 was posterior, whereas that on L5 was anterior. Overall, the back muscles placed great compression forces on all segments, with a force coefficient of 46 Ncm^{-2}.

Conclusion.—This anatomically based model of the lumbar back muscles provides new insights into the actions of the back muscles and the effects of therapeutic exercise on the lumbar spine. In addition to its extensor action, each muscle also generates compression and shear forces. In the upright position, isometric contractions of the back muscles exert an anterior shear force on the L5 segment. These factors must be considered in exercise programs for patients with various injuries.

▶ This is a most difficult paper that examines the effects on all lumbar muscles in upright posture. However, elegant as this study is, it will take some time for the clinical import of the work to be determined.—D.J. Lawrence, D.C.

Age and Gender Related Normal Motion of the Cervical Spine

Dvorak J, Antinnes JA, Panjabi M, Loustalot D, Bonomo M (Wilhelm Schulthess Hosp, Zurich, Switzerland; Yale Univ, New Haven, Conn)

Spine 17:393S–398S, 1992 3–33

Interobserver Repeatability Study

Test	R 2 values	% Diff.
Flex/Ext	0.71	6.6
Lat Bend	0.85	6.3
Rotation	0.84	3.7
Rot/Flex	0.64	6.8
Rot/Ext	0.82	5.6
Average	0.77	5.8

Note: Passive examinations were conducted on 10 random patients by 2 examiners, one after the other. Correlation coefficients were calculated to indicate how reproducible results were with different examiners on the same volunteer.

(Courtesy of Dvorak J, Antinnes JA, Panjabi M, et al: *Spine* 17:393S–398S, 1992.)

Introduction.—For patients with neck pain, measurement of cervical spine motion is a routine part of the clinical examination. There is, however, no standard, noninvasive, repeatable method for measuring cervical spine motion in 3 dimensions. An attempt was made to develop such a method using the CA 6000 Spine Motion Analyzer, to accumulate a data base of normal values and to determine whether there were any age and sex differences in normal subjects.

Methods.—A group of 150 healthy, asymptomatic volunteers of various ages and both sexes were studied to obtain normal values. The measuring device consisted of a linkage device with 6 high-precision potentiometers connected by a series of 7 bars. Measurements were obtained for passive examinations of flexion-extension, lateral bending, rotation, rotation out of maximum flexion, and rotation out of maximum extension. The values for each sex and age group were compared, and a detailed error analysis was done to assess interobserver and intraobserver repeatability, the differences between passive and active tests, and the use of various fixation devices.

Findings.—The average interobserver discrepancy was 5.8%, with larger discrepancies for more complicated motions (table). The average coefficient of variation was 4. Motion tended to decrease with age, particularly in the 30- and 40-year range. Women in their 40s, however, showed a significantly larger range of motion in axial rotation and rotation out of maximum flexion. In corresponding decades of age, significant differences were also noted between gender groups.

Conclusion.—Use of the CA 6000 Spine Motion Analyzer is a reliable and reproducible method for clinical examination of cervical spine motion. Normative values show significant differences between genders and age groups, suggesting that current comparison methods are invalid. The CA 6000 should be used to evaluate motion after soft tissue injuries of the spine, the effects of different treatment methods, the effects of surgery over time, the influence of temporary segmental fixation, and the level of permanent impairment.

A Comparison of the Metrecom Skeletal Analysis System vs Plain Film Radiography in the Measurement of Sacral Base Angle and Lumbar Lordosis

Cowherd GP, Gringmuth R, Nolet P (Downsview, Ont)

J Can Chiropract Assoc 36:156–160, 1992 3–34

Background.—A number of nonradiographic clinical and experimental devices have been introduced for the assessment of spinal position and mechanics. One recently introduced device is a computerized 3-dimensional electrogoniometer, the Metrecom Spinal Analysis System, which is designed to measure the osseous spatial arrangement of the spine, pelvis, and upper and lower limb segments. This system was compared with plain film radiography for measurement of the sacral base angle and lumbar lordosis.

Methods.—The subjects were 15 men with a mean age of 26 years. Subjects had spinal analysis using the Metrecom Skeletal Analysis System, version 1.1, and concurrent lumbar spine radiography. Measurements of the sacral base angle, or Ferguson's angle, and lumbar lordosis by the 2 techniques were compared using Pearson correlation coefficients.

Findings.—The mean sacral base was 39 degrees on radiography vs. 28 degrees by the Metrecom system; the mean lumbar lordotic measurements were 59 degrees and 20 degrees, respectively. Pearson correlation was .236 for the sacral base angle and .519 for the lordosis angle.

Conclusion.—Sacral base and lumbar lordosis measurements made by the Metrecom Skeletal Analysis System show only a weak association with the same measurements made by plain film radiography. There is a statistically significant difference between these 2 measures. Differences in how the angles are calculated raise questions as to whether the same angles are being measured by the 2 techniques.

▶ The Metrecom has widespread use inside and outside the chiropractic profession. Although in some experiments it has had good reliability, in this study it faired only modestly when compared to similar measurements taken from plain film radiographs.—D.J. Lawrence, D.C.

4 Health Problems

Spine

CERVICAL

Hyperextension-Dislocation of the Cervical Spine: Ligament Injuries Demonstrated by Magnetic Resonance Imaging

Harris JH, Yeakley JW (Univ of Texas, Houston; Hermann Hosp, Houston)

J Bone Joint Surg 74-B:567–570, 1992 4–1

Background.—Hyperextension-dislocation (HD) of the cervical spine is enigmatic. No gross displacement appears on lateral radiographs, and conventional imaging techniques do not show ligament damage. The MR images of the cervical spine of adult patients were examined to evaluate damage to the spinal cord in cases of HD.

Methods.—Eight adults with HD and signs of cervical myelopathy underwent MRI. The assessments were done on a GE 1.5-tesla Signa System 3–24 hours after injury, with a standard 5.5-inch circular surface coil. Axial and sagittal T1-weighted images with a repetition time of 800 ms and an echo time of 20 ms were obtained, as well as sagittal T2-weighted and proton-density images with ECG gating and axial and sagittal T2 sequences.

Findings.—In all cases, there was disruption of the anterior longitudinal ligament and annulus of the intervertebral disk. Separation of the posterior longitudinal ligament from the subjacent vertebra was also seen in all patients. Some patients had widening of the disk space, posterior bulging, or herniation of the nucleus pulposus, and disruption of the ligamentum flavum.

Conclusion.—Magnetic resonance imaging confirmed the pattern of injury in acutely injured patients with HD and also clarified the etiopathology of HD. The demonstration of these ligament injuries on MRI, combined with clinical and radiographic findings, is important to patient management.

▶ Drs. Harris and Yeakley discuss an uncommon complication of cervical deceleration injuries. They note one significant point: this injury is hard to identify because there typically is no displacement visible on lateral radiographs, and because conventional images don't assess ligamentous structures very well. As a result, the chiropractor needs to recognize certain clinical signs, notably central cord syndrome after injury involving the face. When such symptoms exist, the chiropractor would be well advised to consider obtaining MR images of the cervical spine. These would demonstrate characteristic findings of damage to the longitudinal ligaments with possible disk disruption. Without these images, it is likely that sprain/strain may be diagnosed, leading to inappropriate therapy.—D.J. Lawrence, D.C.

Cervicogenic Headache: Anesthetic Blockades of Cervical Nerves (C2–C5) and Facet Joint (C2/C3)

Bovim G, Berg R, Dale LG (Trondheim Univ, Norway)

Pain 49:315–320, 1992 4–2

Purpose.—Recently published clinical criteria for cervicogenic headache address the clinical picture but not the underlying etiologic or pathogenetic factors. There is evidence that headache may arise from lesions in the lower cervical levels. Anesthetic blockades of spinal nerves C2 to C5 and facet joint C2/C3 were done to evaluate the possible involvement of these sites in the pathogenesis of cervicogenic headache.

Methods.—The study sample comprised 14 patients with cervicogenic headache (table). The median duration of headache was 4 years. All had blockade of the greater occipital nerve as part of the routine diagnostic workup. Ten had cervical nerve blockages, 8 of the C2 to C5 nerves on separate days. Eleven had facet joint C2/C3 injections; 7 of these also had nerve blockades.

Results.—The C2 nerve blockade resulted in freedom from pain in 5 of 10 patients and thus yielded the most useful information. Only 2 of 9 patients had freedom from pain after C2/C3 facet joint injection. In no case did complete pain relief result from C3 to C5 blockade.

Conclusion.—These results confirm the importance of diagnostic procedures directed toward C2 nerve fibers in cervicogenic headache, and they cast doubt on the value of C4 and C5 nerve blockades. The C3 blockade may be useful in some patients, although these findings showed no complete effect. The potential for leakage of anesthetic from the C2/C3 facet joint must be taken into consideration when this joint is evaluated, because the third occipital nerve runs close to the joint.

▶ This extremely provocative study, albeit without statistically significant results, has helped illuminate the study of cervicogenic headache, which the authors conclude is not an entity but, rather, is probably a reaction pattern with widely divergent causes. The authors suggest (1) that the ability to specifically and exactly inject a facet joint is difficult even with imaging with contrast, and (2) that it is quite likely that escape of anesthetic with perfusion of the surrounding nerves, without actually infusing the facet, is quite possible. Thus, anything but the most fastidious and confirmed infection of the facets is likely to lead to erroneous conclusions.—V.M. Given, D.C., B.A., B.S., M.A.

Main Diagnostic Criteria for Cervicogenic Headache

- Major symptoms and signs
  - Unilateral headache
  - Symptoms/signs of neck involvement
    - Pain precipitated by mechanical pressure to the ipsilateral upper posterior neck region or by awkward head positioning
    - Ipsilateral neck/shoulder/arm pain
    - Reduced range of motion in the cervical spine
- Pain characteristics
  - Non-clustering pain episodes of varying duration (or fluctuating, continuous pain)
  - Moderate, usually non-throbbing pain, starting in the neck and spreading forward
- Other important criteria
  - Anesthetic blockades of the **GON** and/or the **C2** nerve on the symptomatic side abolish pain transiently
  - Female sex
  - History of head and/or neck trauma

(Courtesy of Bovim G, Berg R, Dale LG: *Pain* 49:315–320, 1992.)

Low Energy High Frequency Pulsed Electromagnetic Therapy for Acute Whiplash Injuries: A Double Blind Randomized Controlled Study

Foley-Nolan D, Moore K, Codd M, Barry C, O'Connor P, Coughlan RJ (Mater Misericordiae Hosp, Dublin)

Scand J Rehabil Med 24:51–59, 1992 4–3

Introduction.—Standard treatement of acute whiplash injury with a soft collar and analgesia often is unsuccessful. Because pulsed electromagnetic therapy (PEMT) can promote healing and counter inflammation, PEMT was evaluated in 40 adults with acute "whiplash" injuries of the cervical spine resulting from a rear-end collision.

Study Design.—Either an active PEMT collar generating 27 MHz with a pulse burst width of 60 microseconds and a frequency of 450 per second or a facsimile collar was worn 8 hours per day at home. The patients were advised to mobilize the neck during the 12-week study period, and mefenamic acid was prescribed.

Results.—Actively treated patients had significantly less pain, as determined by a visual analogue scale, after 2 and 4 weeks. The PEMT group members had significantly worse movement scores at the outset, but they improved significantly after 12 weeks. Actively treated patients used significantly less anti-inflammatory medication than did the control patients. Eighty-five percent of the former patients and only 35% of controls believed they were moderately or much improved after 1 month, but 60% of controls believed they had improved at 12 weeks.

Conclusion.—Low-energy, high-frequency PEMT for 8 hours per day is an effective treatment for patients with persistent symptoms of acute whiplash injury.

▶ This study suggests that PEMT is effective for *acute* treatment of whiplash injuries, specifically during the first 4 weeks of care, apparently because there was no significant difference between treatment and control groups at the 12-week interval, and because no data were available for comparison between 4 and 12 weeks.

Although the visual analogue scale seemed to indicate improvement, it is confounding why a similar number of treatments (9 of 20) and control patients (12 of 20) were referred to physical therapy, which was only done if they were "unhappy" with the results of treatment at 4 weeks. This would suggest that although the visual analogue scale was indicating one thing, at least half of all subjects were "unhappy" with the care and the same 4-week interval. It also is unfortunate that the study does not describe the visual analogue range as well as the median scores, because the raw data may also give insight into the "unhappy" outcomes. The study is a promising attempt to show that PEMT is useful in the treatment of acute whiplash injuries (4 weeks); however, extending the study's conclusion that PEMT would be valuable for "acute *and* persistent neck pain" is dubious at best.—V.M. Given, D.C., B.A., B.S., M.A.

Whiplash: General Considerations in Assessment, Treatment, Management and Prognosis

Tarola GA

J Chiroprac 30:63–70, 1993 4–4

Introduction.—Whiplash injury to the neck is a poorly understood, often mismanaged problem. General considerations in the assessment, treatment, and prognosis of whiplash were reviewed.

The Organic Component.—Appropriate treatment should result in full recovery in most cases of uncomplicated soft tissue injuries within 7–16 weeks after injury. With minor trauma, skeletal muscle fibers can regenerate, usually within 6 weeks. In patients with more severe injury, collagen deposition hinders muscle and ligament regeneration. However, collagen has an inherent capacity to contract and remodel 3–14 weeks after injury. Fibroblastic activity and connective tissue healing are reflected in the effects of muscle movement, which is responsible for the development of an orderly fibril arrangement. When motion is introduced appropriately in the first 2 to 4 months after a neuromusculoskeletal injury, the fibroblasts line up and orient themselves in a controlled, efficient matrix, permitting optimal soft tissue healing.

The Inorganic Component.—Progression to chronic pain appears most often to follow a minor-to-moderate nociceptive stimulus that develops into chronic pain because of intrinsic and extrinsic factors. The chronic pain syndrome seems to develop in patients who are predisposed through immature or maladaptive pain and stress coping mechanisms. It is inversely proportional to the intensity of the physical injury. The "late whiplash syndrome," seen in patients more than 6 months after neck injury, consists of headache, neck ache, neck stiffness, depression, anxiety, and social variables. This syndrome has been seen mainly in women aged 21–40 years; it has a poor correlation with physical and radiologic abnormalities.

Conclusion.—In patients with whiplash injury, organic factors include the extent of the true physical injury, preexisting conditions, and aggravating factors. Nonorganic variables are intrinsic or extrinsic. Intrinsic factors are the patient's basic emotional make-up and tendency toward abnormal illness behavior; extrinsic factors are family role reversals, work capacity, life-style changes, financial loss, inappropriate medical management, and litigation. In addition to the organic factors, the physician must recognize and analyze the intrinsic and extrinsic factors involved in optimally treating patients with whiplash injury.

▶ Dr. Tarola presents a thorough discussion of cervical acceleration/deceleration injuries. He emphasizes both the nonorganic and organic components of this injury, and he makes the case that reliance on only the organic, physical, and objective factors will be insufficient to determine prognosis after an automobile accident. He presents protocols that help lay a foundation toward optimizing healing and limiting both disability and chronic pain. This is a prudent and well-thought-out approach to a difficult, yet common, chiropractic complaint.—D.J. Lawrence, D.C.

Cervical Spondylotic Myelopathy

Bernhardt M, Hynes RA, Blume HW, White AA III (Dickson-Diveley Orthopaedic Clinic, Kansas City, Mo; Eisenhower Army Med Ctr, Fort Gordon, Ga; Beth Israel Hosp, Boston)

J Bone Joint Surg 75–A:119–128, 1993 4–5

Introduction.—Cervical spondylotic myelopathy is the most common type of dysfunction of the spinal cord in patients older than age 50 years. Because the presentation of this condition may be subtle and often involves the elderly, it may be underdiagnosed. This underrecognition probably contributes to the number of elderly persons with gait disturbances that result in falls, causing hip fractures, head injuries, and other types of trauma.

Clinical Manifestations.—Difficulty in walking and a stooped, wide-based, sometimes jerky gait are typical of cervical spondylotic myelopathy. Balance is often a problem. Patients may also have loss of dexterity and nonspecific weakness of the upper extremities. Numbness and paresthesias in the upper extremities are not uncommon. Patients may describe an electric shocklike sensation extending through the body with certain neck motions. Bladder incontinence has also been reported, but it is uncommon.

Diagnosis.—Assessment typically reveals lower motor neuron signs at the level of cervical lesions and upper motor neuron signs below the lesions. Upper motor neuron signs occur in both the upper and lower extremities. Upper extremity involvement is often unilateral, whereas lower extremity involvement is usually bilateral.

Pathogenesis.—The pathogenesis of cervical spondylotic myelopathy begins extrinsic to the spinal cord, involves the osseous and soft tissue structures around the cord, and eventually leads to dysfunction of and abnormalities in the spinal cord itself.

Natural History.—In a recent review of the natural history of this condition, it was concluded that not enough information is available to accurately predict when and for whom surgery is absolutely indicated. The spectrum of clinical outcomes varies from minor dysfunction with few neurologic deficits over a long time to acute, catastrophic deterioration in a relatively short time.

Discussion.—Cervical spondylotic myelopathy is the most common type of spinal cord dysfunction in older patients. It is caused by static and dynamic factors involving osseous and soft tissue structures of the cervical spine, resulting in compromise of the space available for the spinal cord or the vascular supply to the cord, or both. The clinical course of this disorder varies greatly. Magnetic resonance imaging and CT after myelography are the best methods of confirming the diagnosis. To facilitate appropriate management before neurologic loss becomes irreversible, myelopathy must be recognized early.

▶ The authors have presented a very thorough review of a condition they believe is underrecognized. Giving close attention to the specific features of the 5 types of cervical spondylotic myelopathy will help obviate misdiagnosis. One interesting procedure presented by the authors is Pavlov's ratio, which is the anteroposterior diameter of the spinal canal divided by the anteroposterior diameter of the vertebral body; a value of .8 or less indicates the presence of a narrow canal with stenosis, increasing the risk of myelopathy. Bernhardt and colleagues do not believe this condition responds well to manipulation, a finding supported by work done by Kirkaldy-Willis and Cassidy.—D.J. Lawrence, D.C.

Seasonal Variation in Neck and Shoulder Symptoms

Takala E-P, Viikari-Juntura E, Moneta GB, Saarenmaa K, Kaivanto K (Inst of Occupational Health, Helsinki, Finland)

Scand J Work Environ Health 18:257–261, 1992 4–6

Background.—There have been few longitudinal studies of neck and shoulder symptoms and associated factors. The seasonal variations in such symptoms were investigated.

Methods.—The study involved women engaged in light sedentary work. Postal surveys were distributed to 380 bank tellers (age range, 20–50 years) in September, December, March, and May. The response rates ranged from 74% to 90%.

Findings.—Statistical analysis of 351 responses revealed a change in the frequency of neck and shoulder symptoms in 40.5% of the subjects from autumn to spring. The frequency of symptoms declined from autumn and winter toward spring. The stability of symptom frequency was positively associated with age (table).

Conclusion.—These findings confirm the fluctuation in neck and shoulder symptoms previously reported. Seasonal variations in symptoms

Odds Ratios (OR) and 95% Confidence Intervals (95% CI) for Mutually Adjusted Effects of 3 Predictors of Neck and Shoulder Symptoms

Predictor contrast	Model1 (8—30 d versus 0—7 d)		Model2 (>30 d versus 0—7 d)	
	OR	95% CI	OR	95% CI
Base-line symptoms				
0—7 d	1.00		1.00	
8—30 d	16.3	4.12—64.5	15.6	1.04—233
>30 d	166	34.3—805	13 900	283—683 000
Age				
Per one year	1.04	0.97—1.12	1.29	1.10—1.50
Season				
Autumn	1.00		1.00	
Winter	0.91	0.47—1.76	0.50	0.17—1.45
Spring	0.28	0.14—0.56	0.07	0.02—0.25

(Courtesy of Takala E-P, Viikari-Juntura E, Moneta GB, et al: *Scand J Work Environ Health* 18:257–261, 1992.)

need to be considered when planning and assessing preventive programs for neck and shoulder disorders.

▶ Although some of the findings in this study (such as an increase in neck disorders in older subjects) are not surprising, the differences in seasonal incidence are in light of the fact that the occupation studied (bank teller) is not subject to a change in work load depending on the time or season of year. The authors offer no clue as to why this might be. When planning programs designed to present future neck pain, this seasonal variation may need to be taken into account.—D.J. Lawrence, D.C.

Klippel-Feil Syndrome

Smith BA, Griffin C (Lackland Air Force Base, Tex)

Ann Emerg Med 21:876–879, 1992 4–7

Background.—Klippel-Feil syndrome, an idiopathic congenital disorder first described in 1912, is characterized by congenital fusion of 2 or more cervical vertebrae. It may also be associated with other organ system anomalies. About half the affected patients display the classic triad of a short neck, limited neck motion, and a low posterior hairline. One boy, 13 years, who was seen after roughhousing with an older sibling, had a hyperflexion injury to the neck. Films demonstrated a 2-mm anterolisthesis at C4-C5, as well as loss of the intervertebral disk space at the C5-C6 level.

Discussion.—It has been speculated that this disorder results from faulty segmentation of the cervical stomites in the third to eighth week of gestation. At affected levels, intervertebral disks are absent. The embryologic insult that precipitates the syndrome may account for other anomalies associated with it. These include urologic abnormalities, deafness, congenital heart disease, and Sprengel's deformity. Congenital neural abnormalities, such as mirror movements, may also be seen. Less commonly reported anomalies are hydrocephalus, hydromyelia, syringomyelia, and meningocele. Other skeletal anomalies, kyphoscoliosis, hemivertebrae, and malformed or cervical ribs, are common. In 1 large series of patients with congenital scoliosis and kyphosis, one fourth also had segmental defects of the cervical spine. The most common lesion in this series was an isolated fusion of C2–C3, but involvement at many levels was not uncommon. The classification of Klippel-Feil syndrome is largely descriptive: type I, extensive cervical and upper thoracic spinal fusion; type II, 1 or 2 cervical interspace fusions, sometimes with associated hemivertebrae and occipitoatlantal fusion; and type III, types I or II with lower thoracic or lumbar spine fusion.

Conclusion.—Congenital fusion of the cervical spine is associated with spontaneous and progressive neurologic problems as well as predisposition to spinal cord injury after relatively minor trauma. In addition, mechanical factors may result in vascular accidents in the CNS. The radiographic abnormalities seen in Klippel-Feil syndrome may stimulate acute pathologic conditions. Thus, further investigation is needed to elucidate the problem.

► Klippel-Feil syndrome involves the fusion of cervical vertebrae. It would be beneficial for chiropractors to keep in mind that the syndrome has a high incidence of other anomalies occurring along with it, with urologic and cardiac abnormalities being among the most serious. The authors present a 3-category classification system: type I involves extensive cervical and upper thoracic fusion; type II has 1 or 2 cervical fusions; and type III adds lower thoracic or lumbar fusions to the cervical involvement. One point for the practitioner to keep in mind is that individuals with this condition are prone to serious neurologic problems after even minor trauma, and that the condition may very well remain silent until the damage has occurred. Therefore, we should recommend protective measures to patients with this syndrome.—D.J. Lawrence, D.C.

Migraine: Theories of Pathogenesis

Blau JN (Natl Hosp for Neurology and Neurosurgery, London)
Lancet 339:1202–1207, 1992 4–8

Introduction.—Migraine is evident only through its effects. Its underlying mechanisms remain uncertain, but migraine manifests itself in complex, sequential patterns of symptoms that differ between and even within individuals. The premonitory symptoms are subtle and can alter mood, behavior, and gastrointestinal activity. Most migraine triggers directly affect the brain. The occurrence of female hormonal triggers also favors a neural mechanism of migraine, but some triggers do affect blood vessels.

Pathogenesis.—A family history of migraine is not uncommon. Some epidemiologic observations would seem to implicate hormonal factors. Vascular theories of migraine have, at various times, implicated both vasoconstricton and vasodilatation. Most of these theories ignore the fact that blood vessels are controlled by nerves or by circulating chemical agents. Among neurotransmitters, a role for serotonin often is discussed. Leão found that a spreading band of cerebral depression migrates across the cortex when a high concentration of potassium is applied, and that reduced blood flow is succeeded by hyperemia. Although a neural theory of migraine cannot omit vascular responses, vascualr phenomena in migraine are believed to be secondary to neuronal activity.

A *Suggestion.*—That women with migraine have fewer electrocardiographic abnormalities and less cerebrovascular disease and ischemic heart disease than others suggests, from a teleologic viewpoint, that migraine may be protective.

▶ Standard theories of migraine pathogenesis have traditionally focused on a vascular etiology, but that does not explain why blood vasculature is controlled by the nervous system. The authors suggest that both vascular and neural etiologies may not be fully explanatory, and they offer more speculation that, in some ways, migraine headache may have teleologic overtones; it may be a protective mechanism. Cardiovascular and cerebrovascular disease occur less frequently in patients who have migraines. It may be that migraine lies on a continuum between normal physiology and permanent dysfunction.—D.J. Lawrence, D.C.

Herniated Cervical Disk Presenting as Ischemic Chest Pain

Mitchell LC, Schafermeyer RW (Carolinas Med Ctr, Charlotte, NC)

Am J Emerg Med 9:457–460, 1992 4–9

Introduction.—Myocardial ischemia must be suspected in any adult who has chest pain; prompt evaluation is imperative. Once this and other life-threatening disorders are excluded, cervical disk disease may be considered the cause of chest pain.

Patients.—Two patients were seen at an emergency department with clinical signs and symptoms consistent with myocardial ischmia, but both were found to have herniated cervical disks. Surgical repair completely eliminated the symptoms. These patients may have neck stiffness with marked spasm of the trapezius or splenius capitus. Palpation over the spinous processes or parasternal region often will produce pain. There may be digital hypesthesia, reduced reflexes, or motor weakness. Stabbing pain is suggestive of disk herniation, especially if reproduced by palpating the chest wall in a patient lacking a history of angina or myocardial infarction. Both patients had a recent history of significant coronary artery disease.

Interpretation.—Pain resembling angina in a patient with a herniated cervical disk may result from constriction of the medial and lateral enteral thoracic nerves.

▶ When a patient has chest pain, the first assumption any prudent physician would make is that myocardial ischemia is present. This article discusses 2 patients in whom the presenting chest pain was caused by cervical disk herniation. The authors suggest that a way to differentiate between them is to note pain radiation; the patient with cervical disk herniation may have pain in the posterolateral neck and scapula, along with numbness in the digits. An examination for stiff neck and pain upon compression is also necessary, but only after the possibility of myocardial involvement has been ruled out. One must also be mindful that there are many additional causes of chest pain that mimic myocardial ischemia, notably those that are gastrointestinal and neuromuscular in nature.—D.J. Lawrence, D.C.

Atypical Chest Pain: Differentiation From Coronary Artery Disease

Richards SD (VA Med Ctr, Mountain Home, Tenn)

Postgrad Med 91:257–268, 1992 4–10

Introduction.—In evaluation of the patient with chest pain, identification of the pain as atypical excludes the possibility of coronary artery disease. An approach to finding the source of chest pain, along with characteristics of ischemic and nonischemic pain, is presented.

Evaluation.—Chest pain may be classified simply by determining whether the discomfort is substernal, whether it is precipitated by exer-

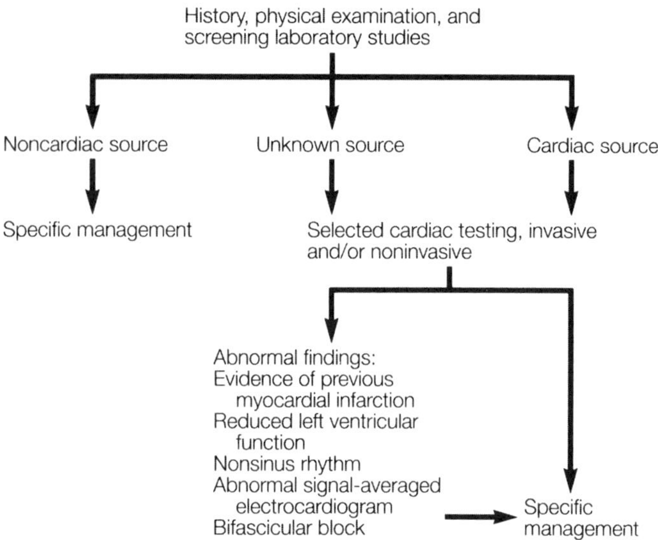

Fig 4–1.—Approach to the evaluation of chest pain. (Courtesy of Richards SD: *Postgrad Med* 91:257–268, 1992.)

tion, and whether it is relieved by nitroglycerin. If the answer to all 3 is yes, it is typical angina; if 2 of 3, atypical angina; and if 1, nonanginal pain. An approach to the evaluation of chest pain with history, physical examination, and laboratory studies is outlined (Fig 4–1).

Characteristics.—Atypical chest pain may result from a variety of factors, including pericarditis, pulmonary disease, aortic dissection, gastrointestinal disorders, chest wall pain, mitral valve prolapse, and psychogenic factors. Characteristically, angina is felt in the center of the chest, behind the sternum, with radiation into the shoulder or arm; atypical pain is often felt in the left submammary area or left hemithorax, and it usually does not radiate. The pain of angina is a tightness, heaviness, or pressure in the chest; atypical pain is usually less profound. Typical angina pain lasts 10–20 minutes and goes away with rest or nitroglycerin. Constant, unabated pain is unlikely to be ischemic. Ischemic pain more commonly occurs with exertion or emotional excitement; gastrointestinal pain may be triggered by eating, and chest wall pain by movement. Angina occurs with other manifestations of myocardial ischemia, which are usually less severe in atypical chest pain. Myocardial infarction usually causes intense pain and radiation, although it may be painless. There may be symptoms of indigestion, or nausea and vomiting may be present. In elderly patients, the diagnosis of infarction may be difficult to make. Noninvasive tests—ECG, echocardiography, and cardiac isoenzyme measurement—are needed for patients with suspected infarction.

Conclusion.—Many patients are seen with atypical chest pain. Correct diagnosis requires an accurate history and an understanding of the prevalence of coronary artery disease in various patient groups. Noninvasive tests may be helpful; only when these results are abnormal or unclear is cardiac catheterization indicated.

▶ The causes of atypical chest pain include pericarditis, pulmonary disease, aortic dissection, gastrointestinal disease, chest wall pain, mitral valve prolapse, and psychogenic factors. Dr. Richards does not list neuromuscular causes as one of the possibilities; however, as was noted earlier, even cervical disk herniation may cause excruciating chest pain. The distinguishing diagnostic features of each of these conditions is well described in this paper, and the approach to evaluation is thorough. Use of these features will help to distinguish cardiac from noncardiac pain, notwithstanding the exclusion of neuromuscular causes of that chest pain.—D.J. Lawrence, D.C.

Cervicogenic Dysfunction in Muscle Contraction Headache and Migraine: A Descriptive Study

Vernon H, Steiman I, Hagino C (Canadian Mem Chiropractic College, Toronto, Ont, Canada)

J Manipulative Physiol Ther 15:418–429, 1992 4–11

Background.—The concept of cervical spine involvement in the etiology of headache is supported by many, but conservative treatment of headache directed at dysfunction of the cervical spine has not been widely reported. The prevalence and nature of findings of cervicogenic dysfunction in subjects with muscle contraction/tension-type (MCH) headaches and common migraine without aura (CM) were surveyed.

Method.—Nineteen subjects with MCH and 28 subjects with CM in a chiropractic outpatient research clinic were assessed with standardized headache history, plain film and dynamic spinal radiographs, motion palpation, and pressure algometry. No therapeutic intervention was undertaken.

Findings.—The most prevalent headache locations for CM were frontal and occipital. Headache was accompanied by neck pain in 90% of the subjects and by upper back pain in 41%. For subjects with MCH, the most prevalent headache locations were occipital and frontal, with neck pain in 100% of the subjects and upper back pain in 27%. Dynamic radiographic studies showed at least 1 significant abnormality of segmental mobility from C1 to C7 in 97% of the patients and abnormalities in 4 or more segments in 43%. Both groups had at least 2 major fixations on motion palpation and at least 1 tender point in the upper cervical region verifiable by pressure algometry. This pattern of cervicogenic myofascial and joint dysfunction in subjects with either CM or MCH headaches is similar to findings in the more narrowly defined category of "cervicogenic" headache. The linking of CM and MCH on the same etiologic spectrum suggests that these 2 headaches are based on a disorder in the cervical spine.

Conclusion.—A high prevalence of neck pain during headache, cervical joint dysfunction and postural malalignment, and myofascial tenderness found in similar levles in subjects with either MCH or CM headaches suggests that the cervical spine plays an important role in causing these headaches. The narrow definition of "cervicogenic headaches" should be reconsidered.

▶ Cervical spine involvement in headache is well accepted but relatively poorly studied. Dr. Vernon, this year's winner of the Researcher of the Year award from the Foundation for Chiropractic Education and Research, looks at the nature of cervicogenic dysfunction in 2 different types of headache and also finds the presence of motion abnormalities, joint dysfunction, and myofascial involvement. This indicates a need for chiropractic intervention in these types of headache, and it was Dr. Vernon who did the seminal work studying chiropractic adjustment as an appropriate and effective therapy for migraine.—D.J. Lawrence, D.C.

Migraine and Tension-Type Headaches: The Questionable Validity of Current Classification Systems

Marcus DA (Univ of Pittsburgh, Pa)

Clin J Pain 8:28–36, 1992 4–12

Background.—The International Headache Society, in an attempt to make the diagnosis of headache more reliable, proposed a classification system providing more specific criteria. It acknowledges that an individual patient may satisfy established criteria for both migraine and tension-type headaches, and it also notes that the features of headache frequently vary in severity at different times. Clinical trials suggest that the migraine-tension dichotomy is artificial, but many specialists still adhere to it.

A *Unified Concept.*—Migraine and tension-type headaches are best viewed as parts of a spectrum. A reasonable single-syndrome approach to benign recurring headaches uses a continuum of severity rather than emphasizing discrete categories of headache. Less severe episodes represent what currently are classified as tension-type headaches; they are characterized by nonthrobbing pain and muscle tenderness, and any associated nausea/vomiting is mild. More severe headaches may be accompanied by a neurologic aura and may be unilateral. Intermediate forms represent what are now called "migraine without aura."

Diagnosis.—Benign recurring headaches involve at least 5 attacks in a 5-year period, each lasting longer than 30 minutes. Exclusion criteria include symptoms of cluster headache, features of cranial neuralgia, and evidence of intracranial pathology. A behavior-oriented approach is helpful in estimating the severity of individual episodes.

► Rather than looking at migraine and tension headache as 2 different clinical entities, there is a developing consensus that these 2 headaches may represent different ends of the same spectrum. Part of this thinking is a result of the overlap of symptoms and therapies shared by these headaches, and part results from the shared pathophysiologic features. The author suggests that, rather than call each headache by its old name, they should all be classified as "benign recurring headache." This does fly in the face of the International Headache Society and its well-accepted classification schema. Before making such a substantive change, more work establishing which pathophysiologic mechanisms are involved must be accomplished.—D.J. Lawrence, D.C.

Complications of Cervical Spine Manipulation: A Case of Locked in Syndrome

Kponkton A, Hamonet C, Montagne A, Devailly JP (CHU Henri-Mondor et Albert-Chenevier, Créteil, France)

Presse Medicale 21:2050–2052, 1992 4–13

Introduction.—The public's current interest in spinal manipulation is a result, in part, of the ineffectiveness of the anti-inflammatory drug therapy commonly prescribed by physicians in the treatment of muscle pain. Whereas manipulation of the lumbar and thoracic spine sppears to cause few serious problems, manipulation of the cervical spine carries an important risk for serious neurovascular injury. A young woman who underwent manipulation of the cervical spine had a severe cerebral neurovascular injury that has left her disabled.

Case Report.—Woman, 29, underwent manipulation of the cervical spine after having had episodic torticollis that did not improve with analgesic drug therapy. The practitioner who performed the manipulation was not licensed for any paramedical discipline. After the third treatment, the patient had a right-sided hemiparesis, which rapidly evolved into a coma. Computed tomography demonstrated cerebellar softening in both hemispheres. Vertebral arteriography did not show dissection of the vertebral artery. She was transferred and underwent emergency decompression of the posterior fossa. The patient gradually regained consciousness after 12 days in a stage III coma. After spending 3 months in the hospital, she was transferred to a rehabilitation service, where she remained for more than a year before being discharged home with part-time nursing care.

► A paper such as this acts as a sobering reminder that complications resulting from cervical spine manipulation are very real and are potentially life-threatening. Excessive rotational force in the cervical spine does carry some risk. By recognizing that risk and by ensuring that patients are tested for potential vertebral artery involvement, we can help to reduce the possibility of "locked-in syndrome" and other cervical involvements.—D.J. Lawrence, D.C.

LUMBAR AND LOW BACK

Chymopapain: A 10-Year, Double-Blind Study

Gogan WJ, Fraser RD (West Palm Beach, Fla; Royal Adelaide Hosp, South Australia)

Spine 17:388–394, 1992 4–14

Introduction.—There has been a need for long-term research comparing the results of chymopapain with those of a placebo. The long-term effects of intradiskal chymopapain were compared with those of intradiskal saline, and delayed adverse sequelae were assessed.

Patients and Methods.—Sixty patients with sciatica resulting from lumbar intervertebral disk herniation were enrolled in the double-blind trial. By random assignment, 30 were given intradiskal chymopapain, and 30 were given intradiskal saline. These patients were followed up for 10 years.

Results.—At the 10-year follow-up, with the patients still unaware of which treatment they received, 80% of those in the chymopapain group considered the injection to be successful, compared with 34% in the saline group. Laminectomy was required in 20% of the patients given chymopapain and in 47% of those given placebo. An independent observer unaware of treatment assignments rated 77% of the patients treated with chymopapain to be at least moderately improved, compared with 38% of the patients treated with saline.

Conclusion.—These findings support the view that chymopapain should be offered to patients with disabling sciatica from a contained disk prolapse when conservative measures have failed. In this study, chymopapain had a therapeutic effect on back pain as well. However, this should not be interpreted to mean that chymopapain necessarily has a treatment effect in patients with disk rupture in whom back pain is the main symptom. It is recommended that, when possible, a decision on the need for surgery should be deferred for 4 to 6 weeks after chemonucleolysis.

▶ For the properly selected patient, consideration of chemonucleolysis may be appropriate before the various surgical options, as a routine procedure. Retrospective studies should compare the long-term outcomes of patients considered to have favorable response both to chemonucleolysis and to surgery in regard to further pain, disability, lost work time, and additional related medical and rehabilitative interventions.—J. Ameen, D.C.

Morbidity and Mortality in Association With Operations on the Lumbar Spine: The Influence of Age, Diagnosis, and Procedure

Deyo RA, Cherkin DC, Loeser JD, Bigos SJ, Ciol MA (Univ of Washington, Seattle; Seattle VA Med Ctr)

J Bone Joint Surg (Am) 74-A:536–543, 1992 4–15

Background.—Morbidity and mortality after lumbar spine surgery have been well characterized for young and middle-aged adults undergoing diskectomy. However, elderly patients often have surgery on the lumbar spine, especially for stenosis. Little information is available on morbidity and mortality after procedures done in older patients or after procedures other than simple diskectomy.

Methods.—The rates of postoperative complications and death recorded in a hospital discharge registry for Washington state from 1986 through 1988 for patients undergoing lumbar spine surgery were analyzed. Excluding those with a malignant lesion, infection, or fraction, 18,122 hospitalizations remained for procedures on the lumbar spine. Eighty-four percent of these involved a herniated disk or spinal stenosis.

Findings.—Morbidity and mortality during hospitalization and after discharge increased with advancing patient age. The complication rate for those aged 75 years or older was 18%. Almost 7% in that age group were discharged to nursing homes. Complications occurred most frequently among patients with spinal stenosis, but according to multivariate analysis, the complications associated with procedures for this condition were primarily related to patient age and type of procedure. Those patients who had had a spinal arthrodesis had more complications, longer hospitalization, and higher charges than those who did not. Overall, surgery for conditions other than a herniated disk were related to more complications and greater use of resources, especially when arthrodesis was done, than was surgery for removal of a herniated disk (Tables 1, 2, and 3).

Conclusion.—Despite study limitations, the data clearly show the importance of patient age, diagnosis, and type of operative procedure in operative morbidity and mortality and use of resources. Such variations are important when clinical decisions are made. Because lumbar spine surgery is almost always elective, patients should be allowed to make informed decisions for or against an operation.

▶ This retrospective research, which covered 2 years and 18,122 hospitalizations for lumbar disk surgery, used a database for the state of Washington. In consideration of the possible national health-care plan and the critical need for cost containment, risk-vs.-benefit assessments appear feasible for all surgeries and hospital procedures through a nationally integrated database. The sensitivity of this study, because of its size, is quite impressive regarding age, complications, and types of operative procedure.—J. Ameen, D.C.

TABLE 1.—Rates of Postoperative Morbidity, Mortality, Placement in a Nursing Home, and Use of Resources According to the Patients' Age and Sex

	No. of Procedures	Complications While Hospitalized *(Per cent)*	Mortality *(Per cent)*	Discharged to Nursing Home† *(Per cent)*	Prolonged Hospitalization (≥10 Days)† *(Per cent)*	Mean Duration of Hospitalization *(Days)*	Mean Hospital Charges *(Dollars)*
Age *(yrs.)*							
18-40	7143	6.4	0.0	0.04	6.8	5.1	3821
41-64	7473	8.7	0.01	0.15	9.6	5.8	4310
65-74	2347	14.6	0.21	1.28	19.5	7.5	5331
≥75	1159	17.7	0.60	6.99	33.1	9.3	6133
Sex‡							
Men	10,610	8.8	0.09	0.22*	8.3*	5.4*	4117*
Women	7512	9.6	0.04	1.36	15.6	6.7	4701
Over-all	18,122	9.1	0.07	0.69	11.3	6.0	4359

Note: All differences between age groups were significant at $P < .001$; between men and women, only differences identified by *asterisks* were significant ($P < .001$).
† Includes only patients who were not admitted from a nursing home.
‡ The mean age of the men was 45.7 years and that of the women was 51.3 years ($P = .0001$).
(Courtesy of Deyo RA, Cherkin DC, Loeser JD, et al: *J Bone Joint Surg (Am)* 74-A:536–543, 1992.)

TABLE 2.—Number and Frequency of Specific Complications After 18,122 Operations on the Lumbar Spine

ICD-9-CM Codes	Description	No. of Patients	Percentage of: All Complications	Percentage of: All Patients
998.8, 998.9, 999.9, E878.8	Unspecified or unclassified complications, reactions, misadventures	446	23.5	2.5
998.2, E870.0	Accidental cut, puncture, or hemorrhage during a procedure	299	15.8	1.6
996.4, 996.6, 996.7	Mechanical, infectious, inflammatory, or other complications of internal prosthetic device or graft	189	10.0	1.0
998.1	Hemorrhage or hematoma complicating a procedure	189	10.0	1.0
997.4	Gastrointestinal complications	169	8.9	0.9
997.5	Urinary tract complications	157	8.3	0.9
997.3, 415.1	Respiratory complications, pulmonary embolism	160	8.4	0.9
997.1, 410.0-410.9, 998.0	Cardiac complications, acute myocardial infarction	91	4.8	0.5
998.5, 999.3	Postoperative infections	69	3.6	0.4
997.0	Central nervous-system complications	60	3.2	0.3
998.3	Disruption of operative wound	23	1.2	0.1
997.2	Peripheral vascular complications (includes phlebitis, thrombophlebitis)	14	0.7	0.1
999.8	Other transfusion reaction (not ABO or Rh incompatibility)	7	0.4	0.04
Several	Other complications occurring in fewer than 5 patients each	21	1.1	0.1
Total		1894	99.9*	10.34†

* Total is slightly less than 100% because of rounding off.
† Total exceeds the percentage of patients who had complications listed in Table 1, because any one patient could have more than one complication.
(Courtesy of Deyo RA, Cherkin DC, Loeser JD, et al: *J Bone Joint Surg (Am)* 74-A:536–543, 1992.)

TABLE 3.—Complications, Duration of Hospitalization, and Charges According to Primary Diagnosis

Primary Diagnosis	No. of Hospitalizations	Mean Age *(Yrs.)*	Complications While Hospitalized† *(Per cent)*	Mean Duration of Hospitalization *(Days)*	Prolonged Hospitalization (≥10 Days)† *(Per cent)*	Mean Hospital Charges *(Dollars)*
Herniated disc	11,914	43.4	5.7	5.2	8.3	3765
Spinal stenosis	3380	65.0	14.4	7.6	18.7	5319
Degenerative changes	1276	49.2	12.7	7.0	13.2	5426
Possible instability	863	45.7	12.8	7.1	14.0	5799
Miscellaneous low-back pain	144	44.3	11.1	6.5	14.6	5141

Note: Significant differences related to diagnosis were found for every variable ($P < .001$). Patients who had a primary diagnosis unrelated to low back pain (e.g., a concurrent morbid condition or complication) are not included.

† Percentages are based on the number of hospitalizations rather than the number of patients.

(Courtesy of Deyo RA, Cherkin DC, Loeser JD, et al: *J Bone Joint Surg (Am)* 74-A:536–543, 1992.)

Outcome Analysis in 654 Surgically Treated Lumbar Disc Herniations

Pappas CTE, Harrington T, Sonntag VKH (Barrow Neurological Inst, Phoenix, Ariz)

Neurosurgery 30:862–866, 1992 4–16

Introduction.—Advances in surgical techniques and methods of patient selection have improved the outcome after lumbar diskectomy. Microdiskectomy has been the technique of choice at the study institution for at least 10 years. The outcomes of 654 consecutive patients treated during a 4.5-year period were reported.

Methods.—The patients underwent a microdiskectomy, a laminectomy plus microdiskectomy, or a decompressive laminectomy with a microdiskectomy for herniated lumbar disks. Approximately one third of the injuries resulted from lifting. Nearly all patients complained of leg pain; 27% reported motor weakness. All were evaluated by CT, MRI, or myelography. To objectively assess outcome, the investigators used the Prolo Functional-Economic Outcome Rating Scale (table).

Results.—Complications developed after surgery in 71 (10.8%) patients. Wound infections above the fascia occurred in 45 patients. One of the 2 arterial injuries resulted in death from complications of abdominal surgery undertaken for repair. Patients who had microdiskectomies had shorter hospital stays than those with more extensive laminectomies. Sixty-one patients required a second lumbar disk operation. As defined by scores on the Prolo Scale, almost 80% of the patients had good outcomes. Those patients with nonindustrial injuries fared better than patients with industrial injuries. Both professionals with legal concerns and laborers with industrial insurance had good outcomes.

Conclusion.—Outcome was good to excellent for most patients undergoing surgical treatment for lumbar disk herniation, whatever technique was used. The Functional-Economic Outcome Rating Scale is confirmed to be a useful tool for the evaluation of spine surgery.

▶ Standardization is sought for the outcome rating criteria and scales for surgical and other interventions. In this retrospective study, the Prolo Functional-Economic scale (see the table) was compared by reference to the Glasgow Coma Scale. The Glasgow scale consists of 3 sections, or items; the Prolo scale consists of two. Of the 645 patients, 10.8% had complications; there was one death. A more sensitive and diversified scale might be more appropriate for postsurgical outcome assessment. Additional criteria, ranging from morbidity and mortality to the duration and long-term cost of rehabilitative and postoperative care, are recommended.—J. Ameen, D.C.

Functional-Economic Outcome Rating Scale

Economic Status

E1: Complete invalid

E2: No gainful occupation including ability to do housework or continue retirement activities

E3: Able to work but not at previous occupation

E4: Working at previous occupation part-time or limited status

E5: Able to work at previous occupation with no restrictions of any kind

Functional Status

F1: Total incapacity (or worse than before operation)

F2: Mild-to-moderate level of lower back pain and/or sciatica (or pain same as before operation but able to perform all daily tasks of living)

F3: Low level of pain and able to perform all activities except sports

F4: No pain, but patient has had one or more recurrences of lower back or sciatica

F5: Complete recovery, no recurrent episodes of lower back pain, able to perform all previous sports activities

(Courtesy of Pappas CTE, Harrington T, Sontag VKH: *Neurosurgery* 30:862–866, 1992.)

The Pathoanatomy and Clinical Significance of the Sacroiliac Joints
Cassidy JD (Royal Univ Hosp, Saskatoon, Saskatchewan, Canada)
J Manipulative Physiol Ther 15:41–42, 1992 4–17

Development and Anatomy.—The sacroiliac joint appears at 10 to 12 weeks' gestation and, at birth, has a thick surface of hyaline cartilage on the sacral side but is poorly developed on the iliac side. The latter aspect of the joint matures into a thin layer of fibrocartilage in the first 3 years of life. After puberty, a ridge develops along the iliac surface with a corresponding depression sacrally. The iliac fibrocartilage tends to degenerate early in life. The joint most often remains patent throughout life.

Clinical Aspects.—The clinical importance of premature osteoarthrosis at this site remains uncertain. No objective means is available for demonstrating involvement of the sacroiliac joints in mechanical low back pain. Nevertheless, these joints are treated to good effect in patients with mechanical back pain. Both manipulation and intra-articular injection therapy have been suggested.

▶ Anatomically staging the typical development and degeneration of the sacroiliac joint is certainly of interest. Osteoarthrosis correctly correlated to age and other factors, patient history, or genetic disposition may differentiate pathogenesis and normal maturation. The age-related exchange of sacroiliac mobility for stability may mediate spinal osteoarthrosis.—J. Ameen, D.C.

Intrathecal Depo-Medrol: A Literature Review
Wilkinson HA (Univ of Massachusetts, Worcester)
Clin J Pain 8:49–56, 1992 4–18

Background.—Intrathecally administered methylprednisolone acetate (IT-MPA) has been reported to have beneficial effects in the treatment of low back pain and "failed back" syndromes, but its use has been largely curtailed because of its potential adverse effects. The available literature on IT-MPA was reviewed and summarized.

Review.—Some reports have shown IT-MPA to be beneficial and safe in patients with low back and, especially, "failed back" problems, including adhesive arachnoiditis. However, other studies have emphasized the potential dangers of the treatment and have advised against its use. Many of these reports implicate the proplylene glycol in the methlprednisolone as being potantially hazardous. Because the literature on this treatment is extensive and conflicting, it is difficult for clinicians to determine the risk/benefit ratio of IT-MPA for patients with "failed back" problems. A literature analysis indicates that reasearch attests to the usefulness and general safety of IT-MPA when used within certain limits. Several studies implicate IT-MPA as a potential cause of arachnoiditis or other neurologic injury, but most of the evidence in such studies is circumstantial, and most complications followed multiple, large-dose, or frequent injections.

Conclusion.—It appears that IT-MPA is of limited usefulness in patients with "failed back" syndromes who have been refractory to most other treatments. Although IT-MPA does have a potential for causing harm, there is no scientific confirmation that IT-MPA used in moderation has actually caused harm to humans or laboratory animals.

▶ A review of the literature challenges the manufacturer's Food and Drug Administration-approved advice against the intrathecal use of Depo-Medrol (methylprednisolone acetate). According to the available literature, the benefit vs. risk, in the prescribing of pharmaceuticals for various purposes is not necessarily represented in the packet-insert, regulatory monographs. Physicians' bias or judgment in following manufacturers' recommendations is seriously questioned. However, application parameters remain discretionary for the "limited but useful role" of this pharmaceutical in the treatment of "failed back" syndromes or adhesive acachnoiditis.—J. Ameen, D.C.

Prognosis in Postoperative Discitis: A Retrospective Study of 111 Cases

Iversen E, Nielsen VAH, Hansen LG (Glostrup Hosp, Denmark)
Acta Orthop Scand 63:305–309, 1992 4–19

Background.—The incidence of postoperative diskitis after lumbar disk surgery varies from .2% to 4%. Radiography characteristically shows blurring of the endplate of the vertebral body, cavitations, narrowing of the disk space, and subsequent healing with new bone formation, fusion, or bony ridging. The postoperative course and long-term prognosis in 111 cases of postoperative diskitis after lumbar disk surgery were compared with those of a matched control group.

Patients.—One hundred eleven patients with postoperative diskitis confirmed by radiography were identified by a retrospective record review. All patients answered a questionnaire concerning postoperative treatment, duration of symptoms, and sick leave, and 53 patients underwent clinical follow-up. Low back pain appeared in these patients at an average of 16 days after surgery. Laboratory findings of elevated erythrocyte sedimentation rate, white blood cell count, and body temperature were not useful in the diagnosis. A control group of 52 patients who were matched for age, sex, and time of operation was selected; 34 patients in the control group participated in the clinical follow-up.

Findings.—The diskitis group had a higher incidence of herniation at the L4–L5 level, a higher incidence of chronic low back pain, and longer sick leave with a greater risk of vocational handicap. Ninety-five of 111 patients with diskitis had low back pain, compared with 38 of 52 control patients. The 2 groups did not differ in the consumption of analgesics, the subjective evaluation of the final outcome, spinal mobility, or neurologic findings.

Conclusion.—The group of patients with diskitis and the individuals in the control group differed substantially in cumulated periods of back pain and the presence of pain at follow-up. There was no difference in the 2 groups in the severity of pain or the consumption of analgesics. Compared with the control group, postoperative sick leave was prolonged in the diskitis group, and the long-term prognosis was worse with greater risk of chronic low back pain.

▶ It is of clinical interest to the chiropractic practitioner that the "cardinal" symptom of postoperative diskitis is low back pain from 0 to 8 weeks after surgery, and that laboratory findings are inconsistent. Plain film radiographs have reliable value. Other symptoms discussed include pain aggravated by movement, referral of pain to the testes, groin, or lower abdominal quadrant, and pain to the lower extremity and, not commonly, true sciatica. The diagnostic value of MRI is also mentioned. Referral for antibiotic therapy is essential if this condition is suspected.—J. Ameen, D.C.

Small Area Analysis of Surgery for Low-Back Pain

Volinn E, Mayer J, Diehr P, Van Koevering D, Connell FA, Loeser JD (Univ of Washington, Seattle)

Spine 17:575–581, 1992 4–20

Background.—The rate at which surgery for low back pain is performed varies widely. Because there is little consensus on the efficacy of surgical procedures for this condition, some of this variability may be accounted for by nonmedical factors. A regression analysis was performed on data regarding surgery for low back pain among the 39 counties in the state of Washington.

Data Analysis.—The data set was the abstracts of all 528,146 patient discharges from nonmilitary short-stay hospitals in Washington in 1985. Of those, 3,929 residents had surgery for low back pain. Six classes of nonmedical factors that could affect surgery rates were postulated: occupation, socioeconomic conditions, neurologic and orthopedic surgeon density, available hospital beds, primary payer, and health-care availability.

Results.—Between the highest and lowest rate of surgery in the 39 counties, there was almost a 15-fold difference. Three explanatory variables were significant: percent in manual occupations, percent receiving food stamps, and hospital occupancy. However, less than 15% of the variability could be explained by those factors.

Discussion.—To address the variability in rates of low back pain surgery, 28 explanatory variables were examined by a statistical model that controlled for spurious association. Despite the thoroughness of this analysis, less than 15% of the variability in the rate of surgery could be accounted for. Therefore, the reason for the major part of this variability has yet to be identified and awaits the quantification of such factors as "physician practice style."

▶ Variation in the regional rates of surgery for low back pain is cited in consideration of outcome variance, little consensus on efficacy, and physicians' discretion. If further investigation will attempt to quantify "physician practice style," then the analysis, having been somewhat without regard for the patient's back condition vs. the postulated so-called nonmedical factors, might benefit to include further distinction, such as the reliability and rate of diagnoses or the virtual diagnoses selected for inclusion. When discussing variable diffusion of medical innovations, preconceptulization, or tolerance for uncertainty, the definition of medical and nonmedical factors needs clarification. This study is at best inconclusive.—J. Ameen, D.C.

Functional Outcomes of Low Back Pain: Comparison of Four Treatment Groups in a Randomized Controlled Trial

Hsieh C-YJ, Phillips RB, Adams AH, Pope MH (Los Angeles College of Chiropractic, Whittier, Calif; Univ of Vermont, Burlington)

J Manipulative Physiol Ther 15:4–9, 1992 4–21

Background.—There are no established appropriate outcome measures for assessing the effect of low back pain treatment. In recent years, functional questionnaires have been used to assess subjective disability. These include the Oswestry Low Back Pain Questionnaire, the Revised Oswestry Low Back Pain Questionnaire (ROLBPQ), and the Roland-Morris Activity Scale (RMAS). The ROLBPQ and RMAS were compared in a prospective, randomized, controlled trial of chiropracic manipulation, massage, corset, and transcutaneous muscular stimulation (TMS).

Methods.—The patients studied were between the ages of 18 and 55 years, and all had had nonspecific low back pain for 3 weeks to 6 months. Eighty-five patients completed the questionnaires. Data on 63 patients who completed the initial and final assessments were analyzed.

Findings.—The ROLBPQ and RMAS both had good internal consistency, with alpha coefficients ranging from .77 to .93. Both showed a significant difference between the chiropractic manipulation and massage groups. Furthermore, RMAS showed significant differences between the chiropractic manipulation and TMS groups, and between the corset and massage groups; the ROLBPQ did not. The RMAS demonstrated that chiropractic manipulation produced better, although not significantly better, results than did corset, possibly because of insufficient sample size and/or treatment duration.

Conclusion.—Both the RMAS and ROLBPQ are reliable for measuring low back pain disability. Chiropractic manipulation provides superior short-term benefit compared with stroking massage and TMS in patients with subacute low back pain. Because it is more sensitive than the ROLBPQ in detecting changes, RMAS appears to be preferable in clinical trials for subacute low back pain.

► The need for standarization of outcome assessment measures cannot be overstated. In comparing 2 low back pain questionnaires, this study suggests a possible differential appropriateness per patient selection. Future clinical trials can also be applied to other populations, such as the postsurgical patient with low back or sciatic pain. These instruments possess greater sensitivity than the Prolo scale used by Pappas (1). The comparison of manipulation and other modalities appears to be inhibited by the small patient sample.—J. Ameen, D.C.

Reference

1. Pappas CTE, et al: *Neurosurgery* 30:862, 1992.

Intrathecal Midazolam for the Treatment of Chronic Mechanical Low Back Pain: A Controlled Comparison With Epidural Steroid in a Pilot Study

Serrao JM, Marks RL, Morley SJ, Goodchild CS (Univ of Leeds, England; York District Hosp, England)

Pain 48:5–12, 1992 4–22

Objective.—Epidural corticosteroid therapy is the most common treatment for chronic mechanical low back pain. The therapeutic effects of intrathecal midazolam were studied in patients with chronic mechanical low back pain.

Patients.—Of 28 patients seeking further treatment for chronic mechanical low back pain, 14 were randomly assigned to epidural injection of 80 mg of methylprednisolone plus intrathecal injection of 5% dextrose, and 14 received epidural injection of normal saline plus intrathecal injection of 2 mg of midazolam. All patients had previously undergone treatments that failed. Pain was assessed before treatment and for 2 months after treatment, using a pain questionnaire, patient pain diaries, visual analogue scores (VAS), and verbal rating scales (VRS) to rate the intensity and unpleasantness of the pain.

Results.—Both midazolam and methylprednisolone injections significantly improved pain intensity up to 2 weeks, but only steroid treatment improved pain unpleasantness up to 2 weeks. At 2 weeks, 9 steroid-treated patients were taking more self-administered analgesic medication, and 5 were taking the same amount, whereas 7 midazolam-treated patients were taking less analgesic medication, 6 were taking the same amount, and only 1 was taking more. At the end of the 2-month study, steroid-treated patients were still taking more or the same amount of self-administered analgesic medication, whereas midazolam-treated patients were still taking less. Seven midazolam-treated patients were still improved, and only 1 was worse, whereas 5 steroid-treated patients were still improved and 3 were worse.

Conclusion.—Intrathecal midazolam is as effective as epidural steroid in the treatment of chronic mechanical low back pain.

▶ The inclusion criteria regarding patient selection for this study are not clear. Patients with disk lesions were excluded, but the parameters for the diagnosis of mechanical low back pain are not fully described. This study is particularly interesting because pain relief exceeds the period of analgesia in the group injected with midazolam. Initial dermatomal changes imply a change in the processing of nociceptive information in the spinal cord. The authors state the possibility of a reversal in neuronal responsiveness, the "so-called neuronal plasticity" associated with chronic pain. Further research on this hypothesis may be enlightening.—J. Ameen, D.C.

Facet Joint Injection and Facet Nerve Block: A Randomised Comparison in 86 Patients With Chronic Low Back Pain

Marks RC, Houston T, Thulbourne T (Dundee Royal Infirmary, Scotland; Ninewells Hosp, Dundee, Scotland)

Pain 49:325–328, 1992 4–23

Objective.—The efficacy of facet joint injection and that of facet nerve block for the management of chronic low back pain were compared in a prospective, randomized study.

Setting.—Eighty-six patients with refractory chronic low back pain received either facet joint injection or facet nerve block using local anesthetic and steroid. The patients in the 2 groups were comparable in terms of demography and clinical data (Table 1). Pain relief was assessed immediately after infiltration and at 1 and 3 months, thereafter.

Outcome.—Overall, the response to facet joint injections was slightly better at every follow-up than was the response to facet nerve block, reaching a weak statistical significance only at 1 month when comparing any positive response with no response at all (Table 2). For both groups, the response was short-lived; at 3 months, only 2 patients treated with facet joint injection and none of the patients treated with facet nerve block had complete pain relief. A history of pain longer than 7 years was the only factor predictive of a positive response to either treatment.

Conclusion.—Facet joint injection and facet nerve block remain equally valuable for the selection of patients for definitive facet treatment, but neither is satisfactory for the treatment of chronic low back pain.

TABLE 1.—Comparability of Study Groups

	Facet joint injection	Facet nerve block
No. of patients	42	44
Age		
Median (years)	44	42
Range	24–58	27–57
Sex		
Male	20	26
Female	22	18
GP referral	12	6
Consultant referral	30	38
Previous spinal surgery	5 (11.9%)	5 (11.3%)
Length of history (years)		
Median	10	7
Range	1.6–35	0.7–25
Dominant pain component		
Spinal	18 (42.8%)	17 (38.6%)
Referred	12 (28.6%)	15 (34.1%)
Equal	12 (28.6%)	12 (27.3%)
Paraspinal tenderness		
None	11 (26.2%)	12 (27.3%)
Lumbosacral only	26 (61.9%)	28 (63.6%)
More extensive/other	5 (11.9%)	4 (9.1%)
Midline tenderness		
None	22 (52.4%)	14 (31.8%)
Lumbosacral only	14 (33.3%)	18 (40.9%)
More extensive	6 (14.3%)	12 (27.3%)
Referred pain below knee	14 (33.3%)	21 (47.7%)

(Courtesy of Marks RC, Houston T, Thulbourne T: *Pain* 49:325-328, 1992.)

▶ The authors are concerned with the relative merit of facet joint injection compared with facet nerve block in the diagnosis or selection of patients with chronic low back pain for definitive facet treatments, such as denervation, surgery, or a "rehabilitation programme." They conclude that neither test is superior. The injections are neither tested nor demonstrated as treatment. The study does not confirm the diagnostic validity of the injections. Table 2 shows higher percentages of patients ($n = 86$) with either no or slight changes in pain severity. There were 22 patients (25.6%) who worsened immediately, with 15 patients (17.4%) remaining unchanged or worsened after 1 month. Would the definitive facet treatments similarly benefit those patients who do not report changes in pain severity after injection? The study by Jackson (1) concludes that injection of intra-articular saline into the facets is as effective as the use of anesthetics and steroids.—J. Ameen, D.C.

TABLE 2.—Reported Changes in Pain Severity After Injection

	Facet joint injection ($n = 42$)	Facet nerve block ($n = 44$)
Immediately after infiltration		
None	15 (35.7%)	20 (45.5%)
Slight	11 (26.2%)	13 (29.5%)
Good	5 (11.9%)	3 (6.8%)
Excellent	11 (26.2%)	8 (18.2%)
Best response in first 2 weeks		
None	14 (33.3%)	17 (38.6%)
Slight	10 (23.8%)	7 (15.9%)
Good	14 (33.3%)	17 (38.6%)
Excellent	4 (9.6%)	3 (6.9%)
Response at 1 month *		
None	18 (42.9%)	29 (65.9%)
Slight	9 (21.4%)	6 (13.6%)
Good	12 (28.6%)	9 (20.5%)
Excellent	3 (7.1%)	0 (–)
Response at 3 months	($n = 41$)	($n = 42$)
None	25 (61.0%)	30 (71.4%)
Slight	7 (17.1%)	6 (14.3%)
Good	7 (17.1%)	6 (14.3%)
Excellent	2 (4.8%)	0 (–)

* $P < .05$.
(Courtesy of Marks RC, Houston T, Thulbourne T: *Pain* 49:325–328, 1992.)

Reference

1. Jackson RP: *Clin Orthop* 279:110, 1992.

The Facet Syndrome: Myth or Reality?

Jackson RP (North Kansas City Hosp, Mo)
Clin Orthop 279:110–121, 1992 4–24

Background.—The lumbar facet joint has traditionally been believed to be an important source of low back pain (LBP). Therefore, a variety of treatments have been directed toward this joint, including anesthetic and cortisone blocks and even denervation procedures. However, there is no conclusive evidence that the facet joint plays any role in the production of LBP.

Discussion.—Patients are generally selected for desensitization or denervation of the facet joint on the basis of clinical findings and facet joint blocks. However, a review of the literature suggests that denervation procedures give generally inconsistent and often poor results, especially over time. The facet syndrome is not well described from a clinical viewpoint, and it may not represent a true disease entity. Even if arthritic, the facet joint appears to make little contribution to persisting LBP.

The facet joint does play an important biomechanical role, and it should, if possible, be used to protect and unload the disk. The facets can slide only so far in extension; at this point, they essentially become fixed in position. In management and rehabilitation, the principle of loading the facet and sparing the disk is currently favored.

Conclusion.—The lumbar facet joints are biomechanically important in that they protect the disk from torsional forces in rotation. However, it does not appear to be a common or apparent source of LBP, and the facet syndrome does not appear to be a reliable clinical diagnosis. Saline injection into the facet is as effective as local anesthetic and steroids in providing temporary pain relief, and a response to facet joint injection does not correlate with or predict clinical results after solid posterior lumbar fusion. More prospective, controlled, and randomized clinical studies of the facet syndrome are needed.

▶ The refutability of the diagnosis of facet syndrome discussed in the introductory and final sections of this article, based on the literature reviewed by the author, is not extensively presented. The biomechanical importance of the facet joints is briefly described. The article elaborates 3 prospective research trials and their outcomes, examining the effect of intra-articular facet injection and using lumbar motion pain assessment (MPA), including analogue pain scales, low back pain questionnaires, pain drawings, and pain and functional assessment (PFA) scales. The reliability and sources of the various assessment scales and instruments were not referenced. The injections of analgesics and steroids did not perform effectively as treatment, were not more effective than saline injections, and did not reliably predict the benefits of facet fusion. The premise for the role of facet joints remains, perhaps, naive. Low back pain may be conferred by heterogeneous biomechanical and proprioceptive functions, rather than by discrete nociceptive loci or synovial innervations.—J. Ameen, D.C.

A Ganglion Cyst in the Lumbar Spinal Canal: A Case Report

Ogawa Y, Kumano K, Hirabayashi S, Aota Y (Kantoh Rosai Hosp, Kawasaki, Japan)

Spine 17:1429–1431, 1992 4–25

Background.—Some reports of ganglion cysts in the spinal canal have appeared in the English language literature. However, there have been no reports of an intraspinal extradural ganglion cyst being demonstrated on MRI.

Case Report.—Man, 23, was seen with low back pain and left buttock pain that had no apparent cause. Routine lumbar spine radiographs were interpreted as normal. Computed tomography revealed a lesion at the left side of the cranial end of the L5 vertebral body in the extradural space. On MRI, the T1-weighted images showed a bulging intervertebral disk at L4–L5. The T2-weighted images showed a smooth oval mass lesion with uniform high-signal intensity at the posterior surface of the L5 vertebral body. Protruding intervertebral disk herniation at L4–L5 was the preoperative diagnosis. Microscopic surgery was performed by using the interlaminar approach at the L4–L5 interspace. The L5 nerve appeared slightly inflamed and was pushed upward by a dark red cystic mass approximately 8 mm in diameter. Needle puncture of the mass produced serous fluid. The cyst was dissected easily from the surrounding tissue and was completely removed by excising its stalk. The fifth lumbar nerve root was decompressed. The intervertrebal disk was almost normal in shape and color.

Conclusion.—This is the first report of MRI of an intraspinal extradural ganglion cyst. In previous reports, myelography or CT after myelography demonstrated an extradural defect but did not show the ganglion cyst itself.

▶ This is the first case ever to demonstrate the presence of an intraspinal extradural ganglion cyst on MRI. The condition itself created low back and buttock pain, some numbness, and a limited straight leg raise. Plain films were normal, but MRI demonstrated the mass. The lesion was best seen on T2-weighted images as an oval mass of uniform signal density. This lesion arose from the posterior longitudinal ligament and was filled with serous fluid.—D.J. Lawrence, D.C.

Rapid Development of a Spinal Synovial Cyst: A Case Report

Cameron SE, Hanscom DA (Madigan Army Med Ctr, Tacoma, Wash)

Spine 17:1528–1530, 1992 4–26

Background.—The development of a synovial cyst appears to be slow and gradual. However, in 1 case, a synovial cyst developed in less than 1 year.

Case Report.—Man, 63, underwent and L5–S1 posterior fusion using facet screws during disk excision surgery 20 years earlier. Nineteen years after this procedure he had pain in both lower extremities. Epidural injections of corticosteroids and nerve root blocks temporarily relieved his symptoms, but they recurred after a few months and became fairly constant. Myelography and CT after myelography showed a synovial cyst from the left L4–L5 facet joint that occupied a large part of the left side of the canal (Fig 4–2). Because the patient's symptoms were incapacitating, surgery was done. The fusion mass at the L5–S1 level was solid. A generous laminotomy at the left L4–L5 was done, and a gray cystic mass was found deep to the ligamentum flavum. After surgery the patient was symptom free.

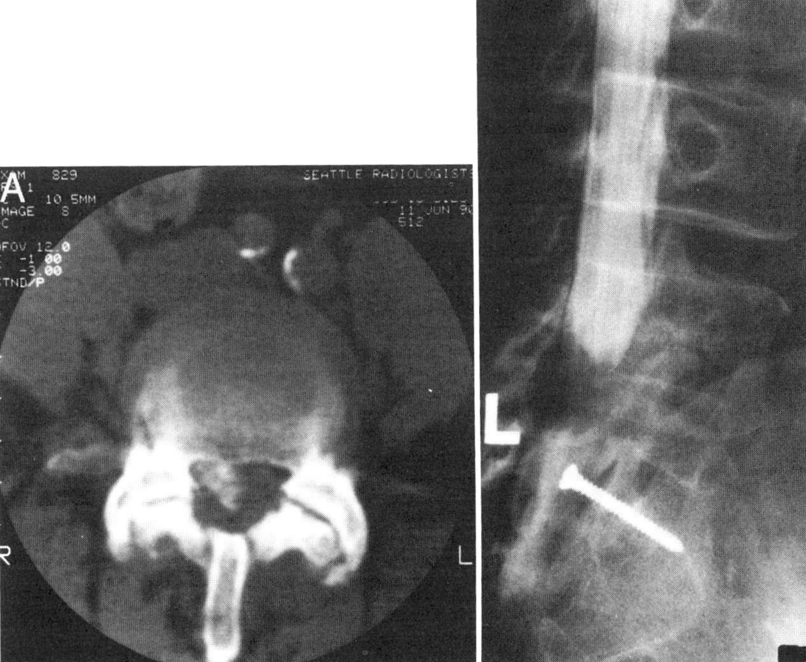

Fig 4–2.—Computed tomogram and myelogram showing a space-occupying mass adjacent to left L4–L5 facet. (Courtesy of Cameron SE, Hanscom DA: *Spine* 17:1528–1530, 1992.)

Conclusion.—In this case, the rapid development of a spinal synovial cyst was captured through imaging techniques. The rate of development of the cyst in this patient was believed to be unusually rapid.

► Spinal synovial cysts occur in conjunction with osteoarthritis; they may be an uncommon cause of nerve root compression. They are usually slow-growing as a result; in this case, the growth was quite rapid. One should suspect cysts when symptoms develop years after fusion, with no known event preceding the onset of the back pain and neurologic sequelae.—D.J. Lawrence, D.C.

The Treatment of the Sacroiliac Joint Component to Low Back Pain: A Case Report

Cibulka MT (Jefferson County Rehabilitation and Sports Clinic, Crystal City, Mo)

Phys Ther 72:917–922, 1992 4–27

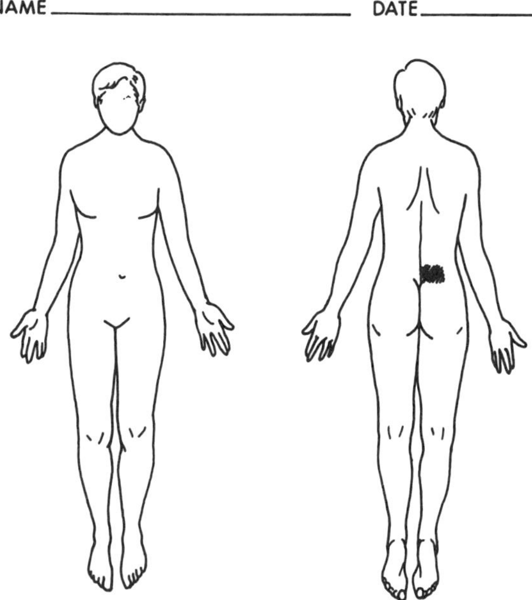

Fig 4–3.—Location of patient's low back pain. (Courtesy of Cibulka MT: *Phys Ther* 72:917–922, 1992.)

Background.—Studies have shown that the sacroiliac joint and limited hip mobility are related. One patient with symptoms and signs of a sacroiliac joint component to low back pain also had asymmetric hip rotation.

Case Report.—Man, 32, had right-sided low back pain without apparent cause. On his initial visit, the patient completed a drawing of his perceived pain (Fig 4–3). He seemed to have sacroiliac joint dysfunction, excessive right hip lateral rotation, and limited right hip medial rotation. The excessive lateral hip rotation was partly attributed to the patient's habit of crossing his right leg over his left while sitting (Fig 4–4). Treatment consisted of a manipulative technique in which the patient was placed supine with the spine laterally flexed to the left. The clinician stood at the patient's right side and threaded 1 arm through the patient's hands, which were clasped behind his neck. The clinician then placed his free hand on the part of the patient's anterior superior iliac spine (AS1S) that was furthest away. A posterior force was then applied to the ASIS while the patient maintained full upper trunk rotation. After treatment, the patient no longer complained of low back pain.

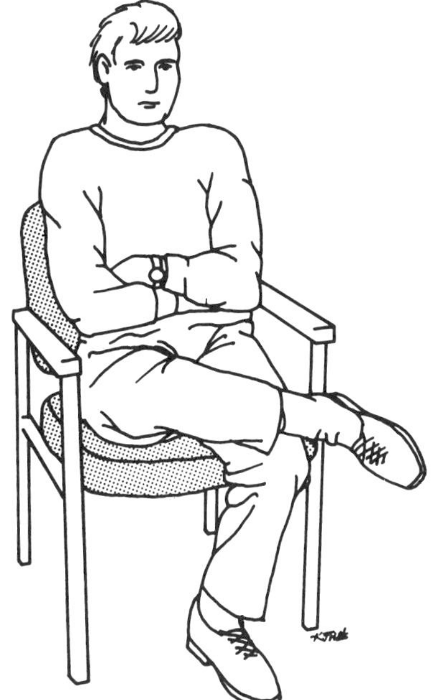

Fig 4–4.—Laterally rotated sitting posture of right hip. (Courtesy of Cibulka MT: *Phys Ther* 72:917-922, 1992.)

Conclusion.—Asymmetric hip rotation may contribute to what is thought to be a sacroiliac joint component to low back pain. Preventing chronic extreme lateral hip rotation during sitting and sleeping and restoring hip rotation in an active and passive range of motion seemed to eliminate the low back pain in this patient.

▶ The author describes a case of sacroiliac syndrome that he believes was caused by excessive right hip rotation. To my knowledge, there are no clinical trials to show that this is a possible cause of the condition; indeed, the debate continues as to whether the SI joints can be a significant source of low back pain. I certainly believe that they can, but the mechanisms remain to be determined. This patient responded nicely to the manipulative therapy, although I wonder how much of a difference the therapy made, considering there are not trials or controls against which to compare it. However, I must acknowledge the author for denoting this point.—D.J. Lawrence, D.C.

Osteochondroma of the Lumbar Spine: An Unusual Cause of Sciatica

van der Sluis R, Gurr K, Joseph MG (St Joseph's Hosp, London, Ont, Canada)

Spine 17:1519–1521, 1992 4–28

Background.—Osteochondroma, a common benign tumor, usually occurs at the end of a long bone. The vertebral column is involved in less than 5% of cases. One patient with right-sided sciatica over the L5 and S1 nerve root distribution was seen with a lumbar osteochondroma.

Case Report.—Woman, 26, had an acute exacerbation of chronic low back and leg pain. She had had aching right-sided lumbar low back pain and intermittent right-sided sciatica for 2 years. Plain radiography revealed a bony mass at the level of the fourth lumbar vertebra on the right side. Computed tomography and MRI demonstrated a mass approximately 2 cm in diameter that was associated with the L4 posterior elements at the level of the L4-5 disk space. An L4–L5 disk herniation was also visualized. At surgery, a large amount of abnormal appearing cartilaginous tissue was found arising from the periphery of the articular surface of the inferior L4 process. The whole section was removed. The extension of the mass appeared to entrap the L5 nerve root. An indentation of the L5 nerve root was relieved when the mass was lifted posteriorly. Additional exploration of the nerve root and L5 disk space revealed disk herniation just medial to the posterior longitudinal ligament. The cartilaginous mass was thought to be responsible for the L5 nerve root compression and S1 symptoms. The L5 nerve root compression may have been partly worsened by the extruded L4-5 disk.

Conclusion.—Osteochondromas do not commonly occur in the vertebral column. In this patient, an osteochondroma and an extruded fragment of the L4–L5 disk resulted in an unusual presentation of right-sided sciatica and low back pain.

▶ This study provides a reminder that not all causes of sciatica and low back pain are the result of disk lesions or muscular causes. In this case, the patient had what appeared to be a rather typical case of sciatica (probably as a result of disk involvement) and had sought care from a chiropractor with little relief. Only after undergoing CT scanning was the tumor identified. Nonresponsive sciatica should be assessed in greater detail if the patient does not respond to standard chiropractic care.—D.J. Lawrence, D.C.

A Clinical Study of Degenerative Spondylolisthesis: Radiographic Analysis and Choice of Treatment

Satomi K, Hirabayashi K, Toyama Y, Fujimura Y (Keio Univ, Tokyo)

Spine 17:1329–1336, 1992 4–29

Background.—There is no consensus on the etiology of degenerative spondylolisthesis (DS). In the belief that DS essentially results from intervertebral disk degeneration, this condition has been treated by using anterior lumbar interbody fusion (ALIF), which decreases the slipping. In elderly patients, who have a high incidence of lateral stenosis and multisegmental spinal instability, posterior decompression is performed, with or without fusion. Diagnostic critieria for selecting the best surgical treatment for DS were investigated by comparing preoperative and post-

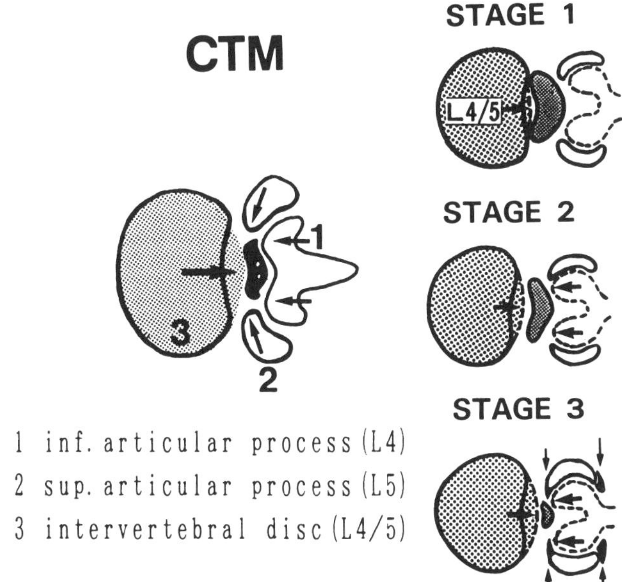

Fig 4–5.—Computed tomography image staging in degenerative spondylolisthesis. Vertical inclination of the articular facets joints is observed in all stages. *Large arrows* point to tissues of compressing dural sac. *Small arrows* indicate osteophytes of superior articular processes of L5. (Courtesy of Satomi K, Hirabayashi K, Toyama Y, et al: *Spine* 17:1329–1336, 1992.)

operative radiographic findings and surgical outcomes in 2 treatment groups.

Methods and Findings.—Surgery was performed in 27 patients by using ALIF and in 14 patients by using posterior decompression. The average degree of recovery was 77% and 56%, respectively. Myelography and CT after myelography demonstrated that anterior shifting of the inferior articular process of the slipping vertebra was the main reason for compression of nervous tissue in the early stages of DS. In the later stages of disease, osteophytes on the superior articular processes of the lower vertebra also contributed to compression. Computed tomography image staging is shown in Figure 4–5.

Conclusion.—Patients in the early stages of DS should be treated by ALIF. In the later stages, patients should be treated with posterior decompression. Computed tomography after myelography can provide the key images used in identifying pathologic processes in DS and in selecting appropriate surgical procedures.

▶ The authors posit that degenerative spondylolisthesis is the result of intervertebral disk degeneration. This is in opposition to the ideas of Finnison (1), who describes a process of lumbar intersegmental instability leading to facet remodeling and possible microfracture at the inferior articular process of the vertebra that ultimately slips anterior. The difference here may be important, because the authors treat spondylolisthesis with anterior lumbar interbody fusion (although they admit to using posterior decompression in elderly patients who also have stenosis and instability). Using CT and myelography, they were able to categorize patients with spondylolisthesis into 3 groups. Earlier stages were best treated by the anterior procedure, although the average degree of recovery was only 77%; the latter stages were best treated with the posterior approach, which had an average degree of recovery of 56%. One has to ask whether the surgical approach is best, given the confusion surrounding the etiology of the condition and the average degree of recovery seen in this study. Nevertheless, the assessment procedure shows great promise as a screening tool for possible conservative care.—D.J. Lawrence, D.C.

Reference

1. Finnison B: *Low Back Pain*, ed 2. Philadelphia, JB Lippincott Co, 1980.

Clinical Efficacy of Spinal Instrumentation in Lumbar Degenerative Disc Disease

Zucherman J, Hsu K, Picetti G III, White A, Wynne G, Taylor L (St Mary's Spine Ctr, San Francisco; SpineCare Med Group, Daly City, Calif)
Spine 17:834–837, 1992 4–30

Introduction.—The inability to run control groups has made it difficult to determine objectively which methods of spinal fusion are most effective in particular clinical situations. There are many theoretical advantages to using lumbar spine instrumentation, but the specific settings where favorable results may be expected are unknown.

Patients.—The results of lumbar fusion were reviewed in 30 patients having posterior lateral fusion and diskectomies without internal fixation; 36 operated on with Knodt rods; 30 receiving Harrington rods; and 30 undergoing variable spine plating. None of the patients had undergone previous surgery, and all had fusions at L3 or L4–S1, using autologous iliac crest bone. Diskectomies were done at 2 or more levels. In all cases the indication was disk herniation, with central back pain exceeding leg pain and a worsening of symptoms occurring with increasing activity.

Results.—There was no apparent advantage to adding internal fixation to posterior latral fusions in these cases. Patients given Harrington rods did worse than when other internal fixation techniques were used or when there was no internal fixation. A significant number of patients who received Harrington rods, Knodt rods, or variable spine plates required reoperation for implant removal.

Conclusion.—It appears advisable to limit the use of lumbar spinal instrumentation to (1) patients with unstable fractures; (2) those with failed fusions and frank instability; (3) situations where immediate stabilization is necessary; and (4) cases where fusion is expected to fail.

▶ There are surprisingly few studies examining the success rates for the use of various lumbar surgical procedures, and in point of fact, there are far more studies showing the benefits of manipulative care. Surgical techniques may involve fusion and diskectomies as noninternal procedures, and Harrington, Luque, or Knodt rods as internal procedures (where a device is implanted). This particular study shows that the procedures that do not involve implantation have superior results. I question whether these procedures were necessary at all; there is so much more evidence for the use of manipulation in patients such as those seen in this study. The patients in this study had disk herniation involving severe back pain with less leg pain, and they also had increased pain on activity. These are prime chiropractic patients, and it is time that the results of chiropractic care are studied against the more invasive surgical techniques, whether they use internal fixation or not.—D.J. Lawrence, D.C.

Microdiscectomy in Treatment of Herniated Lumbar Disc

Postacchini F, Cinotti G, Perugia D (CaHedra di Chiruregia della Mano, Modena; Italy; I Clinica Ortopedica dell ' Universita "La Sapienza," Rome)

Ital J Orthop Traumatol 18:5–16, 1992 4–31

Introduction.—Limited diskectomy involves removal of the ligamentum flavum and, if necessary, a small part of the adjacent laminae, followed by excision of the herniated part of the disk with a limited amount of disk tissue.

Patients.—Lumbar microdiskectomy was performed in 122 patients between 1986 and 1989. Ninety-seven patients had a herniated disk at a single lumbar level, and 4 had herniations at 2 levels of a normal spinal canal. Sixteen patients had root canal stenosis in association with a herniated disk; 5 had isolated nerve root canal stenosis. Limited diskectomy was done in 16 patients with single-level disk herniations in a normal spinal canal. All other patients had complete diskectomy. Sequestered disk fragments were removed in 36 cases.

Results.—More than 90% of patients with a single-level herniation in a normal spinal canal had excellent or good results at final review (table). Only 1 of the 16 patients having limited diskectomy continued to have significant symptoms. Patients with double-level herniations had results only slightly inferior to those achieved by patients with single-level herniations in a normal spinal canal. Almost 90% of the patients with nerve root canal stenosis, either alone or in conjunction with disk herniation, had satisfactory results at final review. Two of 3 patients with diskitis had a satisfactory final outcome.

Results of Surgery

	Patients without complications No. of patients												**Patients with complications No. of patients**											
	Simple herniated disc *				**Double-level herniated disc**				**Nerve root canal stenosis †**				**Missed disc**				**Dural laceration**				**Discitis**			
	E	G	F	P	E	G	F	P	E	G	F	P	E	G	F	P	E	G	F	P	E	G	F	P
At 1 month	28	46	12	1		3	1		4	9	4	1	2	4	1		1	1	1					3
At 3 months	55	22	8	2‡	2	2			9	7	1	1	4	3			2	1				1		2
At final review	56	23	6	2‡	2	2			10	6	2		4	2	1		3				1	1	1	

* Single-level herniated disk in normal spinal canal.
† With or without herniated disk.
‡ At 3 months, 1 underwent reoperation; at final review, both underwent reoperation because of recurrence.
Abbreviations: E, excellent; *G,* good; *F,* fair; *P,* poor.
(Courtesy of Postacchini F, Cinotti G, Perugia D: *Ital J Orthop Traumatol* 18:5–16, 1992.)

Conclusion.—Microdiskectomy is very suitable for patients having single-level unilateral disk herniations, even if sequestered. Patients having this procedure are able to stand sooner and return to work after a shorter period because of less postoperative pain. In the long term, the results are comparable to those of conventional surgery, unless this includes extensive facetectomy.

► The development of microdiskectomy indicates the increasingly "conservative" nature of lumbar disk surgery. The procedure remains fairly controversial, however. Although patients seem to respond well to the procedure over the short term, it fairs no better than other surgical procedures over a longer term. Because it involves less hospitalization than other procedures and allows for return to activity faster than other forms of surgery, it may represent a best option for those who absolutely require surgical intervention. The problem is that there are no real indications for who that individual is, and a course of conservative care certainly seems a more viable first option than surgery.—D.J. Lawrence, D.C.

What Can the History and Physical Examination Tell Us About Low Back Pain?

Deyo RA, Rainville J, Kent DL (Seattle Veterans Affairs Med Ctr; Univ of Washington, Seattle; Tufts Univ, Boston)

JAMA 268:760–765, 1992 4–32

Introduction.—Approximately 70% of adults have back pain at some time. Careful diagnostic evaluation can determine whether therapeutic intervention should be symptomatic, physical measures, or surgery or whether the pain is symptomatic of an underlying disease. The clinical history and physical examination can also influence decisions about diagnostic imaging, laboratory testing, or referral to a specialist. However, in as many as 85% of patients, a definitive diagnosis cannot be made because symptoms, pathologic changes, and imaging results are only weakly associated.

Diagnostic Keys.—Answering 3 basic questions may be useful in evaluation of back pain: (1) Is there a serious systemic disease causing the pain? (2) Is there neurologic compromise that might require surgical intervention? and (3) Is there social or psychological distress that may amplify or prolong pain?

Discussion.—Cancer, spinal infections, compression fractures, and ankylosing spondylitis are among the underlying systemic diseases that may involve back pain. Useful items in the patient history are age, history of cancer, unexplained weight loss, duration of pain, and responsiveness to previous therapy (Table 1). Neurologic compromise most commonly involves herniated intervertebral disk but other causes include nerve root entrapment, spinal stenosis, spinal or paraspinal infections, and neoplasms. Symptoms of sciatica or pseudoclaudication or a history of

TABLE 1.—Estimated Accuracy of the Medical History in the Diagnosis of Spinal Diseases Causing Low Back Pain

Disease to Be Detected	Source, y	Medical History	Sensitivity	Specificity*
Cancer	Deyo and Diehl, 1988	Age ≥ 50 y	0.77	0.71
		Previous history of cancer	0.31	0.98
		Unexplained weight loss	0.15	0.94
		Failure to improve with a month of therapy	0.31	0.90
		No relief with bed rest	>0.90	0.46
		Duration of pain >1 mo	0.50	0.81
		Age ≥50 y *or* history of cancer *or* unexplained weight loss *or* failure of conservative therapy	1.00	0.60
Spinal osteomyelitis	Waldvogel and Vasey, 1980	Intravenous drug abuse, urinary tract infection, or skin infection	0.40	NA
Compression fracture	Unpublished data†	Age ≥50 y	0.84	0.61
		Age ≥70 y	0.22	0.96
		Trauma	0.30	0.85
		Corticosteroid use	0.06	0.995
Herniated disk	Deyo and Tsui-Wu, 1987; Spangfort, 1972	Sciatica	0.95	0.88
Spinal stenosis	Turner et al, 1992	Pseudoclaudication	0.60	NA
		Age ≥50 y	0.90‡	0.70
Ankylosing spondylitis	Gran, 1985	4 out of 5 positive responses§	0.23	0.82
		Age at onset ≤40 y	1.00	0.07
		Pain not relieved supine	0.80	0.49
		Morning back stiffness	0.64	0.59
		Pain duration ≥3 mo	0.71	0.54

* NA indicates not available.
† From 833 patients with back pain at a walk-in clinic, all of whom received plain lumbar roentgenograms.
‡ Authors' estimate.
§ There were 5 screening questions: Was the onset of back discomfort before age 40 years? Did the problem begin slowly? Did the problem persist for at least 3 months? Did you have morning stiffness? Was pain improved by exercise?
(Courtesy of Deyo RA, Rainville J, Kent DL: *JAMA* 268:760–765, 1992.)

numbness or weakness suggest neurologic involvement. A psychosocial history should consider failed previous treatment, substance abuse, depression, or disability compensation. Physical examination findings of fever, tenderness, limited spinal motion and assessment of straight leg raising, dorsiflexion of ankle and great toe, ankle reflexes, and results of sensory examination can aid diagnosis. The reproducibility of such findings can be seen in Table 2. Signs of superficial tenderness, distracted leg raising, or patient overreaction during the examination may suggest back pain as a result of or amplified by psychological distress. Only severe impairments can be detected clinically, and sensitivity is low for disk herniation (Table 3).

TABLE 2.—Reproducibility of Physical Examination Findings

Category	Test	Unit of Measurement	Interobserver Agreement (Statistic)	Source, y
Tenderness	Bone tenderness	Yes/no	0.40 (κ)	McCombe et al, 1989
	Soft-tissue tenderness	Yes/no	0.24 (κ)	McCombe et al, 1989
	Muscle spasm	Yes/no	"Discarded—too unreliable"	Waddell et al, 1982
SLR*	Ipsilateral SLR, inclinometer	Degrees	0.78 to 0.97 (*r*)	Hoehler and Tobis, 1982; Hsieh et al, 1983
	Ipsilateral SLR, goniometer	Degrees	0.69 (*r*)	McCombe et al, 1989
	SLR causes leg pain	Yes/no	0.66 (κ)	McCombe et al, 1989
	Ipsilateral SLR <75° by visual estimation	Yes/no	0.56 (κ)	Waddell et ai, 1982
	Crossed SLR, causes pain	Yes/no	0.74 (κ)	McCombe et al, 1989
Neurologic examination	Ankle dorsiflexion weak	Yes/no	1.00 (κ)	McCombe et al, 1989
	Great toe extensors weak	Yes/no	0.65 (κ)	McCombe et al, 1989
	Ankle reflexes normal	Yes/no	0.39-0.50 (κ)	McCombe et al, 1989; Schwartz et al, 1990
	Any sensory deficit	Yes/no	0.68 (κ)	McCombe et al, 1989
	Calf wasting	Yes/no	0.80 (κ)	McCombe et al, 1989
Inappropriate signs	Superficial tenderness	Yes/no	0.29 (κ)	McCombe et al, 1989
	Simulated rotation or axial loading causes pain	Yes/no	0.25 (κ)	McCombe et al, 1989
	SLR with distraction causes pain	Yes/no	0.40 (κ)	McCombe et al, 1989
	Inexplicable pattern, neurologic examination	Yes/no	0.03 (κ)	McCombe et al, 1989
	Overreaction	Yes/no	0.29 (κ)	McCombe et al, 1989

* *SLR* indicates straight leg raising.
(Courtesy of Deyo RA, Rainville J, Kent DL: *JAMA* 268:760-765, 1992.)

Conclusion.—The 3 questions mentioned in this report and used as the basis for patient history and physical examination may be useful in diagnosing back pain.

▶ The authors provide a lengthy review of the information concerning a wide range of diseases and conditions that may cause low back pain. They look at studies that examine the sensitivity and specificity of the physical examination in diagnosing systemic illness, and they also examine the reproducibility of various parts of the examination (including presence of tender-

TABLE 3.—Estimated Accuracy of Physical Examination for Lumbar Disk Herniation Among Patients With Sciatica

Text	Source, y	Sensitivity*	Specificity*	Comments
Ipsilateral straight leg raising	Kosteljanetz et al, 1984; Hakelius and Hindmarsh, 1972	0.80	0.40	Positive test result: leg pain at <60°
Crossed straight leg raising	Spangfort, 1972; Hakelius and Hindmarsh, 1972	0.25	0.90	Positive test result: reproduction of contralateral pain
Ankle dorsiflexion weakness	Spangfort, 1972; Hakelius and Hindmarsh, 1972	0.35	0.70	HNP† usually at L4-5 (80%)
Great toe extensor weakness	Hakelius and Hindmarsh, 1972; Kortelainen et al, 1985	0.50	0.70	HNP usually at L5-S1(60%) or L4-5 (30%)
Impaired ankle reflex	Spangfort, 1972; Hakelius and Hindmarsh, 1972	0.50	0.60	HNP usually at L5-S1; absent reflex increases specificity
Sensory loss	Kosteljanetz et al, 1984; Kortelainen et al, 1985	0.50	0.50	Area of loss poor predictor of HNP level
Patella reflex	Aronson and Dunsmore, 1963	0.50	. . .	For upper lumbar HNP only
Ankle plantar flexion weakness	Hakelius and Hindmarsh, 1972	0.06	0.95	
Quadriceps weakness	Hakelius and Hindmarsh, 1972	<0.01	0.99	

* Sensitivity and specificity were calculated by reviewers. The values represent rounded averages where multiple references were available. All results are from surgical case series.

† *HNP* indicates herniated nucleus pulposus.

(Courtesy of Deyo RA, Rainville J, Kent DL: *JAMA* 268:760-765, 1992.)

ness, straight leg raise, neurologic examination, and inappropriate signs). Points to ponder: (1) ask key questions; (2) pay attention to the failure of bed rest to relieve pain; and (3) drug use or urinary infection may suggest infection, etc. These recommendations are thorough and should be kept in mind by all physicians treating back pain; the ultimate effect is to help identify nonorthopedic, systemic illness that causes low back pain. Because approximately 20% of back pain arises from a nonspinal structure, this takes on greater importance.—D.J. Lawrence, D.C.

Spinal Mobility and Trunk Muscle Strength in 15-Year-Old Schoolchildren With and Without Low-Back Pain

Salminen JJ, Maki P, Oksanen A, Pentti J (Univ Central Hosp of Turku, Finland; Univ of Jyväskylä, Finland; Turku Regional Inst of Occupational Health, Finland)

Spine 17:405–411, 1992 4–33

Background.—Although some descriptive data on the prevalence of low back pain (LBP) and related factors in young individuals exist, comparisons of studies are difficult because of methodologic differences and, often, poor definitions of LBP. Low back pain was defined exactly in relation to time and localization. Spinal mobility, trunk muscle strength, and early disk degeneration were compared in schoolchildren with recurrent or continuous LBP and in those without LBP.

Methods.—Of 1,503 schoolchildren, 38 (age, 15 years) with LBP and 38 asymptomatic control subjects were selected for spinal mobility and trunk muscle strength testing. The 2 groups were matched for age, sex, and school class.

Observations.—The group with recurrent or continual LBP included 17 boys and 21 girls. The boys in the LBP group were more than 4 cm taller than the boys in the control group. In both girls and boys, sagittal mobility was reduced in lumbar extension and straight leg raising and increased in lumbar flexion. Endurance strength in the abdominal and back muscles was lower than in the control subjects. Seven children had sciatica at some time in addition to recurrent LBP. These subjects had reduced lumbar flexion and side bending compred with those with recurrent LBP without sciatica.

Conclusion.—In this population, there was a subgroup of children with recurrent LBP with a different spinal mobility pattern as well as reduced trunk muscle strength. Without follow-up research, however, it is unknown whether this group is at greater risk of having disabling LBP in adulthood.

▶ Low back pain in the young is relatively uncommon; therefore, large databases of information concerning such pain are lacking. Although certain information was gathered from this study, it cannot as yet be used to predict whether current patients with LBP will continue to have disabling back pain, either now or in the future. Until a longer follow-up can be completed, this information can only be considered demographic in nature.—D.J. Lawrence, D.C.

Do Smokers Get More Back Pain?

Boshuizen HC, Verbeek JHAM, Broersen JPJ, Weel ANH (Univ of Amsterdam)

Spine 18:35–40, 1993 4–34

Background.—Smoking is increasingly implicated as a risk factor for low back pain. This putative association most often is explained by coughing, which increases intradiskal pressures and places added strain on the spine. Other possible mechanisms are a nicotine-induced reduction in vertebral-body blood flow, decreased bone mineral content that lead to microfractures, and a fibrinolytic defect caused by smoking. It also is possible that the apparent association is a result of confounding by other factors.

Methods.—The association between smoking and back pain was examined by reviewing data from an occupational health survey, where it was possible to control for occupation. The study population of 4,054 men aged 25–55 years represented 13 different occupations.

Findings.—The prevalence of back pain differed between smokers and nonsmokers for those working in construction, but not for other occupations. A similar trend was seen for more strenuous occupations requiring regular exertion. In construction workers, back pain increased with the number of cigarettes smoked each day. A more consistent relationship was seen between extremity pain and smoking.

Conclusion.—A relationship between smoking and joint pain in general is more likely than a mechanism involving only the spine.

▶ The 1991 Volvo prize-winning paper, which was written by Michelle Battie and colleagues, demonstrated a direct relationship between smoking and lumbar disk degeneration and low back pain (1). The explanations offered for this finding range from reduced vertebral blood flow to excessive coughing seen in smokers, to decreased mineral content in bone. One other factor not considered in the earlier studies was whether other issues, e.g., economic status or occupation, might confound the findings. With this study's finding that only occupations requiring physical activity have a higher incidence of low back pain, it seems that occupational relationships to smoking do not exist. Although smoking may play a role in the incidence of back pain, it is not as significant a factor as activity, psychological profile, or stress levels; however, any prevention program would do well to include smoking cessation as part of the program for more than the reduction of low back pain.—D.J. Laurence, D.C.

Reference

1. Battie MC, et al: *Spine* 16:1015, 1991.

Initial-Impression Diagnosis Using Low-Back Pain Patient Pain Drawings

Mann NH III, Brown MD, Hertz DB, Enger I, Tompkins J (Vanderbilt Univ, Nashville, Tenn; Univ of Miami, Fla)

Spine 18:41–53, 1993 4–35

Background.—When asked to describe their pain, patients communicate both an understanding of the pain and how they feel about it. Perceptions of pain can be assessed with regard to quality and intensity, whereas reactions to pain are expressed by symptoms such as anxiety, tachycardia, and panic. Past work using pain drawings diagnostically have demonstrated ambiguous patient descriptions of pain.

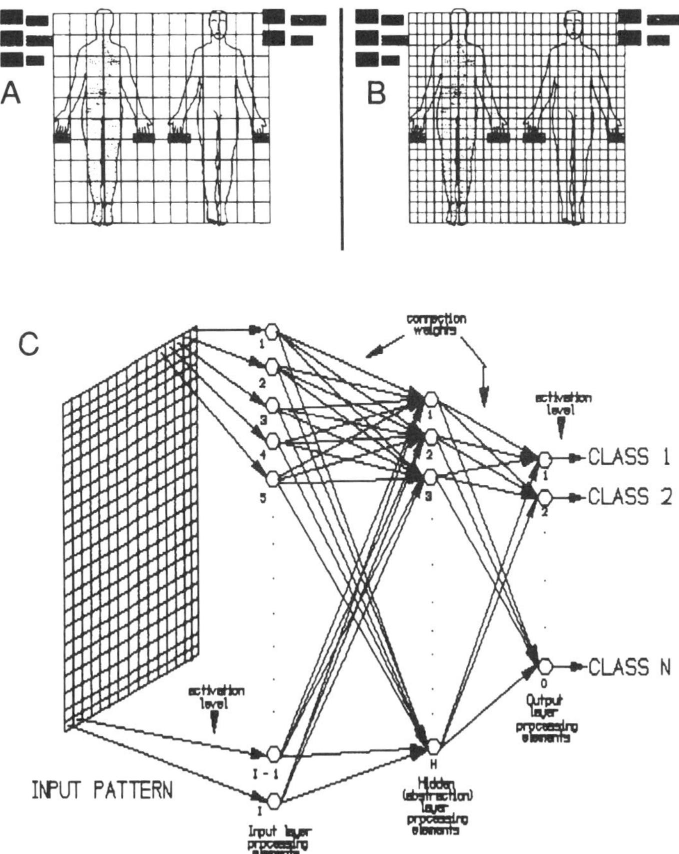

Fig 4–6.—The templates used to create the coarse (**A**) and fine (**B**) granularity ANN input matrixes. **C,** simple figure of the 2-dimensional pattern matrix as applied to an experimental ANN topology. (From Mann NH III, Brown MD, Hertz DB, et al: *Spine* 18:41–53, 1993. Courtesy of Mann NH III, Brown MD: *Orthop Clin North Am* 22:303–317, 1991.)

Patients.—A total of 250 patients were chosen from the files of an orthopedic surgeon specializing in treating low back pain. Fifty patients each had a diagnosis of benign back pain, herniation of the nucleus pulposus, spinal stenosis, serious underlying disease, and psychogenic regional pain disturbance.

Methods.—Patient pain drawings were selected blindly from cases of lumbar spinal disorder and were classified by physicians specializing in low back disorders, discriminant analysis, and computerized artificial neural network (ANN) configurations. Ambiguity was limited by considering only the spatial/anatomic distribution of pain marks. Eight lumbar spine experts experienced in using pain drawings were selected to interpret the drawings. The ANN method began with a set of experimental training patterns derived from empirical patient data and another set based on a general delineation of patient pain marks as reported by an experienced low back pain physician. Trends were sought in these intuitive patterns and were used to construct ANN prototypes designed for data in coarse and fine formats (Fig 4–6).

Findings.—The accuracy of physician ratings averaged 51%. Individual preferences for certain groups of disorders were evident. Computerized methods were 48% accurate, but they classified patients more consistently. The pain patterns predicted by an expert for various diagnostic groups correlated with the patterns generated by the computerized methods. Intraevaluator agreement among both physicians and computers exceeded interevaluator agreement between the physicians and computerized methods. This suggests that the experts relied on some features not used by the computerized methods or not explicitly built into the pain drawings used for computer analysis.

Conclusion.—It appears feasible to establish a computerized system for gaining diagnostic impressions from the pain drawings of patients with low back disorders. The method could aid the triage of patients with low back pain and might enhance the diagnostic competence of physicians.

▶ The use of patient pain drawings is increasing among chiropractic physicians. Because low back pain is such a complex phenomenon, interpretation of the drawings can become cumbersome and difficult. Furthermore, these diagrams often are not able to distinguish between low back pain of musculoskeletal origin or organic origin. In particular, the use of the pain drawing in organic disorders has been ambiguous. The authors of this study attempt to quantify the interpretation of pain drawings by use of computer modeling methods. Four kinds of patients with pain were tested: those with benign back pain; those with herniated nucleus pulposus; those with spinal stenosis; and those with a serious underlying pathology. Spinal experts interpreted the drawings for consistency before modeling procedures. A computerized ANN system was used to study the drawings. The results indicate that it should be possible to develop a system that can make an initial impression of the drawing. The worlds of artifical intelligence systems are providing exciting, but they are not yet at the point where they can replace human intuition—something that may very well be lacking in these diagnostic computer programs.—D.J. Lawrence, D.C.

An 18-Month Follow-Up of a Secondary Prevention Program for Back Pain: Help and Hindrance Factors Related to Outcome Maintenance

Linton SJ, Bradley LA (Örebro Med Ctr, Sweden; Univ of Alabama, Birmingham)

Clin J Pain 8:227–236, 1992 4–36

Background.—Ordinarily, adults spend about one third of their lives at work, making it apparent why work helps shape one's life-style, satis-

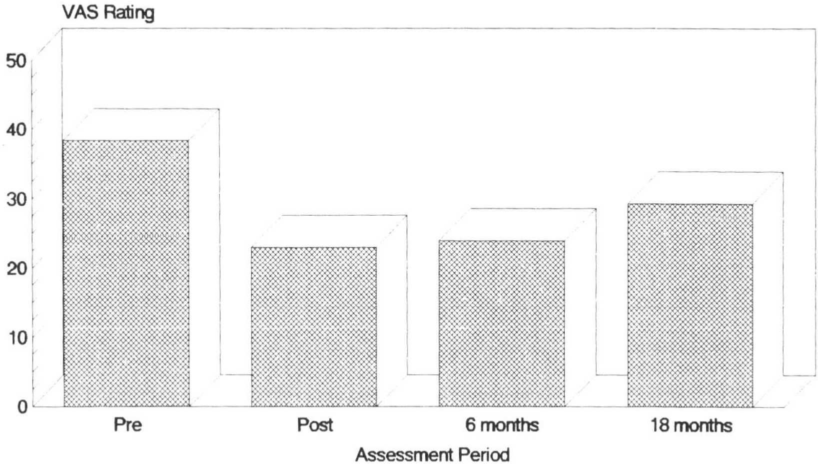

Fig 4–7.—The mean pain intensity ratings for the treatment group over the entire course of the study. *Abbreviation:* VAS, visual analogue scales. (Courtesy of Linton SJ, Bradley LA: *Clin J Pain* 8:227-236, 1992.)

faction, and self-esteem. It also is clear why rehabilitation programs stress return to work as a major goal. Absenteeism is influenced by many factors other than pain that are not addressed by preventive or interventional programs. Secondary preventive efforts seem able to promote improvement at a variety of levels, including pain, mood, sleep, and activity level.

Objective.—Thirty-six subjects participated in an 18-month follow-up study of a secondary prevention program designed for back pain of recent onset to determine whether one's compliance with medical care depends, in part, on the perception that barriers to compliance may be overcome.

Subjects.—The subjects were all women, with a median age of 43 at the start of the program. About two thirds had low back pain, and the others had pain in the upper back or the entire back region.

Methods.—Preventive measures included walking, swimming, cycling, and other exercises, and ergonomic education targeted specifically to high-risk nursing maneuvers, such as lifting patients. Cognitive-behavioral measures focused on ways of controlling pain, solving problems, and using self-rewards to maintain a healthy life-style.

Results.—Pain intensity scores were significantly less at 18 months than at baseline (Fig 4–7). Fatigue also lessened, but an initial lessening of anxiety did not persist. Sleep quality also improved temporarily. Patients became more satisfied with their ability to perform activities of daily living. Depression scores were significantly lower at follow-up, as were helplessness scores. Absenteeism lessened at follow-up, but not to a significant degree. Conservative estimates suggested that employers saved more than the cost of the program.

Implications.—Improvement in absenteeism was most evident in this study when follow-up findings were compared with estimates based on an increasing trend in sick-listing. Problems at work, specifically with support by work supervisors and the work organization, may have interfered with compliance and limited the maintenance of treatment gains.

▶ What factors help or hinder return to work after episodes of back pain? If we can understand those factors in greater detail, we can begin to design more effective prevention programs, so that time and earnings lost from work can be decreased. Studies completed in the recent past indicate that perhaps the most important factor influencing return to work involves satisfaction at work and the support received from superiors (1). The findings of this study support earlier findings; this may indicate that training supervisors may be an important component of prevention programs, and chiropractors involved in work hardening, ergonomics, or prevention programs may want to include supervisory personnel as part of the overall design of the prevention program.—D.J. Lawrence, D.C.

Reference

1. Bigos SJ, et al: *Spine* 16:1, 1991.

Midline Disk Herniations of the Lumbar Spine

Walker JL, Schulak D, Murtagh R (Univ of South Florida, Tampa)

South Med J 86:13–17, 1993 4–37

Introduction.—Up to one third of lumbar disk herniations are in the midline. These herniations presumably cause pain through stretching or injury of the posterior longitudinal ligament. Cauda equina syndrome may develop.

Series.—The results of treating midline disk herniation were examined in 22 patients seen by 4 orthopedic surgeons from 1980 to 1986. The average age was 37 years. All the patients had low back pain. Prolapsed herniation was the most common identifiable type. Thirteen patients underwent open diskectomy, and 4 had chemonucleolysis.

Results.—Three patients had persistent sensory loss during an average follow-up of 34 months, but none had a persistent motor or bowel/bladder deficit. Patients involved in workman's compensation or legal claims had a poorer overall outcome. Four patients required reoperation. The final outcome in the 6 patients having spinal fusion did not differ significantly from those in the other patients.

Diagnosis.—Low back pain and sciatica were nearly universal in these patients, but only about one fourth had cauda equina syndrome. Myelography was more reliable than CT alone in detecting midline herniations. A focal midline and ventral defect indenting the dural sac by more than 2–3 mm distinguishes midline herniation from a more diffusely bulging disk.

▶ Midline disk herniations, although accounting for up to one third of lumbar prolapses in some studies, are less well understood than the more typical posterolateral or posteromedial prolapse. Typical symptoms of this prolapse include low back pain (rarely with sciatica) and, reportedly, the presence of cauda equina syndrome. This study attempted to identify those symptoms in greater detail. It found that only 27% of subjects *did* have the cauda equina syndrome, whereas all had back pain and nearly all had sciatica. This is in contradiction to standard information on the subject. In addition, myelography appears to be a more reliable procedure than CT in detecting these disk lesions, as opposed to the use of CT in posterolateral prolapses. A lesson to remember from this study is that patients with low back pain and sciatica, and with a straight leg raise that causes pain but with no radiation, even in the absence of cauda equina syndrome, should be considered candidates for a midline prolapse. Few data are available concerning the chiropractic management of this condition, a point not considered by the author of this paper, as his concern was with respect to several surgical procedures. A course of flexion/distraction therapy may be warranted in these cases.—D.J. Lawrence, D.C.

Classification of Nonspecific Low Back Pain. I. Psychological Involvement in Low Back Pain: A Clinical, Descriptive Approach

Coste J, Paolaggi JB, Spira A (Ambroise Paré Hosp, Boulogne, France; Bicêtre Hosp, Le Kremlin-Bicêtre, France)

Spine 17:1028–1037, 1992 4–38

Purpose.—Some classification system for low back pain (LBP) is needed for diagnostic as well as therapeutic purposes. A new approach consists of identifying clinical subtypes of LBP and examining the relationships between clinical presentation and the existence of a psychiatric disorder.

Methods.—The study sample consisted of 330 unselected outpatients with localized nonspecific LBP. Most were self-referred to the rheumatology clinic at Ambroise Paré Hospital. The 180 women and 150 men had a mean age of 49 years. Forty-four percent had been symptomatic for 90 days or longer, and 11% were receiving compensation. All subjects underwent a detailed clinical assessment, physical examination, and psychiatric interview based on the *Diagnostic and Statistical Manual of Mental Disorders, Third Edition* (DSM-III) classification. Clinical subtypes of LBP were sought by use of multiple correspondence and cluster analyses.

Findings.—Forty-one percent of subjects had an axis I DSM-III diagnosis, most commonly anxiety disorder, mood disorder, and depression. Correspondence analysis suggested the existence of a "psychological pain" syndrome, with symptoms including diffuse back pain; impossibility of assessing the intensity of pain on a pain scale; aggravation of pain by changing climate, domestic activities, and psychological factors; and back dysesthesias. Cluster analysis suggested a 4-group classification of LBP. The first cluster was characterized by a high frequency of mechanical features and possible physical signs and a low frequency of "nonorganic" signs; the fourth was characterized by uncommon mechanical features and physical signs and frequent "nonorganic" signs; the second and third were characterized by intermediate findings. The prevalence of psychiatric disorders was 26% in the first cluster and 58% in the fourth. A further 3-cluster structure emerged on cluster analysis of patients with psychiatric disorders only.

Conclusion.—Cluster analysis has provided support for the concept of a 4-group classification of patients with LBP based on the existence of mechanical and psychiatric syndromes. This is a descriptive model that does not address any etiologic or pathophysiologic hypotheses. The clinician should remember that many patients with LBP have psychiatric disorders and that treating the psychiatric syndrome may decrease the back pain.

▶ The authors suggest that there are 4 general groups of patients with low back pain, based on mechanical and psychological syndromes. These groups consist of (1) purely mechanical low back pain, (2) mechanical pain with little associated psychological factors, (3) mechanical pain with psychiatric disorder, and (4) purely psychogenic pain. Knowing the group to which a patient belongs will have ramifications for the type of therapeutic intervention a doctor chooses to use. For example, one might expect purely psychogenic pain to respond poorly to manipulation, but well to psychiatric counseling.—D.J. Lawrence, D.C.

Classification of Nonspecific Low Back Pain: II. Clinical Diversity of Organic Forms

Coste J, Paolaggi JB, Spira A (Ambroise Paré Hosp, Boulogne, France; Bicêtre Hosp, Le Kremlin-Bicêtre, France)

Spine 17:1038–1042, 1992 4–39

Introduction.—There is a growing consensus among clinicians and researchers that some widely acceptable diagnostic classifcation of low back pain (LBP) is needed. In a companion article, the relationship between clinical presentation of LBP and the existence of a psychiatric disorder was examined. The results of an analysis done to identify clinical subgroups of "purely organic" LBP are now presented.

Methods.—A detailed assessment, physical examination, and psychiatric interview of 330 consecutive adults with localized nonspecific LBP revealed that 41% of patients had an axis I *Diagnostic and Statistical Manual of Mental Disorders, Third Edition* (DSM-III) diagnosis. The remaining 194 patients, who were considered to have purely organic LBP, underwent cluster analysis. The most important factors of the previous multiple correspondence analysis and 2 standardized continuous variables, the duration of LBP and the number of previous attacks, were used to provide this precise analysis of the clinical diversity of organic LBP.

Findings.—The analysis suggested a 7-cluster population structure. The first 4 appeared to be well-differentiated clinical entities. The first was characterized by sudden onset, pain increased by movement and relieved by lying down, and limited movements on physical examination; the second was characterized by insidious onset, moderate or mild pain, and increased pain on sitting or standing; the third was characterized by a chronic condition after acute episodes, with limitation of passive movements; and the fourth was characterized by older patients and "mechanical" symptoms, as well as by limitation of passive movement. The other 3 clusters were less well-defined, including the largest one, which was characterized by sudden onset and aggravation by impulsion and lifting. The 7 clusters showed no satisfactory correlation with any existing "pathoanatomic" classification or hypotheses.

Conclusion.—Several subgroups of patients with LBP with different clinical presentations have been identified, and these classifications suggest there are various etiologic or pathophysiologic patterns of LBP and, possibly, more specific management strategies. Establishment of a clinical classification of LBP will require more comprehensive descriptions and evaluation of clinical symptoms and syndromes.

▶ The authors of this paper apply their experimental procedures to the pain from organic (not psychiatric) causes and develop a classification system that lists 7 classes resulting from organic and mechanical causes. The class to which the patient is assigned will affect the types of therapy he or she receive. Some classes involve the intervertebral disk, whereas others involve stenosis of the canal. It obviously is important to know which class the patient is in, because some patients may positively respond to manipulation (for example, patients with disk involvement), whereas others have been shown not to do so (for example, those with lateral recess stenosis.)—D.J. Lawrence, D.C.

A 1- to 4-Year Follow-Up Review of Treatment of Sciatica Using Chemonucleolysis or Laminectomy

Javid MJ (Univ of Wisconsin, Madison)

J Neurosurg 76:184–190, 1992 4–40

Background.—Laminectomy for the removal of herniated lumbar disks was first introduced in 1934. In 1964, a new approach to treating herniated nucleus pulposus with chemical hydrolysis using chymopapain, "chemonucleolysis," was developed. However, the use of chemonucleolysis decreased dramatically in the United States after catastrophic neurologic complications were reported. The procedure is currently being done successfully and with increasing frequency in other parts of the world, especially in Europe, where only experienced surgeons with proper training perform it. The comparative effects of chemonucleolysis and diskectomy were investigated.

Methods.—One hundred seventy-eight consecutive patients with sciatica who did not respond to conservative treatment were studied. None had had laminectomy or chemonucleolysis or spinal stenosis. In patients with radiologic evidence of an extruded migrated disk, a laminectomy was done. The remaining patients were given a choice of chemonucleolysis or laminectomy, which was subsequently performed on 106 and 72 patients, respectively.

Outcomes.—At 6 weeks, substantial postoperative improvement was recorded in 82.7% of patients undergoing chemonucleolysis and 92.5% of those undergoing laminectomy. At 6 months, the rates were 92.8% and 89.7%, respectively. Most patients in both groups had improved neurologic signs. One to four years after surgery, follow-up questionnaires indicated that the overall success rate was 86.5% for chemonucleolysis and 83.8% for laminectomy. Success rates for both procedures were lower in patients who received workers' compensation. There were no significant differences in improvement in neurologic symptoms or signs between the 2 treatment groups. At follow-up, 85.1% of the chemonucleolysis group and 78.5% of the laminectomy group were employed.

Conclusion.—The routine use of postmyelography CT is recommended to achieve the best results and eliminate inappropriate candidates for chemonucleolysis. When used properly, chymopapain chemonucleolysis is a suitable alternative to surgical diskectomy.

▶ There is another way to look at the results of this paper, and that is to note that approximately 10% of the patients in this study did not achieve any improvement postoperatively, regardless of whether they had laminectomy or chemonucleolysis. Over time, this figure increases even further, to approximately 15% four years after surgery. I'm left with the belief that other interventions need to be considered—that the record of chiropractic care in patients with similar conditions would yield results equal to or higher than those achieved here, but at lower cost and at lower risk of complication or neurologic sequelae.—D.J. Lawrence, D.C.

Diagnosing Instability

Pope MH, Frymoyer JW, Krag MH (Univ of Vermont, Burlington)
Clin Orthop 279:60–67, 1992 4–41

Background.—Although the definition of segmental instability remains enigmatic, a workable definition is that instability is synonymous with a loss of motion segment stiffness, such that force applied to that motion segment creates more displacement that would occur normally. For clinical reasons, the following qualifying criteria should be added: the condition causes pain, may result in progressive deformity, and places neurologic structures at risk. Many important clinical experiments have been done, and certain conclusions were drawn from the extensive literature.

Discussion and Conclusions.—Although changes in single radiographs accompany degeneration, the relationship of those changes to the working definition of instability and low back pain is unclear. Instant center computations are sensitive to error, which limits their usefulness as a measure of instability. Abnormal kinematics that are mainly shear along the anteroposterior axis can be identified. Abnormal coupling of spinal motion is observed in patients with and without low back pain, but the patterns that occur are often paradoxical and have little relationship with clinical symptoms. Instability has not been predictably found in patients with isthmic spondylolisthesis. Patients fulfilling the clinical criteria for degenerative segmental instability have no predictable patterns of abnormal motion. Palpation has not been proved as a diagnostic method. Immobilization by external skeletal fixation is probably useful in some patients, but it needs further verification. Direct skeletal measures, currently under investigation, are somewhat invasive but have the potential for yielding very accurate data with little disruption of normal motion patterns. It is hoped that such data will help establish objective kinematic-based criteria to define instability.

► Dr. Pope provides keys to diagnosis of instability in the spine. These include radiographic techniques, motion and palpation assessment, and newer procedures, such as the use of motion transducers and light-emitting diodes, which is seen in the WATSMART 3-dimensional system. Although all these procedures have helped us gain information regarding spinal instability, its definition remains enigmatic.—D.J. Lawrence, D.C.

Effect of Cervical Spine Motion on the Neuroforaminal Dimensions of Human Cervical Spine

Yoo JU, Zou D, Edwards WT, Bayley J, Yuan HA (State Univ of New York, Syracuse)

Spine 17:1131–1136, 1992 4–42

Objective.—Patients with cervical degenerative arthritis and herniated nucleus pulposus are prone to the common sequela of nerve root impingement within a stenotic neuroforamen. Assessment of the injury, selection of a maneuver to elicit symptoms, and selection of a position of immobilization position for management rely on the understanding of the effects of cervical position on foraminal size. A biomechanical study of cadaver cervical spines was done to measure the variations in neuroforaminal size as a function of cervical position.

Methods.—Fresh-frozen cervical spine specimens from 5 adult cadavers were tested using combinations of flexion-extension and rotational position. Normal cervical spine loading was simulated with 10 pounds of axial loading. A set of precisely graded circular probes was used to measure directly the C5–C7 foramina.

Findings.—Compared with neutral position, the foraminal diameter was reduced by 10% at 20 degrees of extension and by 13% at 30 degrees of extension. In contrast, diameter was increased by 8% at 20 degrees of flexion and by 10% at 30 degrees. Foraminal size decreased with ipsilateral 20-degree roation and increased with contralateral rotation, but these differences were not significantly different from the mean. Compared with sagittal position with no axial rotation, there was no change in foraminal size with combinations of flexion or extension position with axial rotation. The mean change in foraminal diameter was 1.4 mm from 30 degrees of extension to the same amount of flexion.

Conclusion.—Studies in cadaver cervical spines reveal that foraminal area is decreased with extension and ipsilateral rotation. The diagnosis of spinal stenosis may be established by provocative maneuvers of flexion, extension, and rotation. These findings imply that patients managed by conservative means should be immobilized in a flexed position, rather than an extended one, to decrease nerve root impingement.

▶ We have long known that in flexion the intervertebral foramen will open up, and in extension it will close down. What may not always be appreciated is to what extent it opens or closes. It may reduce by as much as 13% in extension, while opening up to 8% in flexion. When pathology such as disk herniation is present, this becomes of clinical import, and therapy and rehabilitation should therefore use flexed procedures to minimize the effects of IVF encroachment.—D.J. Lawrence, D.C.

THORACIC

The Natural History and Long-Term Follow-Up of Scheuermann Kyphosis

Murray PM, Weinstein SL, Spratt KF (Dept of Orthopedic Surgery/SGHST, Sheppard Air Force Base, Tex; Univ of Iowa Hosps and Clinics, Iowa City)

J Bone Joint Surg (Am) 75–A:236–248, 1993 4–43

Introduction.—Scheuermann, in 1921, described a form of fixed dorsal kyphosis consisting of wedged vertebrae with disordered vertebral end-plates. The cause remains uncertain, but a wide range of theories have been proposed involving increased growth hormone release, defective collagen formation, juvenile osteoporosis, strenuous manual work, trauma, vitamin A deficiency, epiphysitis, emotional stress, and osteochondrosis.

TABLE 1.—Characteristics of Scheuermann Kyphosis According to Selected Criteria

Criterion	No. of Patients	Apex of Curve* T1-T8	T9-T12	Chi² Test	Degrees of Freedom	P Value	Magnitude of Curve* ≤65 Degrees	66-85 Degrees	>85 Degrees	Chi² Test	Degrees of Freedom	P Value
Sex				0.065	1	0.80				1.59	2	0.46
Male	37	57	43				43	32	24			
Female	17	65	35				41	47	12			
Marital status				0.33	1	0.57				5.54	2	0.07
Single	8	75	25				38	13	50			
Married	44	57	43				46	41	14			
Smoking				3.24	2	0.20				17.5	4	0.002
Never	19	68	32				58	21	21			
Quit	20	65	35				10	70	20			
Yes	15	40	60				67	13	20			
Pain medication				0.92	1	0.34				5.61	2	0.07
No	30	67	33				50	23	27			
Yes	24	50	50				33	54	13			
Level of activity on job				0.39	1	0.54				2.28	2	0.32
Active	19	53	47				47	42	11			

(continued)

Table 1 *(continued)*

Passive	16	69	31				63	19	19			
Not applicable†	19											
No. of sick days/yr. due to low-back pain				0.94	2	0.63				6.95	4	0.14
None	29	59	41				48	28	24			
1 to 3	7	43	57				57	43	0			
4 or more	7	43	57				14	57	29			
Not applicable†	11											
Tenderness of spine				0.000	1	1.00				0.75	2	0.69
No	28	61	39				39	36	25			
Yes	25	60	40				48	36	16			
Location of pain				4.31	2	0.12				11.6	4	0.03
No pain	14	79	21				29	21	50			
Back	36	56	44				50	39	11			
Lower extrem.	3‡	25	75				25	75	0			
Back and lower extrem.	1‡											

* Values are percentages, with the exception of those for χ^2 test, degrees of freedom, and *P* value.
† Data on patients for whom the criterion was not applicable were not included in the calculations.
‡ Counts were combined across some categories of data for the purpose of calculating the χ^2 test.
(Courtesy of Murray PM, Weinstein SL, Spratt KF: *J Bone Joint Surg (Am)* 75-A:236–248, 1993.)

TABLE 2.—Data on the 52 Patients Who Underwent Pulmonary Function Testing

Variable	No. of Patients	Mean and Standard Dev.	Min.-Max. Values (Range)	Predicted Value (*Per cent*)
Lung mechanics				
Forced vital capacity (*L*)	49	4.14 ± 1.30	1.29-7.63	96
Forced expiratory volume (FEV_1) (*L*)*	49	3.10 ± 1.05	0.83-6.39	98
Forced expiration flow*	49	2.61 ± 1.30	0.39-6.42	79
$FEF_{25\text{-}75}$ (*L/sec.*)				
FEF_{max} (*L/sec.*)	49	9.17 ± 3.17	1.68-17.74	113
Lung volume				
Total lung capacity (pleuth) (*L*)*	47	7.09 ± 1.68	3.12-11.00	116
Inspiratory capacity (*L*)*	48	3.32 ± 1.04	1.36-5.05	115
Thoracic gas volume (pleuth.) (*L*)	48	3.84 ± 1.15	1.02-6.93	118
Expiratory reserve volume (*L*)	48	1.15 ± 0.69	0.03-2.97	79
Reserve volume (pleuth.) (*L*)*	47	2.76 ± 0.85	1.05-4.67	133
Slow vital capacity (*L*)	47	4.47 ± 1.36	1.51-7.68	104
Resisted air volume (*cm H_2O/L/sec.*)*	44	1.05 ± 0.69	0.18-2.88	—
Specific conductance air volume (*sec./cm H_2O/L^2*)	44	0.38 ± 0.36	0.07-1.99	—
Diffusing capacity				
Diffusing lung capacity (*ml/min./mm Hg*)*	47	29.79 ± 8.98	13.39-49.00	106
Alveolar volume (*L*)*	47	6.14 ± 1.37	3.38-8.97	98
Diffusing lung capacity/alveolar volume	47	4.84 ± 0.83	3.29-6.88	107

* Various measures of pulmonary function were often highly correlated. To avoid overlap in the results, only variables that were less linearly correlated with one another were used. These variables are marked with an *asterisk*.

Note: Not all patients had all tests.

Abbreviations: FEF, forced expiratory flow; *FEV_1,* forced expiratory volume in 1 second; *Pleuth,* pleuthesmography.

(Courtesy of Murray PM, Weinstein SL, Spratt KF: *J Bone Joint Surg (Am)* 75-A:236–248, 1993.)

Series.—Sixty-seven patients with Scheuermann kyphosis, whose mean angle of kyphosis was 71 degrees, were followed for an average of 32 years after diagnosis. The findings were compared with those in 34 age- and sex-matched control subjects. A single questionnaire was used to acquire data on demographics, health, activity, self-esteem, pain, and the social and work histories using visual analogue scales.

Findings.—Work histories were comparable in the 2 groups. Activity at work did not differ according to the location of the apex of the curve (Table 1). Pain did not interfere with patients' lives more than was found for control subjects. Patients had more medical illness than control subjects, but men and smokers were more prevalent in the study group. There was no group difference in the limitation of recreational activity by back pain. Self-consciousness was not more prominent in study subjects. Restrictive lung disease tended to occur in patients whose kyphosis exceeded 100 degrees and in those in whom the apex of the curve was in thoracic segments 1 through 8 (Table 2).

Conclusion.—Patients with Scheuermann kyphosis may have some functional limitations, but the disorder does not interfere with their lives to a major degree. These unoperated patients adjusted reasonably well to their condition.

▶ One cannot help but be impressed by a study with a time frame running out to 48 years, but the information gleaned here substantially adds to our understanding of the implications of Scheuermann's disease. One thing appears certain: outside of experiencing pain, there is little difference between those who have the disease and anyone else. Even functional studies of the lung, long believed to be a sequela of Scheuermann's disease, were found to be essentially normal. None of the subjects in this study underwent surgery, and the authors contend that the use of surgery should be reexamined. The use of bracing and manipulation may prove beneficial to these patients and should be studied in great detail.—D.J. Lawrence, D.C.

Thoracic Spine Fracture in a Football Player: A Case Report

Elattrache N, Fadale PD, Fu FH (Univ of Pittsburgh, Pa)

Am J Sports Med 21:157–160, 1993 4–44

Case Report.—Football player, 22, described back pain and stiffness since a tackling injury 24 hours before. An axial impact to the head and shoulders had resulted in compression and flexion of the back. An "electric shock" sensation had radiated from the midscapula area to the lower back on impact. The patient had resumed playing after a few minutes. The paraspinous muscles in the interscapular region were in spasm, and point tenderness was noted at the T8 and T9 levels. Radiographs showed anterior compression fractures of these vertebrae with a 40% loss of vertebral height. Computed tomography showed the fractures to be limited to the anterior parts of the vertebral bodies. An extension thoracolumbar spinal orthosis was fitted for 12 weeks, after which sports activity was resumed. After 2 years, the patient was playing professional football.

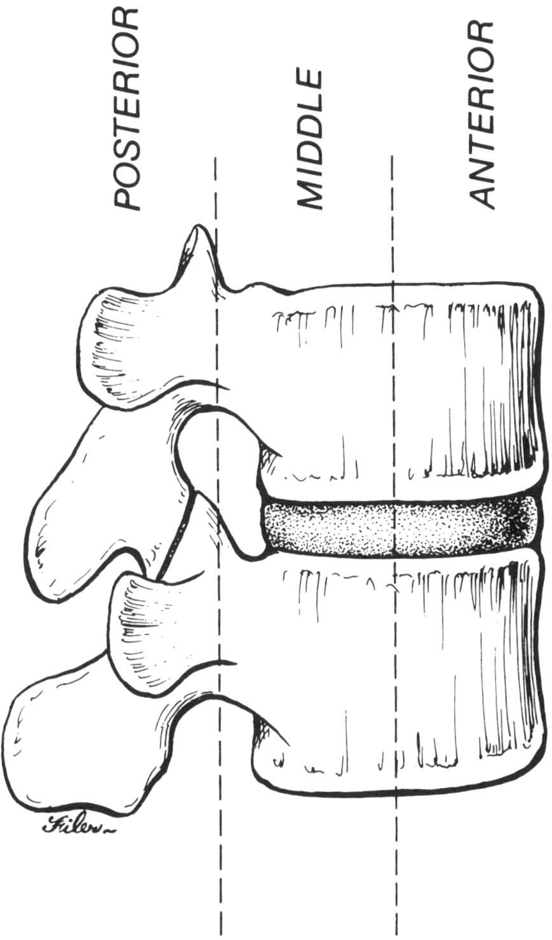

Fig 4–8.—Anterior, middle, and posterior columns of the spine. (Courtesy of Elattrache N, Fadale PD, Fu FH: *Am J Sports Med* 21:157–160, 1993.)

Mechanisms.—Even though "spearing" is illegal, the thoracic spine is at risk when an axial load is absorbed from the shoulder region with some degree of forward or lateral flexion of the spine. The anterior column fails under axial loading, whereas the middle column is somewhat protected (Fig 4–8). The spine generally remains mechanically stable.

Diagnosis.—Diffuse back pain and stiffness may be present, but there may be no impressive physical findings. Distal neurologic impairment is rare, but its absence does not exclude significant bony injury. Lateral radiographs may show anterior wedging of the vertebral body, whereas the anteroposterior view shows an irregular lateral cortex resulting from end-plate collapse. Lateral wedging may or may not be present.

Management.—The stable bony architecture permits nonoperative treatment in a plastic jacket or extension brace for 12 weeks. Bracing is indicated if the loss of vertebral body height exceeds 50%, but the risks of late kyphosis and chronic back pain are increased. More severe compression fractures may require late surgical stabilization.

▶ As the recent injury to hockey star Wayne Gretzky attests, injuries to the thoracic spine, although uncommon, do occur. In Gretzky's case, there was injury to the thoracic disks; in this report, the injury is a compression fracture of both T8 and T9. Although compression fractures are not uncommon, we are accustomed to seeing them more in the elderly and not in an active, young athlete. Such fractures result from axial compressive injury. Initial suspicion of this injury may be delayed as a result of the nonspecific nature of the ensuing complaints. Treatment consisted of an extension thoracolumbar orthosis, which was worn for 12 weeks.—D.J. Lawrence, D.C.

Comparison of Three Noninvasive Methods for Measuring Scoliosis

Pearsall DJ, Reid JG, Hedden DM (Queen's Univ, Kingston, Ont, Canada)

Phys Ther 72:648–657, 1992 4–45

Background.—An erect posteroanterior radiograph of the full spine is needed to evaluate scoliosis accurately. The Cobb method calculates an angle of lateral curvature within the affected part of the spine, but this method is incomplete; it does not fully describe the 3-dimensional geometry of the spine and associated deviations. The Scoliometer® (SCOL) is a specially designed inclinometer that presumably is sensitive to rota-

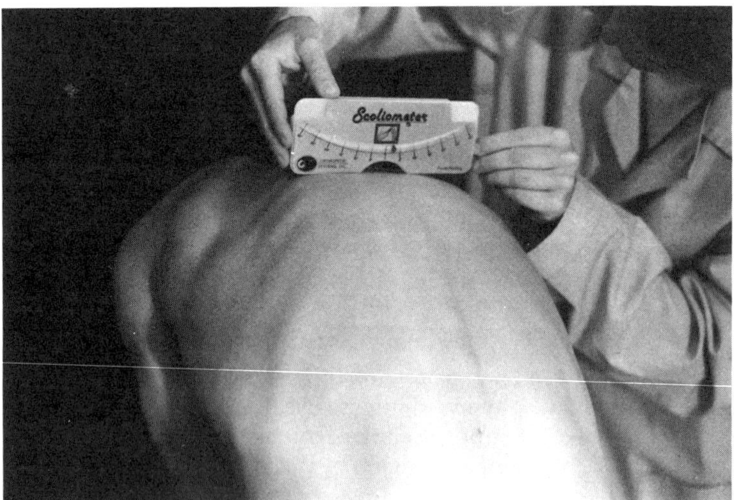

Fig 4–9.—Scoliometer® measurement of axial trunk rotation with subject in the forward-bending position. (Courtesy of Pearsall DJ, Reid JG, Hedden DM: *Phys Ther* 72:648–657, 1992.)

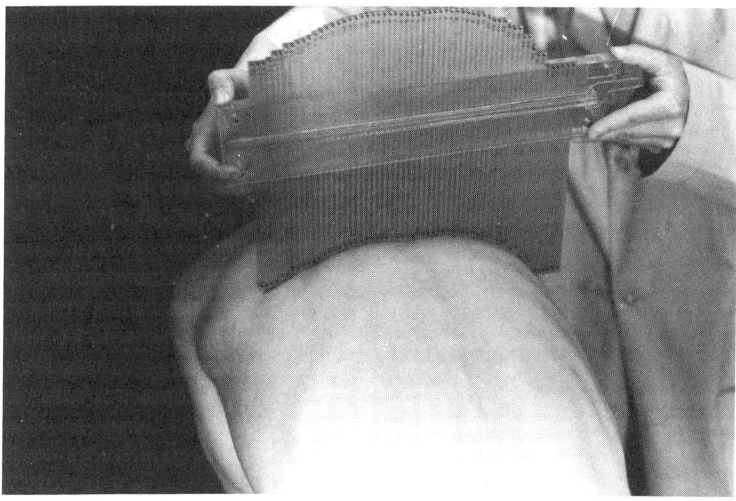

Fig 4–10.—Back-contour device measuring axial trunk rotation with subject in the forward-bending position. (Courtesy of Pearsall DJ, Reid JG, Hedden DM: *Phys Ther* 72:648–657, 1992.)

tional deformities (Fig 4–9). The back-contour device (BCD) (Fig 4–10) consists of a frame and a series of moveable rods that may be used to record the contour of the opposing back surface in the forward-bending position. More elaborate methods, such as the integrated shape imaging system and Raster stereography, also have been used.

Objective.—Fourteen subjects with idiopathic adolescent scoliosis participated in a study comparing 3 methods of assessment: the SCOL, the BCD, and moiré topographic imaging (MTI)—1 of the more elaborate methods. Posteroanterior radiographs were obtained to determine Cobb angles.

Findings.—In the thoracic and lumbar regions, values of axial trunk rotation (ATR) obtained with the SCOL and BCD methods correlated closely (table). Neither of these measurements, however, related well to MTI measurements. The SCOL and BCD measurements correlated especially closely in the thoracic region. Except for MTI values, ATR measurements in the thoracic and lumbar regions together correlated poorly with Cobb-angle measurements. In the thoracic region alone, all ATR measurements correlated with Cobb-angle values to a significant degree. No such correlation was evident within the lumbar region.

Implications.—Measurements of ATR reflect the severity of lateral scoliotic curvature most accurately in the thoracic spine. Noninvasive indicators are less useful in evaluating the lumbar spine. Radiography re-

Pearson Product-Moment Coefficient Correlation Matrices of Axial Trunk Rotation Measurements According to Method and Region

(a) Thoracic and lumbar regions ATR values (n=24)

	SCOL	BCD	MTI
SCOL	1.00		
BCD	0.87†	1.00	
MTI	0.02	0.26	1.00

(b) Thoracic region ATR values (n=12)

	SCOL	BCD	MTI
SCOL	1.00		
BCD	0.91†	1.00	
MTI	0.58*	0.71†	1.00

(c) Lumbar region ATR values (n=12)

	SCOL	BCD	MTI
SCOL	1.00		
BCD	0.62*	1.00	
MTI	0.11	0.28	1.00

* $df = 22, P < .005$.
† $df = 10, P < .005$.
‡ $df = 10, P < .025$.
(Courtesy of Pearsall DJ, Reid JG, Hedden DM: *Phys Ther* 72:648–657, 1992.)

mains necessary for an accurate clinical diagnosis of the scoliotic condition of the entire spine.

▶ The authors raise an interesting point concerning the use of x-ray film in scoliotic children: it can only be used to a certain extent because of the exposure to radiation. Is it possible to develop a noninvasive procedure that does not require great cost or exposure to harmful ionizing radiation? If so, the impact on scoliosis monitoring could be dramatic. Three such devices do exist: the Scoliometer, which is essentially an inclinometer; the back-contour Device, which allows a series of moveable pieces to mold the position of the back surface; and moiré topography, an opaque overlapping line system used to produce a 3-dimensional image of the back. The authors set out to compare these techniques against each other and against Cobb's angle. Moiré topography had the highest correlation, although all 3 seemed to work well in the thoracic spine; all three fared poorer in the lumbar spine. The design allowed comparisons among the 3 modalities; in this study, moiré topography did not correlate well to the other 2 devices. Finally, it is important to note that these devices really require further refinement; although they work well with measurements of angular trunk rotation, they do not correlate as well to Cobb's measure and, therefore, are less valuable. They represent potentially effective methods for scoliosis screening as a result.—D.J. Lawrence, D.C.

Thoracic Disk Herniation
Wilson TA, Branch CL Jr (Wake Forest Univ, Winston-Salem, NC)
Am Fam Physician 45:2162–2168, 1992 4–46

Introduction.—Thoracic disk herniation is rare, accounting for only .5% to 1.5% of ruptured disks. The diagnosis and treatment of thoracic disk herniation was studied, 2 representative case patients were examined.

Diagnosis.—The neurologic findings of thoracic disk herniation are highly variable. Sensory signs include hyperalgesia, hypalgesia, or analgesia. The symptoms include numbness, paresthesia, or dysesthesia. Sensory signs and symptoms are usually seen in the distribution of the affected nerve root or the distal spinal cord. Abnormal motor findings from lateral corticospinal tract involvement are common. Weakness of 1 or both legs, increased muscle tone, and exaggerated stretch reflexes and extensor plantar responses are all characteristic of upper motor neuron dysfunction. Magnetic resonance imaging is becoming the diagnostic procedure of choice.

Treatment.—Symptomatic thoracic disk herniation may be managed nonsurgically with limited activity, physical therapy, bracing, nonsteroidal anti-inflammatory agents, and transcutaneous electric stimulation. Surgical intervention is indicated for thoracic disk herniation with significant static myelopathy or progressive neurologic deterioration.

Case 1.—Man, 56, with a 3-month history of progressive bilateral dysesthesias in the legs and abnormal gait was referred for evaluation of possible peripheral neuropathy. Physical examination showed weakness in the right lower extremity, hyperactive reflexes, and upgoing toes. Magnetic resonance imaging revealed a large herniation of the thoracic disk at T5-T6. The herniated disk was removed via a posterolateral approach. The patient's strength in the right leg returned to normal, his gait improved, and his lower extremity dysesthesias disappeared.

Case 2.—Woman, 36, had back pain radiating to the left anterior chest, which had started after she unloaded groceries from her car and which had not improved with bed rest, analgesics, and physical therapy. Physical examination showed moderate paraspinous muscle spasm in the midthoracic region. Neurologic examination was normal except for a hyperpathic band just below the nipple on the left. Computed tomographic myelography revealed a herniated thoracic disk at T5-T6, mostly on the left side. She improved with continued conservative therapy.

▶ Thoracic disk herniations are rare and may have varying presentations, making misdiagnosis quite common. They seem to occur most frequently in the third to fifth decade of life, more often in men and generally below the level of T8. Contrast T1-weighted MRI is the best imaging modality to demonstrate findings. There is little information within the chiropractic literature regarding manipulative approaches to management. Further studies should be done, but patients for such studies may be hard to locate.—D.J. Lawrence, D.C.

Diagnostic Findings in Painful Adult Scoliosis
Grubb SA, Lipscomb HJ (North Carolina Spine Ctr, Chapel Hill)
Spine 17:518–527, 1992 4–47

Objective.—The diagnostic findings were reviewed in a group of 55 adults having both scoliosis and pain. The mean age at initial contact was 53 years; nearly 80% of the patients were women. The mean duration of pain was 12 years.

Findings.—Forty-nine percent of scoliotic curves were classified as being of adult degenerative onset, whereas 44% were idiopathic. All degenerative curves were lumbar, whereas the idiopathic curves were more variable. A majority of idiopathic patients had primarily mechanical back complaints, whereas those with degenerative-onset scoliosis chiefly had symptoms of spinal stenosis. The latter patients tended to have myelographic defects within the primary curve, as well as abnormal—although not always painful—disks throughout the lumbar spine. Idiopathic patients had defects most frequently in a compensatory lumbar or lumbosacral curve. All these patients had at least 1 abnormal, painful disk on diskography. Nearly 80% of idiopathic patients had abnormal, painful disk in other areas than in the compensatory curve.

Conclusion.—Adults with idopathic scoliosis frequently have pain-producing changes in area of the spine that would not routinely be included in the area of fusion. Structural problems must be evaluated to avoid surgery that could promote progression, but they should not be the only consideration when determining treatment.

▶ Pain is not a common symptom of adolescent juvenile scoliosis, but it may be more common when the scoliosis is present in the adult. There also appears to be a substantial percentage of adult scoliotic patients who have disk abnormalities, although these disk involvements are not always the cause of pain.—D.J. Lawrence, D.C.

Extravertebral

Achilles Tendon Ruptures: Making the Diagnosis
Hamel R (Santa Rosa, Calif)
Physician Sportsmed 20:189–200, 1992 4–48

Causes.—Achilles tendon rupture is the most common major tendon rupture in the lower extremity in active individuals. This tendon is the largest in the body. Rupture occurs more often with fatigue, usually as a result of abnormal force or force from an abnormal direction. An explosive jump or a move that suddenly forces the ankle into plantar flexion—as in tennis and basketball—can totally rupture the Achilles tendon.

Warning Signs?—It is not clear that real warning signs of impending rupture exist. The tendon may ache or feel stiff for some time before rupture takes place. Chronic tendinitis or tendinosis may weaken the tendon, making it more vulnerable to injury. Older age probably is a factor in injury. Injections such as steroid treatment may weaken the Achilles tendon.

Diagnosis.—Pain need not be present in patients with Achilles tendon rupture. Complete ruptures are often less painful than partial tears. The ability to plantar flex the foot does not always rule out total tendon rupture. The most reliable measure for rupture is the Thompson test. Magnetic resonance imaging may demonstrate a light break in the dark tendon area, but such imaging is very costly.

Management.—Most physicians treat partial ruptures by cast immobilzation. Some prefer surgery for complete ruptures, followed by casting or bracing. An active athlete may be a better candidate for surgery than an elderly individual. The site of rupture also is a factor; surgery probably is indicated for tears 2 to 6 cm above the calcaneal attachment, an area of low blood supply. Usually, 6 to 12 months are needed for the tendon to regain its strength. Typically, the tendon is immobilized for 6 weeks after surgery.

Prevention.—Potentially vulnerable individuals can take measures to prevent Achilles tendon rupture by controlling their body weight, wearing proper shoes, and warming up before exercising. Completing rehabilitation will lessen the risk of recurrent injury.

▶ Nearly one quarter of complete achilles tendon ruptures are mistaken for incomplete tears. To distinguish between the two, Ms. Hamel suggests noting the amount of pain; a complete rupture is usually *less* painful than a tear. The Thompson test is believed to be the most reliable test for establishing the diagnosis. It is performed by flexing the knee and then squeezing the calf; if the foot fails to flex, it indicates a ruptured tendon. The reliability of this test has not been established, however. One might consider imaging procedures such as MRI, although the costs really aren't justified.—D.J. Lawrence, D.C.

Myofascial Release Technique and Mechanical Compromise of Peripheral Nerves of the Upper Extremity

Leahy PM, Mock LE III (Colorado Springs, Colo)

Chiroprac Sports Med 6:139–150, 1992 4–49

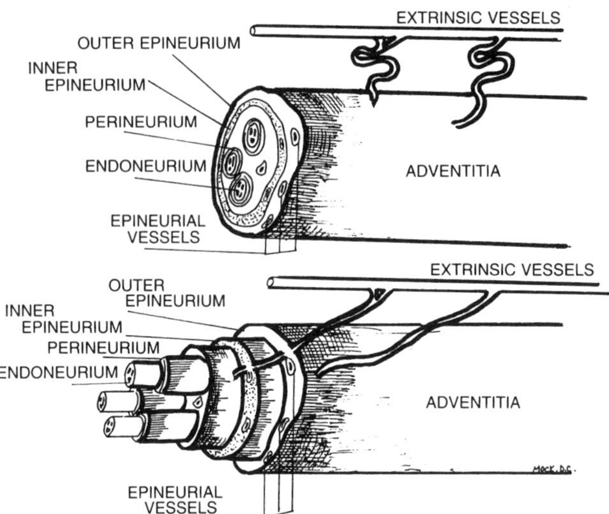

Fig 4–11.—Diagram of the sliding phenomenon in which the epineurium, perineurium, and endoneurium glide within the moving extremity. (From Leahy PM, Mock LE III: *Chiroprac Sports Med* 6:139–150, 1992. Courtesy of Totten PA, Hunter JM: *Hand Clinics* 7:505–520, 1991.)

Introduction.—Peripheral nerve entrapment, compression neuropathy, and traction neuropathy are frequent disorders that tend to occur when constant, repeated motions are performed over a long period. Peculiar postures, exposure to high-frequency vibration, and direct trauma also may produce these disorders. Carpal tunnel syndrome is 1 of the most common conditions affecting workers in the United States. These disorders may be included in the category of cumulative trauma disorder.

Mechanisms.—Several supportive tissue sheaths of the peripheral nerve system provide physiologic support to nerve fibers during gliding

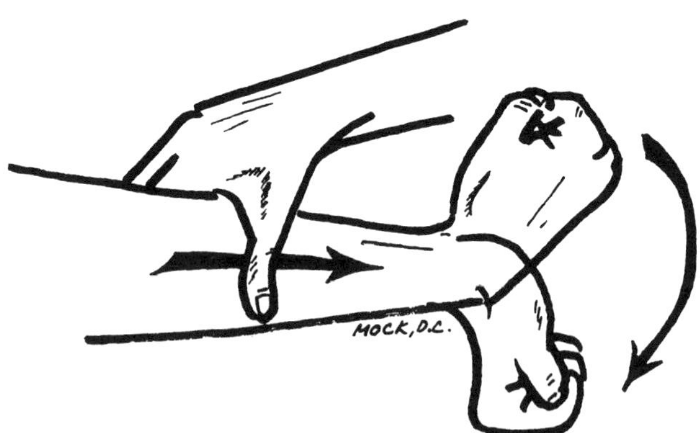

Fig 4–12.—Diagram of the application of MRT to an area of adhesion over the wrist flexors. (Courtesy of Leahy PM, Mock LE III: *Chiroprac Sports Med* 6:139–150, 1992.)

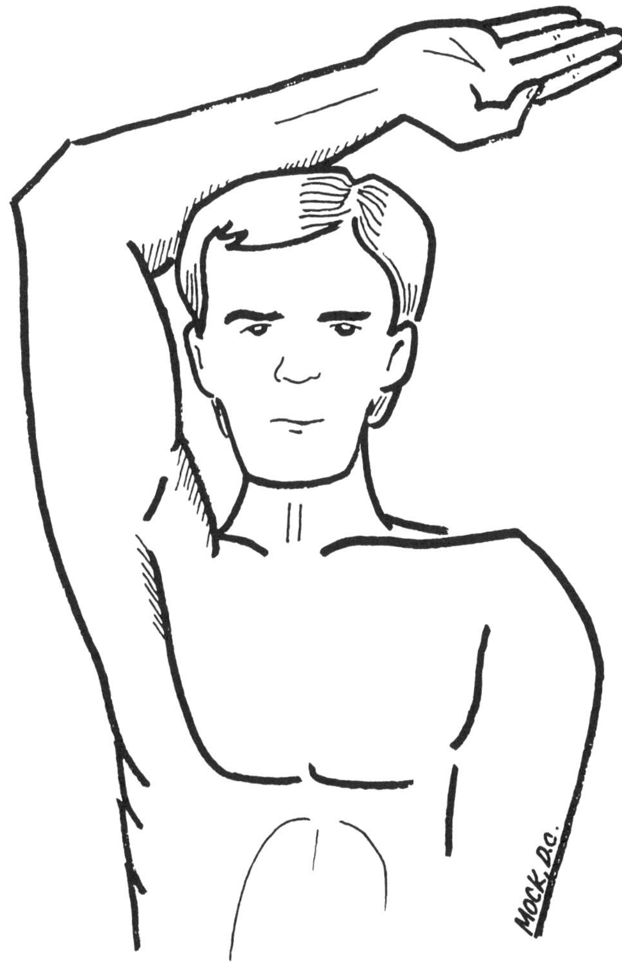

Fig 4–13.—Destination of the active movement of the patient's arm when applying MRT to the subscapularis. (Courtesy of Leahy PM, Mock LE III: *Chiroprac Sports Med* 6:139–150, 1992.)

(Fig 4–11). A long-forgotten injury may produce long-standing traction or tension on a nerve, culminating in nerve fixation. Chiropractic sports medicine deals with the ways that fibrous adhesions may interfere with the performance of a joint system.

Diagnosis.—The symptoms of entrapment neuropathy in the upper extremity generally develop gradually; pain and paresthesias are most frequent. Weakness usually is a very late finding. The dominant extremity most often is the first to be affected, and it is the one most severely involved. The patient's description of sensory change should give the first indication of where entrapment is located.

Management.—The skillfull palpator will be able to feel an adhesion break as a limb is drawn under the contact. Myofascial release treatment (MRT) may be very painful, but pain can be minimized by working very slowly and by using a broad, flat contact. A lubricant is helpful. One should always work in the direction of blood flow so as not to damage veins. Techniques of MRT are illustrated in Figures 4–12 and 4–13. It is best to work longitudinally along the fibers. Three to 5 passes are made over each area to the limit of patient tolerance at each visit. Because MRT is not a long-term measure, it does not require maintenance treatment. Most often, 3 to 10 treatments will suffice. The patient usually does not have to miss work.

▶ The authors provide a detailed discussion of the etiology, diagnosis, anatomy, and treatment for peripheral neuropathies, especially carpal tunnel syndrome. Their approach uses myofascial release procedures that remove fibrotic adhesions to restore function. These procedures are well demonstrated in this paper, which is a nice touch because their approach differs from standard chiropractic management of this condition. The procedures do, however, remain open to some controversy, because they have not yet been adequately tested in randomized controlled fashion. The basis for doing so is established by clinical presentations like the ones described in this study.—D.J. Lawrence, D.C.

Lack of Scientific Evidence for the Treatment of Lateral Epicondylitis of the Elbow: An Attempted Meta-Analysis

Labelle H, Guibert R, Joncas J, Newman N, Fallaha M, Rivard C-H (Univ of Montreal, Quebec, Canada)

J Bone Joint Surg 74–B:646–651, 1992 4–50

Background.—There is continued debate concerning the best treatment for lateral epicondylitis (LE), or "tennis elbow," because it is empiric and based on personal experience. The current literature was reviewed to determine whether there was scientific evidence to support any particular treatment method.

Methods.—The English and French literature from 1966 through 1990 was searched. A total of 185 articles were found, 78 of which covered treatment. Of the studies that used concurrent control groups, only 18 were randomized and controlled. The method of Chalmers et al. was used to grade these studies for scientific validity.

Findings.—The mean score of the articles was 33%; the lowest-scoring study had a score of 6% and the highest a score of 73%. Because a score of at least 70% is needed for a valid trial, none of the current methods of treatment had sufficient scientific support. Methodologic differences precluded quantitative meta-analysis, but a qualitative review underscored the importance of the syndrome's natural evolution and the placebo effect of all treatments.

Conclusion.—There is insufficient scientific evidence to support any of the current treatment methods for acute LE. Studies of the topic are fraught with methodologic problems, and treatment groups have been small. Improvement is seen in almost all studies, suggesting that the condition improves spontaneously with time. Well-designed controlled studies are needed.

► Of all the clinical trials for treatment of LE, only one was found to meet the standards for a valid clinical trial. The implications of this are frightening: How are we to determine standards of care for certain conditions in light of the lack of rigorous scientific research? Similar studies have been done for low back pain, and they have had similar (although slightly better) results. One major problem of practitioners and researchers is not taking the natural history of a disease into account, i.e., would the condition have resolved on its own in the same time frame that the response occurred in the research? For that reason alone, 60 papers had to be excluded from this study. We cannot allow standards of care to be set solely by consensus; some scientific research *must* support ethical and appropriate standards of care. Much as everyone may be tired of hearing it, more studies are required—for tennis elbow as much as for low back or neck pain.—D.J. Lawrence, D.C.

Anterior Shoulder Dislocations
Yu J (Loma Linda Univ, Calif)
J Fam Pract 35:567–576, 1992 4–51

Introduction.—The shoulder capsule is largely responsible for maintaining a stable shoulder. The fibrous glenoid labrum and the rotator cuff muscles help maintain the humeral head in the glenoid fossa, regardless of position. The deltoid, triceps, and biceps muscles also help stabilize the shoulder. Traumatic dislocations often are associated with fracture or other complications mandating a long period of immobilization. The resultant scar formation may contribute to greater stability and minimize the risk of recurrent dislocation.

Postreduction Management.—Many studies have been done to determine the effectiveness of immobilization in preventing recurrent dislocation (table). In general, immobilization for 3 weeks appears to be best for primary anterior shoulder dislocation. Longer immobilization may be appropriate for the young and for athletes. It is important to strengthen the subscapularis, a major factor in preventing anterior laxity of the shoulder. Rehabilitative measures may enhance muscle strength and help regain mobility after a period of rest and immobilization.

Complications.—Osseous complications of anterior shoulder dislocation include features of the shoulder girdle, including the humeral head and surgical neck. Fractures of the anterior glenoid rim dispose the patient to recurrent dislocation. Rotator cuff tear is another complication of shoulder dislocation. Nerve injuries are relatively infrequent and tend

Studies Showing the Impact of Age and Treatment on the Rate of Recurrence of Shoulder Dislocations

Study	Total Patients	Impact of Age on the Recurrence of Dislocation		Impact of Treatment on the Recurrence of Dislocation	
		Age (y)	% Recurrence	Treatment	% Recurrence
MacLaughlin and Cavallaro	101	<20	90	Sling and swathe 3+ wk	0
		20–40	60	Sling and swathe 2–3 wk	1
		>40	10	Sling and swathe 1–2 wk	6
				Sling and swathe 0–1 wk	14
Rowe and Sakellarides	324	<20	94	Sling 3–6 wk	37
		20–40	74	Sling 1–3 wk	46
		>40	14	No treatment	70
				Sling and swathe 3–6 wk	33
				Sling and swathe 1–3 wk	26
Kazar and Relovszky	566	<20	46	Immobilized 15 d	4.5
		21–30	31	Immobilized 8–14 d	6
		31–40	6	Immobilized 0–7 d	16
		>41	<6		
Hovelius	63	<20	90	Immobilized >20 d	75
		20–25	65	Immobilized 10–20 d	87
		>25	50	Immobilized <10 d	68
Kiviluoto et al	53	16–20	56	Immobilized 3 wk	22
		21–30	26	Immobilized 1 wk	56
		>30	<8		

Yoneda et al	104	21.5	17.3	Sling and swathe 5 wk, then limited exercise 6 wk	17.3
Henry and Genung	121	19 (average)	—	Immobilized	90
				Not immobilized	85
Simonet and Cofield	116	<20	66	Immobilized, then activity restricted 6 wk	44
		20–40	40		
		>40	0	No activity restricted	85
Hovelius	254	12–22	55	Age <22 y	
		23–29	37	Immobilized 3–4 wk	64
		30–40	12	Mobilized early	58
				Mixed treatment	17
				Age 23–29 y	
				Immobilized 3–4 wk	58
				Mobilized early	47
				Mixed treatment	17
				Age 30–40 y	
				Immobilized 3–4 wk	63
				Mobilized early	33
				Mixed treatment	20
Wheeler et al	38	—	—	Immobilized 3 wk, then 3 mo physical therapy and activity restriction	92

(Courtesy of Yu J: *J Fam Pract* 35:567–576, 1992.)

to occur with severe dislocations. Vascular injuries are rare and usually occur in elderly individuals who may have abnormal vessels.

Surgery.—Surgery is chiefly done to prevent recurrences of anterior shoulder dislocation or, in rare cases, to reduce an otherwise unreducible dislocation. The procedures include shortening of the subscapularis tendon, alteration of bone stability, and anterior capsulorrhaphy. Arthroscopy may be a useful intermediate step in very high-risk patients and elite athletes.

▶ Age is the best determinant in the prognosis of a patient who has had an anterior shoulder dislocation, both in terms of treatment time and recurrence. The authors recommend an immobilization period of approximately 3 weeks, except in the young (in this study, defined as those aged 20 years or younger). For the young, the period of immobilization is increased from 6 weeks to 3 months, to allow for tendon healing. The rehabilitation offered by Dr. Yu involves gravity and antigravity exercise; it might be made much stronger with the addition of careful chiropractic mobilization directed at the healing shoulder.—D.J. Lawrence, D.C.

Collagen Type III in Rotator Cuff Tears: An Immunohistochemical Study

Kumagai J, Uhthoff HK, Sarkar K, Murnaghan JP (Ottawa Gen Hosp, Ont, Canada; Ottawa Civic Hosp, Ont; Canada; Univ of Ottawa, Ont, Canada)

J Shoulder Elbow Surg 1:187–192, 1992 4–52

Background.—Indefinite conservative management is the rule for elderly patients with a rotator cuff tear. Surgery generally is performed only when pain persists with a significant loss of function. The interval from diagnosis to surgery may vary widely. Experimentally, collagen type III predominates in the elderly stages of sound healing and later is replaced by collagen type I as the scar matures.

Objective.—Four surgically removed specimens were obtained from patients aged 63 to 71 years with complete rotator cuff tears to relate the time of preoperative conservative management to the distribution of collagen types. Conservative treatment had been given for 3 months to 3 years.

Findings.—Studies with the peroxidase-antiperoxidase method and monoclonal antibody against human collagen type III demonstrated type III collagen throughout the tendon proper, often in association with proliferating fibroblasts. Type III collagen was abundant only in the perivascular spaces of the thickened bursal wall extending over the margins of the tear. Vascular proliferation was less evident in the substance of the tendon, where type III collagen was related more to proliferating cells.

Conclusion.—The presence of collage type III indicates a need to attempt repair at the site of a rotator cuff tear. The duration of symptoms preoperatively has no substantial effect on collagen formation. It may be that transformation to type I collagen occurs after surgery, or that bridging of the wound is needed for this to take place. Type I collagen is necessary for tensile strength to develop in the tendon.

▶ Incomplete rotator cuff tears are frequent athletic injuries that are effectively treated by conservative means. This study shows that even with successful conservative care, some granulation tissue (made up of collagen type III) will be present after cessation of symptoms. This apparently is independent of the time frame for conservative care and, in some instances, even for surgical repair. Dr. Kumagia postulates that the presence of type III collagen indicates a need for continued repair at the site and that it may be possible to transform it into type I collagen (seen in normal tissue) by surgery. It may be possible to do the same via more conservative, manipulative methods.—D.J. Lawrence, D.C.

Idiopathic Osteonecrosis of the Hip

Thorkeldsen A, Cantillon V (Anglo-European College of Chiropractic, Bournemouth, England; Cork Chiropractic Clinic, Ireland)

J Manipulative Physiol Ther 16:37–42, 1993 4–53

Introduction.—Hip pain is frequent in chiropractic patients, with or without degenerative joint disease. Pain may be a result of osteonecrosis or avascular necrosis of the hip, even if radiographs are negative.

Case Report.—Man, 77, reported constant dull, deep pain in his left hip and leg. Pain had occurred intermittently in the hip for 3 years and had become worse in the past year, increasingly limiting movements. A restricted adductor gait was evident, and the patient could not stand or walk without support. The gluteal and thigh muscles on both sides were atrophied, and the left hip muscles were in spasm. There was no Achilles reflex on the left side. Radiographs showed that both femoral heads were deformed and flattened and the superior joint spaces were markedly narrowed. Patchy sclerosis and cystic change were evident in both femoral heads and acetabule. Earlier films showed changes of moderate degenerative joint disease with no evidence of osteonecrosis in either hip.

Classification.—Stage 0 osteonecrosis of the hip is a preclinical and preradiographic stage. Stage 1 osteonecrosis is suspected in a painful hip with limited motion but normal radiographs. The first signs of sclerosis and osteopenia are seen in stage 2 cases. Stage 3 is characterized by the "crescent" sign and by flattening and collapse of the articular surface of the femoral head (Fig 4–14). The joint space is preserved, but in stage 4, articular cartilage is progressively lost, and osteophytosis is noted in the femoral head and acetabulum. There may be bony debris within the joint capsule. The most revealing views are the lateral "Lauenstein" or "frog-

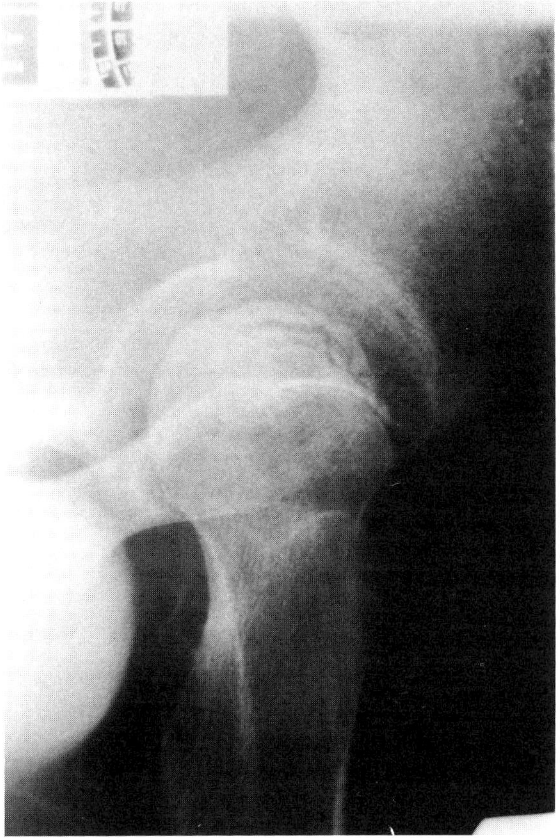

Fig 4–14.—In this frog-leg view, the irregular radiolucent line parallel to the articular surface of the femoral head represents fracture of the cancellous subcortical bone and is called the "crescent" sign. The fracture involves primarily the superior and anterior aspects of the femoral head. (Courtesy of Thorkeldsen A, Cantillon V: *J Manipulative Physiol Ther* 16:37–42, 1993.)

leg" projection and a 30-degree anteroposterior cephalad angulated spot view.

Treatment.—Surgery usually is necessary to avoid femoral head collapse and joint incongruity. Core decompression is most effective when done at an early stage. If surgery is not planned, weight bearing should be avoided until symptoms resolve; an individualized, progressive weight-bearing regimen can then begin.

▶ Idiopathic osteonecrosis of the hip may be exceedingly difficult to identify, because it may not cause altered radiographic findings and, unlike necrosis (where the cause is known), the patient has no underlying problem. What causes the interrupted blood flow to the hip is not known, but it may involve altered fat metabolism or past trauma. The predominant symptom is hip pain on weight-bearing, which is later followed by loss of motion. The disease develops in 5 stages, only some of which are radiographically evident. Bone scintigraphy will identify early changes with far greater sensitivity than plain film radiographs. Unfortunately, therapy is surgical intervention. No protocols for a strict conservative approach exist.—D.J. Lawrence, D.C.

Avascular Necrosis of the Femoral Head: An Unusual Complication of an Intertrochanteric Fracture

Shih L-Y, Chen T-H, Lo W-H (Veterans Gen Hosp; Young-Ming Med College, Taipei, Taiwan)

J Orthop Trauma 6:382–385, 1992 4–54

Introduction.—Intertrochanteric fractures of the femoral head are common, especially in the elderly. The major treatment problems are continued fracture instability and the complications of fixation that result, including nail penetration and bending or breakage of an implant. The relationship between fracture and avascular necrosis of the femoral head (ANFH) remains uncertain.

Series.—A review of 1,800 intertrochanteric fractures of the femur treated at a veterans' center between 1980 and 1989 revealed 6 cases of ANFH.

Clinical Details.—The 6 men had an average age of 46 years. None had a history of alcoholism, steroid therapy, or metabolic problems related to avascular necrosis. All the patients had a type I intertrochanteric

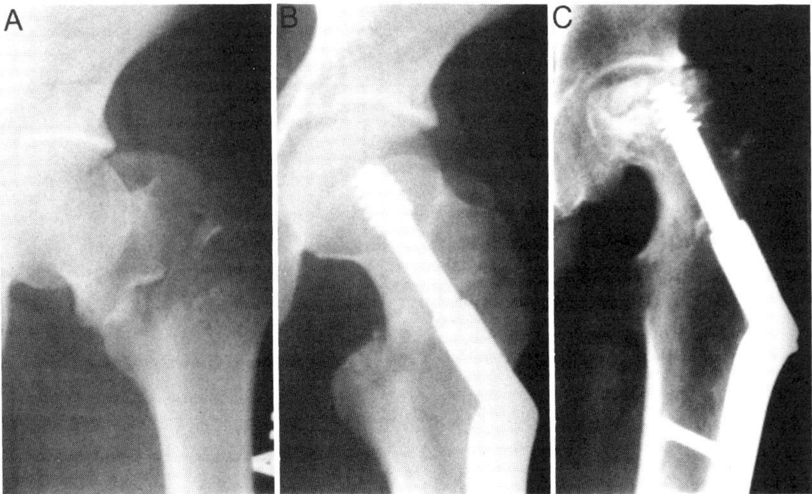

Fig 4–15.—**A,** radiograph on admission showing rotational displacement of the fracture fragment. **B,** radiograph after open reduction and internal fixation. **C,** radiograph 14 months after surgery showing ANFH. (Courtesy of Shih L-Y, Chen T-H, Lo W-H: *J Orthop Trauma* 6:382-385, 1992.)

fracture, with the fracture lines extending upward and outward from the lesser trochanter. All fragments were displaced initially. Four patients had closed reduction and internal fixation with a sliding hip screw-plate. Two underwent open reduction and internal fixation with a screw-plate. Rotational instability was evident in 4 cases. The injured hip began aching 12 to 56 months after injury, when radiographs showed stage III avascular necrosis in 1 case, stage IV changes in 3, and stage V disease in 2. Four of the patients had bipolar endoprostheses inserted; 2 underwent total hip replacement. All were relieved of pain and had improved function. The resection specimens exhibited complete ANHR.

Discussion.—High-energy injury with initial displacement of the fracture fragments may compromise the blood supply and thereby lead to ANFH (Fig 4–15). Young patients with proximal, high-energy injuries should be closely followed, even if healing is uneventful. Rotational instability also may dispose patients to the development of ANFH.

▶ Avascular necrosis, although not an uncommon clinical diagnosis, is not a usual complication of an intertrochanteric fracture. The authors found 6 such cases in a 5-year period, in patients ranging in age from 19 to 67 years. Chiropractors should be mindful of the possible development of necrosis after these types of fracture. In patients in whom pain persists for long periods after fracture, scout hip films might be worth considering.—D.J. Lawrence, D.C.

Femoral Neck Stress Fracture Presenting as Low Back Pain

Hubka MJ, Cassidy JD, Dust W (Los Angeles College of Chiropractic, Whittier, Calif; Royal Univ Hosp, Saskatoon, Sask)
J Can Chiroprac Assoc 36:217–221, 1992 4–55

Introduction.—Femoral neck stress fractures in young adults usually produce pain in the groin or anterior thigh. The symptoms often are mild, and low back pain may point to a lumbar spinal disorder, rather than hip pathologic abnormalities.

Case Report.—Woman, 39, an aerobics instructor, had suddenly had intense low back pain develop 3 months earlier, with no apparent cause. She was treated for urinary tract infection 6 weeks later, but left flank pain and pain in the left lower back and left lower abdominal quadrant persisted. Sharp lower back pain was accompanied by aching in the left anterior thigh. Pain worsened on prolonged standing and walking, but it was temporarily relieved by 2 hours of aerobic exercises. Left sacroiliac joint syndrome was diagnosed, but the patient's condition failed to improve on current treatment and manipulation. Radiographs subsequently showed a subcapital stress fracture of the left femur (Figs 4–16 and 4–17). Internal fixation was carried out 4½ months after the onset of symptoms. After 2 months, the patient was able to walk without pain or a limp and had full

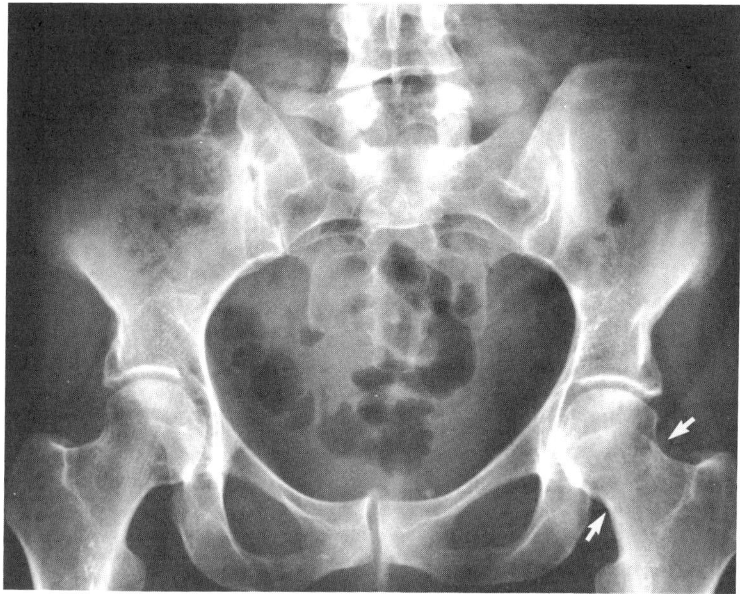

Fig 4–16.—Anteroposterior pelvic x-ray film shows linear, ill-defined sclerotic zone in the subcapital region of the left femur (*arrows*). (Courtesy of Hubka MJ, Cassidy JD, Dust W: *J Can Chiroprac Assoc* 36:217–221, 1992.)

hip movement, with only slight pain at extreme external rotation. The fracture was healing.

Discussion.—Femoral stress fractures are seen in young individuals engaging in sustained strenuous activity and also in older individuals with osteopenic bone exposed to repeated but minimal stress. Patients usually have no obvious deformity apart from an antalgic limp, and initial x-ray films may be unremarkable. If pain persists, the patient should be placed on crutches or bed rest, and radiography should be repeated in 10–14 days, when endosteal or subperiosteal callus may be present. Treatment is by internal fixation with pins or cannulated screws.

▶ The authors correctly note that it is often possible to overlook hip pathology, because it rarely has actual hip pain as a symptom. With regard to hip fracture, failure to diagnose may lead to the development of avascular necrosis. The combination of groin, thigh, and trochanteric pain, perhaps with low back pain as well, should alert us to the possibility of hip pathology.—D.J. Lawrence, D.C.

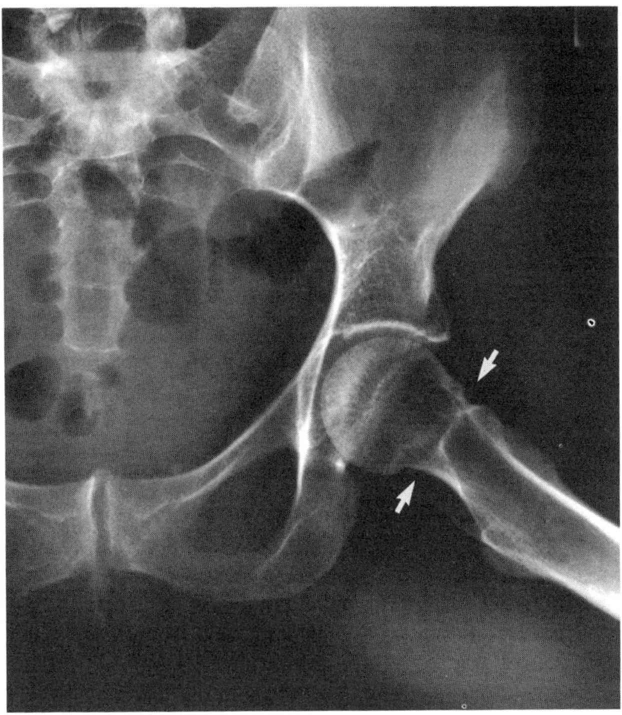

Fig 4–17.—An oblique view of left hip shows discontinuity in cortex and linear density across the femoral neck (*arrows*). (Courtesy of Hubka MJ, Cassidy JD, Dust W: *J Can Chiroprac Assoc* 36:217-221, 1992.)

Sciatica Due to Piriformis Pyomyositis: Report of a Case
Chen W-S (Chang-Gung Mem Hosp, Kaohsiung, Taiwan)
J Bone Joint Surg (Am) 74–A:1546–1548, 1992 4–56

Introduction.—Lumbar disk herniation is the usual cause of sciatica. Piriformis muscle syndrome is one of the less frequent causes, and this diagnosis most often has been made after excluding other causes of sciatica.

Case Report.—Man, 42, had paresthesia develop in the left gluteal region, radiating along the posterolateral thigh and calf to the dorsolateral aspects of the foot. The symptoms, which included a tingling feeling, were worse on walking, sitting, and bending forward. The straight leg raising and Lasègue tests were positive at 60 degrees. A sensory deficit was noted along the dorsolateral aspects of the thigh, leg, and foot; and the ankle and toe extensors were very weak. A diagnosis of piriformis muscle syndrome was made. The patient became febrile and had leukocytosis develop with a leftward shift. Studies with CT showed swelling of the piriformis muscle with an area of attenuation but no lumbar spine lesion.

Surgical exploration revealed a swollen, inflamed piriformis muscle which yielded purulent fluid. The piriformis tendon was incised to relieve compression of the sciatic nerve. Culture of the purulent material yielded *Staphylococcus aureus,* and cephalosporin was given for 3 weeks. The fever subsided, and sciatic pain was absent after 1 week. Extensor muscle weakness lasted 3 months longer, but the patient eventually resumed full normal activity and had no motor or sensory deficit and no limitation of hip motion.

Discussion.—An enlarged piriformis muscle may push the sciatic nerve anteriorly or entrap it against the gemellus superior muscle. In this case, pyomyositis of the piriformis muscle caused it to swell, displacing the sciatic nerve and entrapping it. Either CT or MRI may allow an early diagnosis of suppurative inflammation in a deep-seated muscle.

Arteriovenous Malformation of the Spine as a Cause of Scoliosis

Hains F, Dzus AK, Cassidy JD (Canadian Mem Chiropractic College, Toronto; Royal Univ Hosp, Saskatoon, Sask)

J Can Chiroprac Assoc 36:205–212, 1992 4–57

Introduction.—Scoliosis is frequent in patients having spinal vascular malformations. It may be secondary to neurologic damage that produces muscle imbalance or to impairment of the blood supply to osseous structures, leading to vertebral body asymmetry.

Case Report.—Girl, 14 years, had been recognized as having scoliosis 2 years previously. A 33-degree right thoracic curve was treated with a Milwaukee brace, but the curve had progressed. The curve was accompanied by a 2.5-cm rib hump, and a left thoracolumbar curve with a 1.5-cm transverse process hump also was noted. A left trunk shift of 2 cm was present. The patient had 2 large café-au-lait spots but no other signs of neurofibromatosis. The x-ray films showed a 37-degree right thoracic curve and a 54-degree left thoracolumbar curve (Fig 4–18).

Bracing was discontinued. The patient had back pain after activity, and the scoliosis progressed. The right fibula appeared gracile (Fig 4–19), but workup at a neurofibromatosis clinic showed no evidence of the disease. After 6 months, a myelogram and CT scan showed an expanded cord between T2 and T8, and an MR study suggested an arteriovenous malformation (Fig 4–20). Spinal angiography confirmed an intramedullary malformation at T4–T6. The plan was to embolize the malformation if the scoliosis continued to progress or if the patient's neurologic status deteriorated.

Discussion.—Patients with a spinal arteriovenous malformation tend to have their condition deteriorate slowly and in a step-like manner. Direct compression of the spinal cord or increased venous pressure within the cord may be responsible. The malformations may cause spinal deformity. An idiopathic curve usually progresses less rapidly as spinal maturity nears; however, in this patient, the curve continued to progress rap-

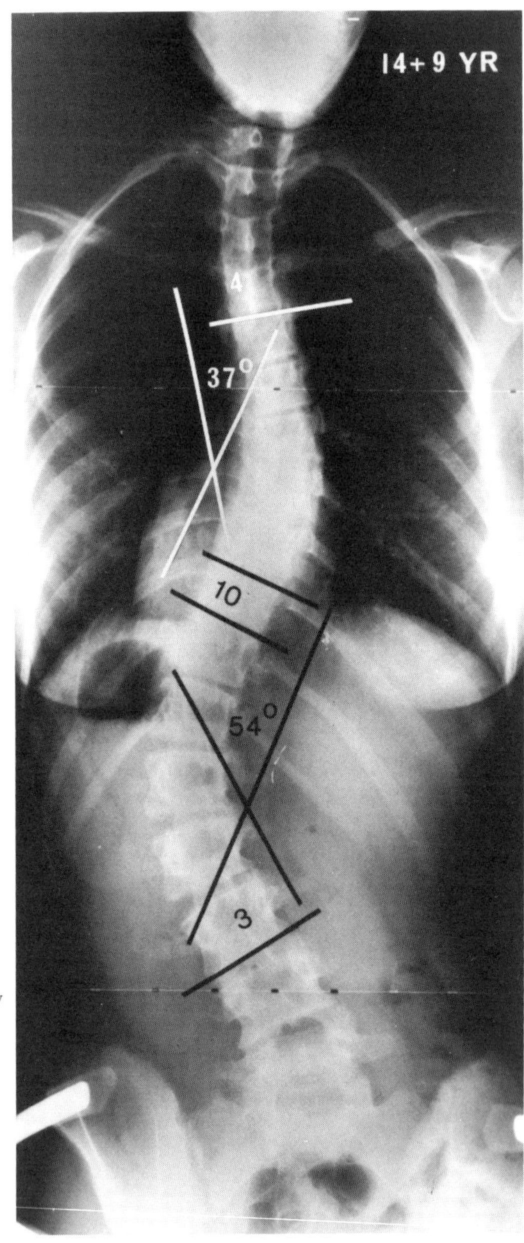

Fig 4–18.—Posteroanterior view of scoliosis shows 37-degree right thoracic curve measured from T5 to T10 and 54-degree left thoracolumbar curve measured from T11 to L3. (Courtesy of Hains F, Dzus AK, Cassidy JD: *J Can Chiroprac Assoc* 36:205–212, 1992.)

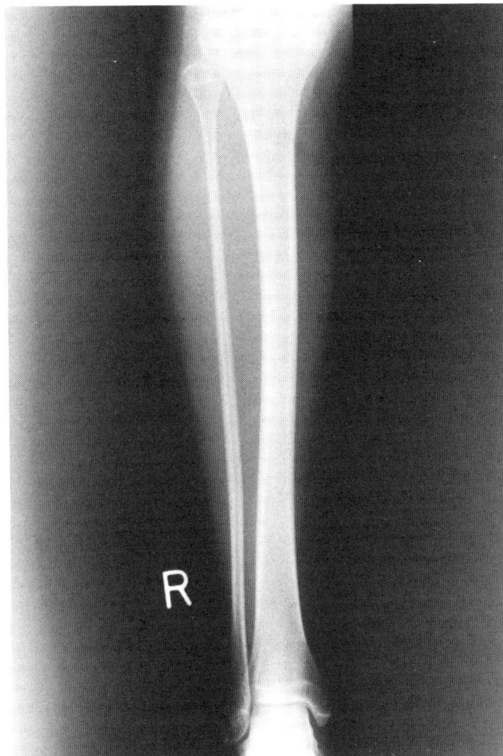

Fig 4–19.—Anteroposterior radiographic view of right tibia and fibula shows gracile fibula. (Courtesy of Hains F, Dzus AK, Cassidy JD: *J Can Chiroprac Assoc* 36:205–212, 1992.)

idly. Surgery or embolization is indicated at an early stage, but there is a high risk of creating further neurologic deficit during surgery, especially in cases of intramedullary malformation.

▶ Here we have a 13-year-old girl who had what appeared to be idiopathic scoliosis. After being fitted for a brace, her curvature continued to progress, and she began to demonstrate neurologic signs. Magnetic resonance imaging and other imaging techniques were able to demonstrate an arteriovenous malformation as the cause of her worsening condition. Never assume that what appears to be a "standard" patient is indeed just that. This is like looking at the world while wearing blinders; you will miss a lot of the view. Failure to diagnose this situation may have had profound effects of the young girl. Whenever a scoliotic teen shows developing neurologic signs and symptoms, signals ought to go off and further imaging should be mandatory.—D.J. Lawrence, D.C.

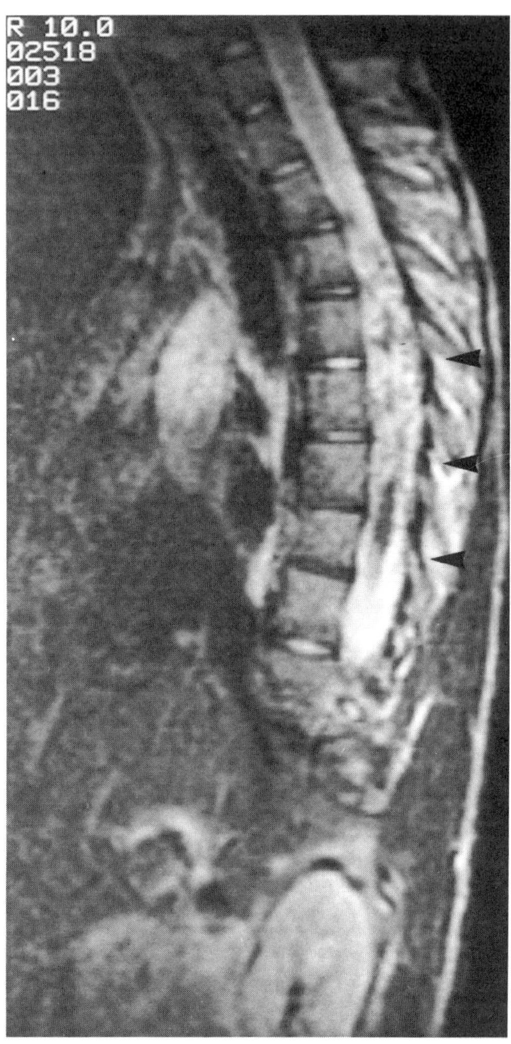

Fig 4–20.—Sagittal-section thoracic MRI scan shows mixed signal intensity within enlarged cord (*arrowheads*). This suggests a spinal arteriovenous malformation, most likely intramedullary. (Courtesy of Hains F, Dzus AK, Cassidy JD: *J Can Chiroprac Assoc* 36:205-212, 1992.)

Osteoid Osteoma: A Case Report

Towne KJ (Luedtke-Storm-Mackey Chiropractic Clinic, SC, New Glarus, Wis)
J Chiroprac 29:35–38, 1992 4–58

Introduction.—Osteoid osteoma is a benign neoplasm of bone that produces increasingly severe, aching pain unrelieved by rest or exercise. A majority of patients have dramatic relief at night when aspirin is taken. Male patients aged 11-26 years predominate. The tibia and femur are

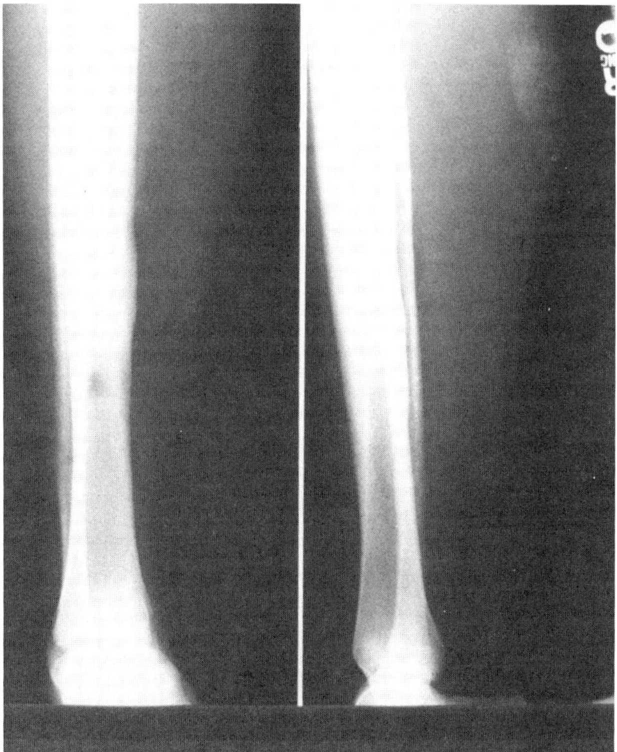

Fig 4–21.—Right tibia of a man, 19, demonstrating regional sclerosis associated with osteoid osteoma. (Courtesy of Towne KJ: *J Chiroprac* 29:35–38, 1992.)

most frequently involved. Complete removal of the nidus assures a very good prognosis.

Case Report.—Man, 19, had low back pain, right leg pain, and muscle cramping. He periodically had to lift heavy objects at work and had to stand for long periods. The leg pain was much worse at night, but aspirin provided significant relief. An elevation was palpated at the anteromedial aspect of the right tibia, and the right gastrocnemius and soleus muscles were hypertonic. Radiographs reactive sclerosis with eccentric cortical thickening (Fig 4–21). A bone scan confirmed osteoid osteoma, and the nidus was excised. The patient recovered well and no longer has pain at night.

Conclusion.—When x-ray films suggest osteoid osteoma but a nidus is not clearly seen, a bone scan or CT study may confirm the diagnosis. Recurrences are rare after complete excision of the nidus.

▶ Dr. Towne discusses a virtual textbook case of osteoid osteoma. One point to remember is that the presence of long bone night pain, especially when relieved by aspirin, should signal to the chiropractor the suggestion of this tumor. With muscle cramping present, it may be possible to confuse the presence of the tumor with a more benign muscular problem.—D.J. Lawrence, D.C.

Acute Carpal Tunnel Syndrome Due to Pseudogout

Rate AJ, Parkinson RW, Meadows TH, Freemont AJ (Wythenshawe Hosp, Manchester, England)
J Hand Surg (Br) 17B:217–218, 1992 4–59

Case Report.—Woman, 82, had had a week of pain and paresthesias in the median nerve area of the right hand. Anti-inflammatory therapy had been ineffective. The patient had a history of Crohn's disease and had had hip arthroplasty for osteoarthritis several years previously. Fever of 37.5°C was present. Tenderness and swelling were present over the carpal tunnel, and sensation was diminished in the median nerve distribution. Active finger flexion was painful and limited, and passive extension was actively resisted. Radiography showed calcification in the triangular fibrocartilage. Surgical exploration showed the median nerve to be flattened and atrophic. Florid synovitis involved the flexor tendons and wrist joint, and the tissues were heavily calcified. Flexor tenosynovectomy was done. The histologic diagnosis was acute pseudogout; there was no evidence of infection. Pain was relieved after surgery, but numbness persisted 6 months later.

Discussion.—Acute carpal tunnel syndrome most often is associated with fractures about the writs. Gout is a rare cause, along with tumoral calcinosis and acute hemorrhage. Delay in decompressing the median nerve in acute cases may predict a poor outcome. It may be difficult to distinguish between pseudogout and septic arthritis. Cases such as this one call for urgent nerve decompression combined with arthrotomy and irrigation.

▶ Not all causes of carpal tunnel syndrome are the result of tightness in the flexor retinaculum. Rate and colleagues discuss acute carpal tunnel syndrome that they suspected was the result septic arthritis causing compression. In fact, it was caused by pseudogout and was ultimately operated. More common causes of carpal tunnel syndrome include tight retinaculum, swelling from strain or sprain, and fracture of rheumatoid arthritis. Rapidly occuring symptoms of carpal tunnel involvement should signal a more acute problem.—D.J. Lawrence, D.C.

Thickening of the Synovium of the Digital Flexor Tendons: Cause or Consequence of the Carpal Tunnel Syndrome?

Lluch AL (Hosp Sant Pau, Barcelona)

J Hand Surg (Br) 17B:209–212, 1992 4–60

Introduction.—Surgery for carpal tunnel syndrome frequently reveals fibrous thickening about the flexor tendons. Some surgeons consider this to represent tenosynovitis and to be a cause of median nerve compression; however, both the epineurium and synovium exhibit histologic changes that do not resemble true tenosynovitis. Vascular proliferation, edema, perivascular round-cell infiltration, and deposition of collagen fibers are recognized in these cases.

Objective and Methods.—An attempt was made to produce carpal tunnel syndrome in rabbits by using a wire suture to approximate the radial and ulnar walls of the carpal canal, thereby reducing the volume of the carpal tunnel. On the other side, the suture was tied without tension. The animals were killed 1, 2, and 3 weeks after the procedure.

Findings.—Fibrous tissue proliferation was apparent macroscopically about the flexor tendons when the carpal volume was reduced, but it was not apparent in the control extremity. New small arteries, venules, and capillaries were observed, and there was an exudate containing neutrophils and monocytes around the vessel walls. Fibrosis was most extensive when compression had been present for longer periods.

Pathogenesis.—A decrease in volume of the carpal tunnel causes the pressure to rise and results in deterioration of the endothelial lining of venules and capillaries, increased vascular permeability, and edema formation. Leukocytes adhere to the vessel walls and migrate extravascularly, after which some of them transform into fibroblasts and deposit collagen. The outcome is fibrosis of the synovium of the flexor tendons (Fig 4–22).

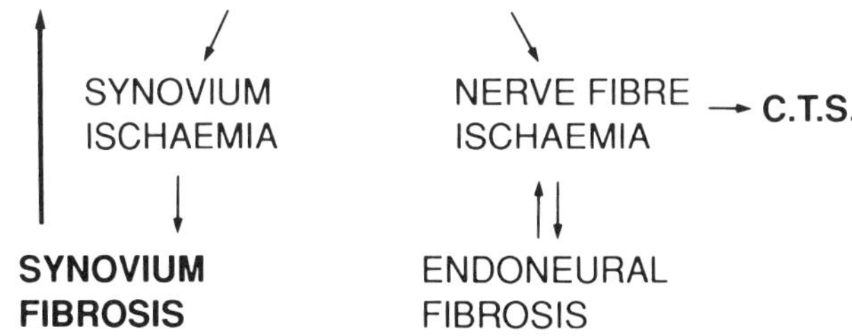

Fig 4–22.—*Abbreviation:* *CTS,* carpal tunnel syndrome. Schematic representaton of changes occurring when intracarpal pressure increases. (Courtesy of Lluch AL: *J Hand Surg (Br)* 17B:209–212, 1992.)

Conclusion.—Edema and fibroblastic proliferation are reactions to local ischemia, rather than causes of carpal tunnel syndrome.

▶ As noted in the previous abstract, carpal tunnel syndrome can be the result of a number of different causes, but all of them eventually compress the median nerve. Because thickening of the flexor tendons is often seen in patients who have the condition, could it be that this either is the cause or contributes to the cause? If so, it would require alterations in standard therapies for the condition. Lluch decided that the thickening is a *consequence* of the syndrome, not its cause. We need not alter our therapy to take this into account.—D.J. Lawrence, D.C.

Scapholunate Failure: A Long Term Clinical Follow-Up

Mior SA, Dombrowsky N (Canadian Mem Chiropractic College, Toronto)

J Manipulative Physiol Ther 15:255–260, 1992 4–61

Background.—"Carpal instability" has become a catch-all term to describe any loss of normal alignment of carpal structures, but Mayfield suggests that injuries of the wrist should be considered as part of a continuum of mechanical dysfunction. In a study of a patient with rotary subluxation of the carpal scaphoid, the anatomy, biomechanics, diagnosis, and treatment of scapholunate failure were examined.

Case Report.—Man, 43, had progressive right wrist pain of 6 weeks' duration with an onset attributed to difficulties pull-starting a motor. There was moderate effusion over the area of the right scapholunate articulation and moderate limitation of range of motion by pain on ulnar deviation and flexion. The wrist was treated for a second-degree sprain with electric stimulation and gentle long axis mobilization, and it was supported by taping and a wrist orthotic. The right wrist also had a 10-year history of recurrent pain resulting from a forced hyperdorsiflexion injury that had been treated with cortisone injections, a carpal tunnel release, and chiropractic manipulation to the wrist. There was slow improvement until the wrist injury was reaggravated. After the reinjury, the scapholunate articulation was very painful and was associated with crepitation. Radiographs revealed disassociation of the scapholunate joint and a rotary subluxation of the scaphoid, which was treated with a customized wrist orthotic and monitoring. A radioscapholunate fusion was performed almost 2 years after the injury; 6 years later, he had nearly constant pain, loss of all ranges of motion at the wrist except for about 15 degrees of dorsiflexion, and permanent work disability. Radiographs revealed collapse of the radiocarpal joint and moderate degenerative changes, especially at the scapholunate articulation.

Roentgenographic Findings.—Typical roentgenographic findings in rotary subluxation of the carpal scaphoid include widening of the gap between the scaphoid lunate in the anteroposterior projection, foreshortened appearance of the navicular with an associated ring, and vertical position of the scaphoid greater than 70 degrees.

Conclusion.—As illustrated by this patient, stabilization and other conservative care can reduce symptoms but do not deal with underlying pathology. In this patient, long-standing disassociation required triscaphoid fusion that ultimately failed. Early recognition of characteristic x-ray findings, with appropriate stabilization, may prevent the carpal joint from further collapse.

► The scaphoid bone is the most frequently fractured bone in the wrist; rarely, it will undergo rotary subluxation, creating a carpal instability. The scapholunate ligament helps to provide stability to the surrounding articulations, and if it is disrupted, as it was in this case, disassociation may occur. Radiographic evidence of this injury includes widening of the gap between the scaphoid and the lunate on anteroposterior plain films (the "Terry Thomas sign" [1]), vertical position of the scaphoid, and a shortened appearance of the bone with an associated ring sign. Failures, as seen in this case, are not amenable to conservative care.—D.J. Lawrence, D.C.

Reference

1. Frankel VH: *Clin Orthop* 129:321, 1977.

Sacral Neurofibroma in a Chiropractic Patient Presenting With Low Back and Leg Pain

LuBow RR, Kent C (New Milford, NJ; ICA Council on Imaging)

ICA Review 48:53–57, 1992 4–62

Introduction.—Spinal abnormalities occur in 60% of patients with neurofibromatosis. A patient with a history of neurofibromatosis who sought chiropractic care for low back and leg pain was examined. A large sacral neurofibroma was revealed by MRI.

Case Report.—Man, 52, received an incidental diagnosis of neurofibromatosis 10 years earlier, when his son was found to have the same condition. Before the diagnosis, the patient had been asymptomatic. In addition to the characteristic café-au-lait spots, the patient had a 5-year history of a "tingling sensation" in his left leg. He was seen with moderate low back pain and stiffness, as well as severe sciatica in the left leg. Plain radiographs of the lumbosacral spine and a myelographic study, obtained during neurologic consultation, were judged normal.

When the patient sought chiropractic care, MRI examinations were ordered and revealed a large sacral neurofibroma on the left posterior sacrum and another in the left foot. The patient declined surgery recommended by the neurology team. Clinical findings, with the exception of an unexplained white blood cell count of 21,000, were consistent with the working diagnosis of neurofibroma-induced mechanical disturbance. Conservative chiropractic care, designed to correct the lesions associated with the vertebral subluxation complex, were then initiated. Eight weeks later, after 3 visits per week, the patient was free of pain. At 18-month follow-up, he reports only a mild stiffness 90% of the time. Occasional exacerbations appear to be triggered by a specific traumatic event.

Conclusion.—A careful study of MRI studies showed the relationship of adjacent spinal nerves to the tumor. Because the pattern of pain was nondermatomal in distribution, no reflex changes had occurred, and the pinwheel examination was normal, chiropractic care was appropriate as a first option.

▶ Neurofibromatosis is rarely seen in a chiropractic setting, but as primary-care physicians, we should be familiar with its presenting symptoms and signs. In this paper, the radiographic findings of the condition are also discussed, and the author provides a detailed description of the therapy he chose to use in managing the patient's pain. Case reports are important to the profession because they provide a barometer of the full spectrum of chiropractic diagnosis and therapy.—D.J. Lawrence, D.C.

Effect of Osteopathic Medical Management on Neurologic Development in Children

Frymann VM, Carney RE, Springall P (Osteopathic Ctr for Children, La Jolla, Calif; Timao Found for Research and Development, San Diego, Calif; Springall Academy, La Jolla, Calif)

J Am Osteopath Assoc 92:729–744, 1992 4–63

Objective.—Manipulative osteopathic treatment was investigated in children to determine whether it influences neurologic development.

Subjects.—Forty-three children aged 18 months to 12 years, some of whom had neurologic deficits, were followed up for 3 years. Six to 12 osteopathic manipulative treatments were directed to areas of impaired physiologic motion with the goal of reducing the influence of somatic dysfunction on cerebral function.

Assessment.—Houle's Profile of Development was used to estimate neurologic developmental status. This profile evaluates sensory performance, manual competence, mobility, and spoken language.

Findings.—Neurologic performance significantly improved after treatment in children with defined neurologic problems, and to a lesser extent in those given a medical or structural diagnosis (Fig 4–23). Improvement continued to occur over several months of observation.

Conclusion.—The use of osteopathic manipulative treatment (when indicated) in pediatric patients was supported. Children with neurologic problems have exhibited significantly improved sensory and motor functions.

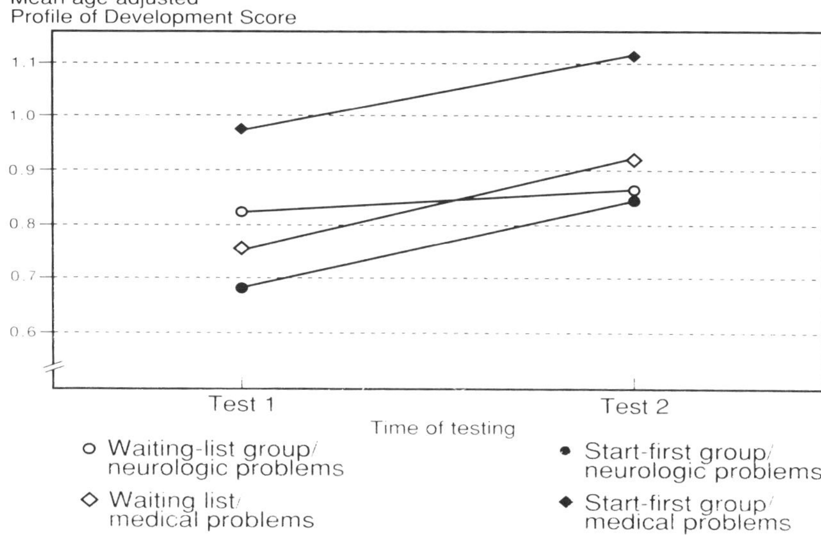

Fig 4–23.—Comparison of changes in average total Profile of Development scores between first and second testings for children classified by research group, waiting-list (wait) or start-first (start), and by type of problem, neurologic (neuro) or medical (med). Test 1 for the wait subgroups is pretest, and test 2, post-test with treatment between the 2 testings. (Courtesy of Frymann VM, Carney RE, Springall P: *J Am Osteopath Assoc* 92:729–744, 1992.)

▶ Let me quote from the introduction to this paper: "This study was designed to test the clinical view that intervention directed toward removal or reducing the influence of somatic dysfunction permits neurologic development and performance to progress to a child's optimum potential." If we substitute the word "subluxation" for the words "somatic dysfunction," we are provided with a chiropractic rationale for taking pediatric cases, something which has become quite controversial during the past year. Exciting as this may be, there are some concerns in this work. The 2 groups tested are not the same; the medical group included children with medical or structural problems but without somatic dysfunction, and the neurologic group included children with known problems such as behavioral problems or developmental delays. No real meaningful comparisons can be made here. Other methadologic problems also exist, and although both groups responded to therapy, there is no control to examine their results against. There may certainly be important roles for osteopathy or chiropractic to play in managing children, but this paper will do little to assuage any concerns other healthcare professional may have.—D.J. Lawrence, D.C.

Special Topic: Knee

A Prospective and Blinded Investigation of Magnetic Resonance Imaging of the Knee: Abnormal Findings in Asymptomatic Subjects

Boden SD, Davis DO, Dina TS, Stoller DW, Brown SD, Vailas JC, Labropoulos PA (George Washington Univ, Washington, DC)

Clin Orthop 282:177–185, 1992 4–64

Purpose.—With recent improvements in MRI technology, its diagnostic accuracy in pathologic conditions of the knee joint has increased to about 90%. However, the issue of specificity—that is, the incidence of false positives—remains unknown. The incidence of abnormal knee MRI findings was documented in asymptomatic volunteers.

Methods.—The study sample comprised 74 volunteers with an average age 34 years. None had any history of knee pain, swelling, locking, or giving way or any knee injury or surgery. Each subject had multiplanar MRI scans of 1 knee. The scans were intermixed with 26 scans from symptomatic patients and were then reviewed in independent and blinded fashion by 3 radiologists.

Results.—A meniscal abnormality consistent with the presence of a tear was found in 16% of the asymptomatic subjects. This finding increased with age, from 13% in subjects younger than 45 years to 36% in those older than 45 (table). Another meniscal abnormality was present in an additional 30% of volunteers—this consisted of a linear area of increased signal, not communicating with a meniscal edge and not believed to represent a tear. There were no ligamentous abnormalities and only a few cases of mild degenerative changes. There was an 8% incidence of popliteal cyst.

Conclusion.—A high incidence of abnormal knee MRI findings was demonstrated in asymptomatic subjects. The findings emphasize the difficulty of relying on diagnostic tests alone, with no clinical correlation. It

MRI-Evident Meniscal Signal (Grade 1 and 2) in Asymptomatic Subjects

	Age (Years)							
	16–25	*(n = 14)*	*26–45*	*(n = 49)*	*46–65*	*(n = 11)*	*All*	*(n = 74)*
Location	*No.*	*%*	*No.*	*%*	*No.*	*%*	*No.*	*%*
Medial								
Anterior	1	7	6	12	3	27	10	14
Posterior	8	57	28	57	8	73	44	59
Lateral								
Anterior	4	29	9	18	3	27	16	22
Posterior	4	29	13	27	6	55	23	31

(Courtesy of Boden SD, Davis DO, Dina TS, et al: *Clin Orthop* 282:177–185, 1992.)

is vital to have access to clinical data when reading MRI scans of the knee.

▶ Previous research has demonstrated a high incidence of apparent disk bulging in asymptomatic patients, casting questions regarding the sensitivity and specificity of the procedure. In this study, the sensitivity (percent of false negatives) and specificity (incidence of false positives) for MRI in asymptomatic knees is examined. There was still a relatively high percentage of abnormalities consistent with meniscal tear; this percentage increased with the age of the patient (13% in patients younger than age 45 years, and 36% when older than 45 years). This would indicate that positive MRI findings require correlation with clinical signs, particularly in the older patient complaining of knee pain. One possible bias in this study is that patients were recruited to represent a broad spectrum of age ranges, reflective of a typical practice; however, the abnormal findings are age dependent, which weakens the power of the study.—D.J. Lawrence, D.C.

Effects of Tibial Rotations on Patellar Tracking and Patello-Femoral Contact Areas

Hefzy MS, Jackson WT, Saddemi SR, Hsieh Y-F (Univ of Toledo, Ohio; Med College of Ohio, Toledo)

J Biomed Eng 14:329–343, 1992 4–65

Introduction.—The patellofemoral syndrome, characterized by pain in the anterior part of the knee, is consistently found in runners, but its actual cause is not well understood. Common to most proposed explanations is abnormal patellar tracking. Few studies have been done to discern a complete 3-dimensional picture of patellar tracking.

Objective.—The effects of tibial rotation on patellofemoral kinematics and contact areas were examined under physiologic loading conditions of the knee-extension exercise.

Methods.—A motion-tracking device that uses electromagnetic technology to determine the precise position and orientation of a sensor with respect to a source was used. Geometric data describing the patella, tibia, and femur were acquired using a 3-dimensional digitizer and tracker system (3-space). The kinematic and geometric data were then combined, and coordinate transformations between different coordinate systems were calculated to determine the relative positions of the femur, tibia, and patella (Figs 4–24 and 4–25). Experiments were done using fresh human cadaveric lower extremities.

Findings.—Tibial rotations produced significant differences in patellar tilt, patellar rotation, and patellar medial-lateral shift. The extent of the total contact area at a given knee flexion angle did not change significantly with tibial rotation, but the medial and lateral components of total contact areas were altered. Medial femoral contact increased with in-

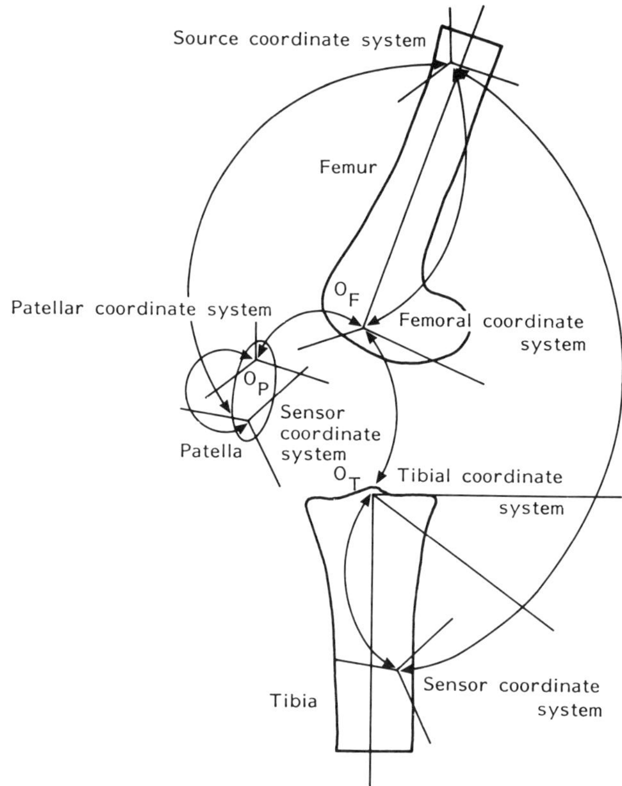

Fig 4–24.—Transformations among different sets of coordinate systems of axes used in analysis. The following systems of axes are identified: source coordinate system located within the source; sensor coordinate systems located within each sensor; and 3 bony coordinate systems of axes—the tibial, femoral, and patellar coordinate systems of axes. (Courtesy of Hefzy MS, Jackson WT, Saddemi SR, et al: *J Biomed Eng* 14:329-343, 1992.)

ternal tibial rotation at all felxion angles, while lateral femoral contact increased with external tibial rotation. Kinematically, the patella shifted medially on internal tibial rotation and tilted more medially near full extension, thereby increasing medial contact and reducing lateral contact.

Implications.—Differences in reported findings may relate to the use of differing techniques, variations in the degree of applied load or in the time of load application, biological differences between specimens, and measurement errors. Internal tibial rotation forces the patella to tilt medially, increasing medial patellar and femoral contact. The findings may explain why "runner's knee" is associated with rotatory changes in the tibia secondary to increased pronation of the foot.

▶ This elegant and difficult study used mathematical modeling drawn from cadaveric lower limbs to determine how the patella interacts with the tibia

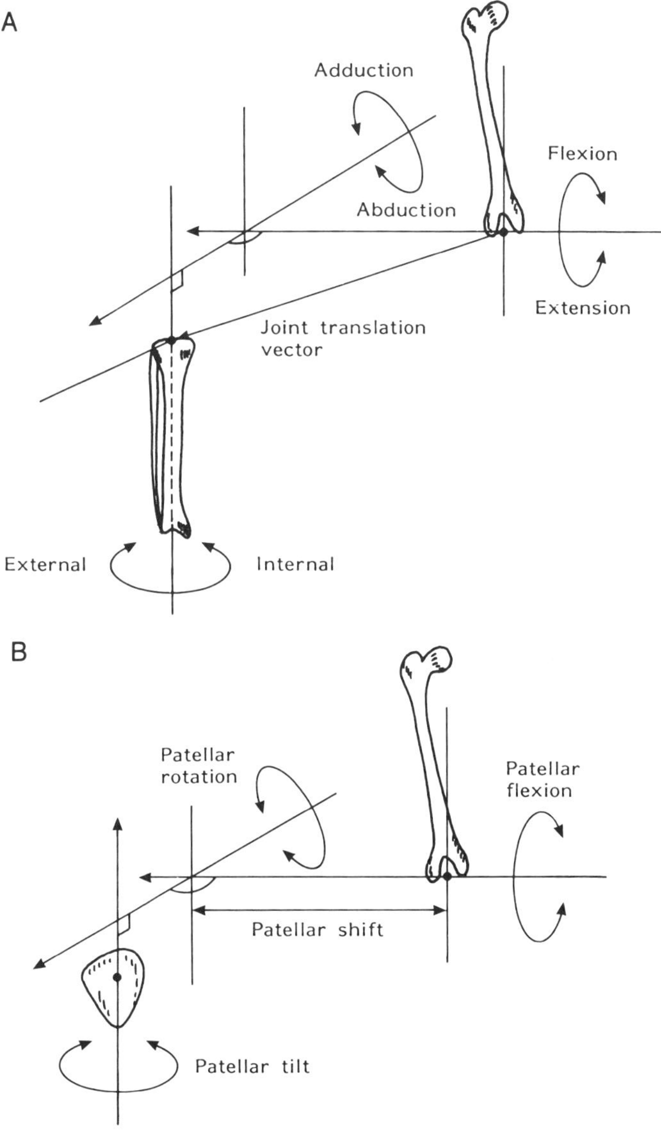

Fig 4–25.—Two joint coordinate systems used to describe 3-dimensional motions of tibiofemoral joint (**A**) and patellofemoral joint (**B**). (Courtesy of Hefzy MS, Jackson WT, Saddemi SR, et al: *J Biomed Eng* 14:329-343, 1992.)

when the latter rotates. The intent was to draw conclusions regarding patellar tracking problems in addressing the diagnosis of chondromalacia. The problem is that chondromalacia patellae is a pathologic diagnosis, not a clinical one; whether this is an appropriate diagnosis is still argued today. If the roughening of the undersurface of the patella does occur, there should be some way to assess how and in what situations the patella comes in contact with the tibial groove. This study does that, and it also examines patellar tracking. A significant finding is that patellofemoral contact forces are increased when foot pronation occurs, because the latter will cause tibial rotation. Reduction of foot pronation should be considered in the runner with pronated feet.—D.J. Lawrence, D.C.

Stress Fracture in the Medial Femoral Condyle: A Case Report
Lafforgue P, Acquaviva P-C (Centre Hospitalier, Marseille, France)
Acta Orthop Scand 63:563–565, 1992 4–66

Introduction.—In the absence of radiographic changes, a patient with suggestive symptoms and a medial condylar scintigraphic hot spot generally has osteonecrosis diagnosed. Magnetic resonance imaging (MRI) has recently proven of value in the diagnosis of osteonecrosis of the knee and occult intraosseous fractures. A patient had a stress fracture of the medial femoral condyle that was recognized only on MRI.

Case Report.—Woman, 88, had pain in the medial aspect of her right knee. She had tenderness of the medial femoral condyle, with pain on passive flexion but no effusion. Plain x-ray films were normal 2 weeks after the onset of symptoms and showed only slight mottled sclerotic changes at 5 weeks. Radionuclide bone scanning showed an intense hot spot in the right medial femoral condyle. The MRI, done to confirm the provisional diagnosis of osteonecrosis, showed a horizontal, sharply defined linear band within the medial condyle. This, along with an ill-defined halo of low-high signal on T1/T2 sequences, was considered

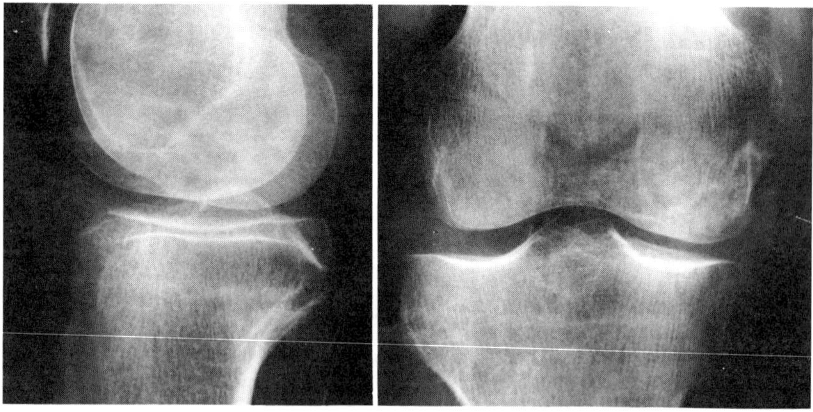

Fig 4–26.—X-ray films 5 weeks after onset of pain show moderate and nonspecific mottled sclerotic changes in the medial femoral condyle. (Courtesy of Lafforgue P, Acquaviva P-C: *Acta Orthop Scand* 63:563–565, 1992.)

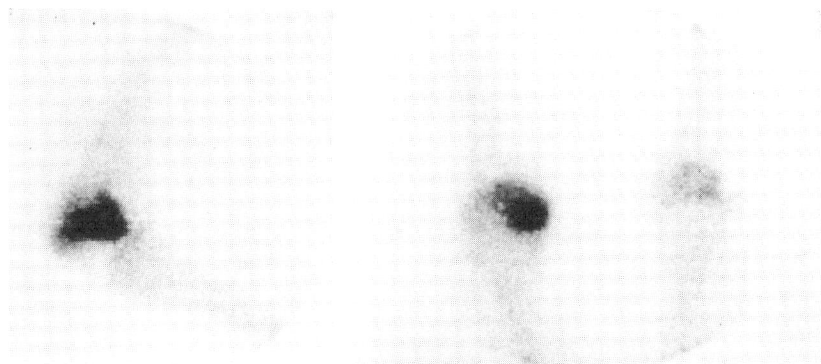

Fig 4–27.—Radionuclide bone scans show intense hot spots in the medial femoral condyle. (Courtesy of Lafforgue P, Acquaviva P-C: *Acta Orthop Scand* 63:563–565, 1992.)

typical of stress fracture, given the lack of an osteonecrotic lesion (Figs 4–26, 4–27, and 4–28). Bed rest and calcitonin therapy resulted in complete resolution of pain within 3 weeks.

Conclusion.—In this case, MRI demonstrated a stress fracture of the medial femoral condyle in a patient whose clinical and scintigraphic findings suggested spontaneous osteonecrosis. In contrast to the images in this patient, the MRI appearance of osteonecrosis is a variable-signal lesion surrounded by a well-defined margin within a more diffuse area of altered signal.

▶ Stress fractures are often difficult to diagnose, because they often are not seen on intake radiographs. Although scinitigraphy may demonstrate hot spots, the finding may indicate osteonecrosis as well as fracture. Magnetic resonance imaging is much more sensitive. The characteristic appearance is

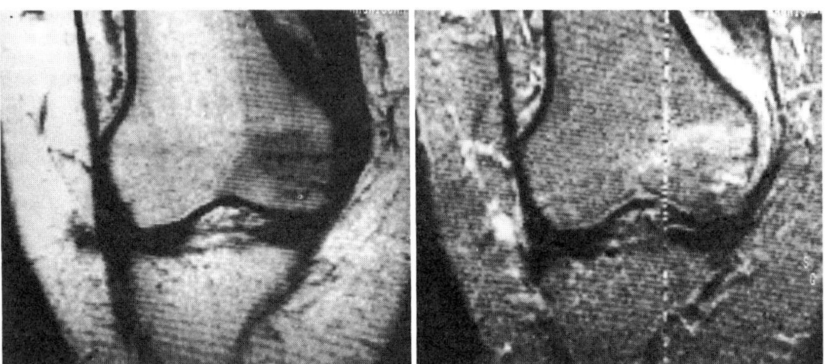

Fig 4–28.—Magnetic resonance imaging. **Left,** T1 sequences (TR 450 ms/TE 28 ms) show low-signal, horizontal, sharply defined line surrounded by more diffuse area of low signal. **Right,** both T1 lesions have high signal on T2 examination (TR 1,800 ms/TE 120 ms). (Courtesy of Lafforgue P, Acquaviva P-C: *Acta Orthop Scand* 63:563–565, 1992.)

a linear band in the condyle, with low signal intensity on T1-weighted images, but high intensity on the T2-weighted images. It is likely that the diagnosis of osteonecrosis in the knee is often made incorrectly in lieu of stress fracture; judicious use of MRI is a new tool to help distinguish the two.—D.J. Lawrence, D.C.

Normal Limits of Knee Angle in White Children: Genu Varum and Genu Valgum

Heath CH, Staheli LT (Univ of Washington, Seattle; Children's Hosp and Med Ctr, Seattle)

J Pediatr Orthop 13:259–262, 1993 4–67

Introduction.—Knee angle progresses from bowlegs in infancy to knock knees in early childhood. Data on normal limits are available for Chinese children but not for white children. Such data could be collected by plain film radiography, but this would be expensive and expose the children to radiation.

Methods.—To establish normal limits for tibiofemoral angle, measurements of knee angle and intermalleolar (IM) or intercondylar (IC) distance were obtained in 196 white children. The children ranged in age from 6 months to 11 years. Knee angle measurements were made photographically. Two axes were drawn for each lower extremity, one connecting the anterior supcrior iliac spine and the center of the patella and the other connecting the patella and a point halfway between the medial and lateral malleoli.

Findings.—Based on pooled data for both sexes, there was a trend from extreme bowlegs before age of 18 months to maximal knock knees at 4 years, after which knee angle progressed gradually toward neutral. The greatest mean varus of 16 degrees was noted at 6 months of age, whereas a maximum valgus of 9 degrees was noted at 4 years. This was the only age at which there was a significant sex difference, with girls tending to be more knock-kneed. A similar course of development was reflected by measurement of IC or IM distance.

Conclusion.—Age-specific ranges of normal for knee angle were established in developing white children. At none of the ages studied did normal knee angle include any amount of varus, with even 11-year-old children having at least 2.5 degrees of valgus. Bowlegs in children older than 2 years of age is abnormal. The need for treatment of extreme valgus or varus was not addressed.

▶ Normal limits for knee angles in children have not been adequately established, leaving confusion concerning how much genu varum or valgum is present before a pathologic condition is suggested. Intercondylar and intermalleolar measurements, along with knee angle measurements, were made on a group of children to help set those norms. There may be some room for error here, because 2 of these measures involved the use of a tape measure; this increases the risk of low intrarater reliability, which in fact was not assessed by this study. However, given the shortcoming, the values obtained indicate that up to 12 degrees of valgus is normal, although this is age dependent (with small infants generally showing varus angulation up to age 2 years); up to 8 mm for intermalleolar distance and 3 mm for intercondylar distance is normal. With these norms in place, a standard is set for identification of pathology. Screening procedures can now be accomplished with greater accuracy.—D.J. Lawrence, D.C.

Long Patellar Tendon: Radiographic Sign of Patellofemoral Pain Syndrome: A Prospective Study

Kannus PA (President Urho Kaleva Kekkonen Inst, Tampere, Finland)

Radiology 185:859–863, 1992 4–68

Introduction.—Patellofemoral pain syndrome is a common musculoskeletal disorder in physically active people that progresses rapidly to a chronic state. There is great confusion as to the definition of this syndrome and the radiologic criteria for "pathologic" position of the patella. Studies of this syndrome must be prospective to define the study group adequately, must include only unilateral cases to allow comparison with the healthy knee, and must use only a few well-established radiologic criteria.

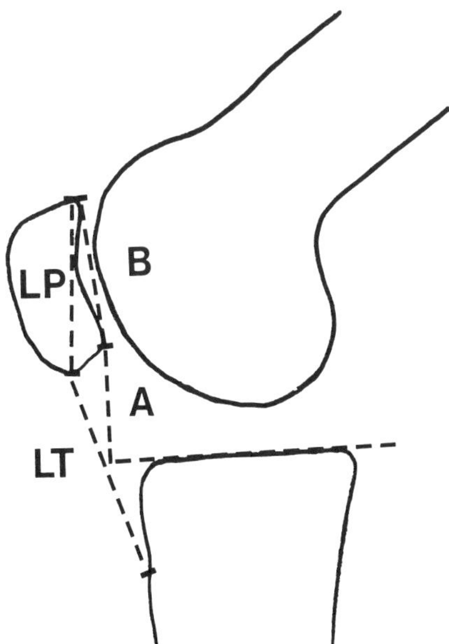

Fig 4–29.—Methods of measuring height of patella on lateral x-ray film. The Insall-Salvati index is the ratio of the length of the patellar tendon (*LT*) to the greatest diagonal length of patella (*LP*). The Blackburne-Peel index is the ratio of the shortest distance between the lower pole of the patellar articular cartilage and tibial plateau (*A*) to the articular length of patella (*B*). (Courtesy of Kannus PA: *Radiology* 185:859–863, 1992.)

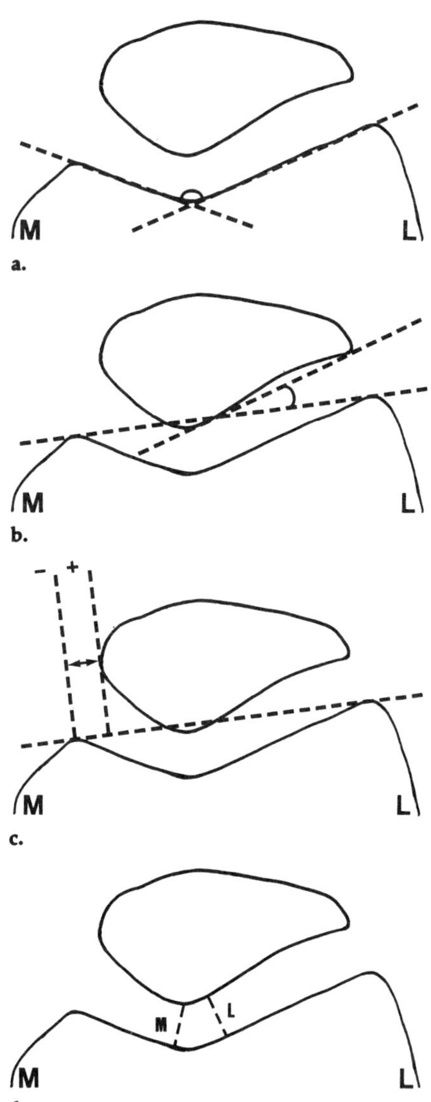

Fig 4–30.—Methods of determining shape of interchondylar sulcus and mediolateral position of patella to demonstrate possible patellofemoral incongruence and lateral patellar tilt. *L*, lateral side of the knee; and *M*, medial side of the knee. **a,** sulcus angle. **b,** lateral patellofemoral angle (LPA). According to Laurin et al., in normal knees, LPA always opens laterally; in chondromalacia, 10% of the patients show parallel lines (0 degrees); and in recurrent dislocation of the patella, 60% of the patients show parallel lines, and in the other 40%, LPA opens medially in evidence of lateral patellar tilt. **c,** lateral patellofemoral displacement (LPD), expressed in millimeters. According to Laurin et al., in normal knees, LPD is always 0 or negative (negative indicates medial displacement). Thirty percent of patients with chondromalacia and 53% of patients with recurrent dislocation of the patella have positive LPD values. **d,** Patellofemoral index. This index is defined as the relationship between relative thickness of medial (*M*) and lateral (*L*) patellofemoral compartments (*M/L*). Measurement *M* is the shortest distance between the medial femoral groove and the junction of the medial and lateral patellar facets. Measurement *L* corresponds to the shortest distance between lateral patellar facet and lateral femoral condyle. According to Laurin et al., in all normal knees, PFI is 1.6 or less, but in 93% of patients with chondromalacia and all patients with recurrent dislocation of patella, PFI is greater than 1.6. Laurin et al. regard PFI as a good indicator of lateral "mini-tilt" of patella. (Courtesy of Kannus PA: *Radiology* 185:859-863, 1992.)

Methods.—Patellar position was assessed prospectively in 45 consecutive patients with unilateral patellofemoral pain syndrome. The subjects were 24 women and 21 men; 28 were recreational athletes, and 17 were competitive athletes. None of these subjects had any signs or symptoms of patellar instability at their first examination. Using standardized anteroposterior, lateral, and tangential x-ray films, the investigators calculated 6 measures of patellar position in each knee: ratio of the patellar tendon to the greatest diagonal length of the patella (Fig 4–29), sulcus angles, lateral patellofemoral angle, lateral patellar displacemant, patellofemoral index (Fig 4–30), and knee angle.

Findings.—On comparison with the healthy knees, the patellar tendons in the symptomatic knees were significantly longer, whereas the patellar lengths were equal. This was confirmed for all measures of patellar height. The sulcus angle, lateral patellofemoral angle, lateral patellar displacement, patellofemoral index, and knee angle were not significantly different between the 2 groups.

Conclusion.—Patella alta is closely related to idiopathic patellofemoral pain syndrome. Because it alters the contact area of the patellofemoral joint, patella alta could be an important causal factor. Patellofemoral incongruence and lateral patellar tilt do not appear to play an important role.

▶ Patellar pain syndrome (a more acceptable term these days than chondromalacia patellae) is a poorly understood clinical entity. The causes advanced as factors in its etiology include trauma, overuse, congenital abnormalities, increase Q angle, malalignment in the extension process of the knee, and patella alta. Based on the results of this study, patella alta must be seen as at least a contributory factor to the disease. Great care was taken in matching patient populations and to ensure comparison within patients (only 1 knee of the subject was affected, leaving the other as a matched control). The study also took into account the shape of knee and tibiofemoral region; these were found to be similar between the experimental and control groups. The chief factor appears to be a long patellar tendon, which allows the patella to ride high. Management of patients with patellar tracking disorders will need to include examination for this finding and therapy should be altered accordingly.—D.J. Lawrence, D.C.

When to Prescribe a Knee Brace

Zachazewski JE, Geissler G (Massachusetts Gen Hosp, Boston; Harvard Univ, Cambridge, Mass)

Physician Sportsmed 20:91–99, 1992 4–69

Introduction.—Wearing a knee brace during activity to stabilize an injured knee or to prevent knee injury may or may not be effective. Before the availability of today's knee brace, athletic directors and players taped knees to achieve mechanical stability. The various types of knee braces are reviewed along with their degree of benefit to the active athlete.

Effectiveness.—Prophylactic braces have been available for about 15 years. Their primary use focuses on protecting the medial collateral ligament (MCL) in the event of a lateral blow or lowering the valgus stress to the normal knee (Fig 4–31). Functional braces attempt to stabilize the unstable knee and to allow maximum function, whereas rehabilitative braces absolutely immobilize the knee after injury or surgery.

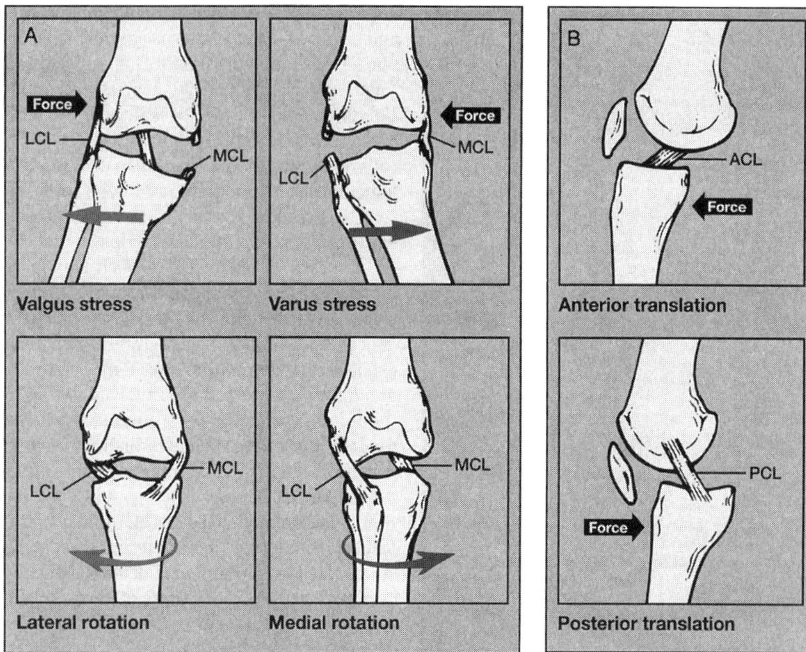

Fig 4–31.—Braces are used to stabilize the knee from abnormal rotation or translation (**A, B**). (Courtesy of Zachazewski JE, Geissler G: *Physician Sportsmed* 20:91-99, 1992.)

Results.—Prophylactic braces may or may not work; both positive and negative results have been reported. Thus, clinicians should use prophylactic braces only if the individual athlete appears to benefit from a particular device design. For functional braces, again clinicians should consider the differing outcomes of studies with a host of device types. Extrapolating the results of reported trials with functional braces to high-velocity, high-force actual sports activities may not work. Clinicians should consider that the main benefit often is psychological rather than medical or mechanical. Patients must understand that use of the brace requires their full compliance. They should sign an informed consent agreement stating that the patient completely understands that the risks and benefits of the knee brace depend on proper use of the brace. Selection of the correct device requires knowledge of the athlete, the sport, the cost effectiveness of the respective devices, their durability, and their fit and comfort.

Conclusion.—Complete brace treatment also includes simultaneous rehabilitation and conditioning, activity modification, and possible surgical intervention. Realistic expectations must accompany the therapy outline.

▶ This paper provides a basic set of guidelines to aid the clinician who is selecting the appropriate knee brace for his or her patients. Of special interest in this study is a short discussion of the ethical and legal issues surrounding bracing, which raises the important yet little considered question of liability when prescribing a brace to a team athlete based on position or relative risk. The suggestions concerning informed consent should be followed; in some states, this is required. To the authors list of points for the informed consent form, I would also add a statement concerning the benefit of the brace. Although short, this paper contains a host of worthy recommendations and information.—D.J. Lawrence, D.C.

Difficult Reductions in Traumatic Patellar Dislocation

Roger DJ, Williamson SC, Uhl RL (Albany Med College, NY)

Orthop Rev 21:1333–1341, 1992 4–70

Introduction.—Unreduced patellar dislocations are commonly reduced in the emergency department with the use of analgesics, sedation, and knee extension with medial force to the patella. However, there have been patellar dislocations that could not be reduced in this way, frequently requiring open reduction instead.

Patients.—Two patients with patellar dislocation that did not respond to conventional reduction maneuvers are reported. In the first case, a medially directed force was unsuccessful; it seemed only to increase the tension of the extensor mechanism (Fig 4–32). Downward pressure was then applied to the lateral aspect of the displaced patella, resulting in unlocking of the patella from the lateral femoral condyle (Fig 4–33). In the second case, a lateral radiograph demonstrated a full 90-degree internal rotation deformity of the patella. Again, a lateral and downward force against the lateral aspect of the patella reduced the rotational component of the dislocation. This allowed reduction of the rotational deformity with a medially directed force.

Conclusion.—Unreducible patellar dislocations can involve varying degrees of internal rotation of the patella. In some cases, the medial facet or anterior surface of the patella may be locked into the lateral aspect of the lateral femoral condyle. This dislocation, which may be reduced by a downward force on the lateral aspect of the patella, should

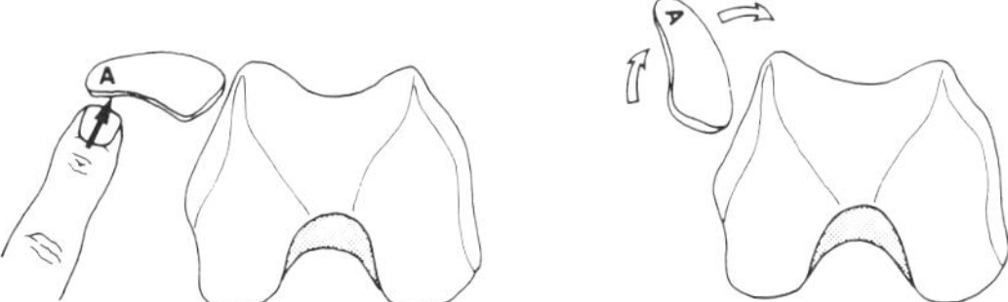

Fig 4–32.—Medially directed pressure applied to the patella from the lateral side in this case will increase the amount of internal rotation and accentuate the deformity. This reduction maneuver is unlikely to be successful in reducing this type of patellar dislocation. (Courtesy of Roger DJ, Williamson SC, Uhl RL: *Orthop Rev* 21:1333–1341, 1992.)

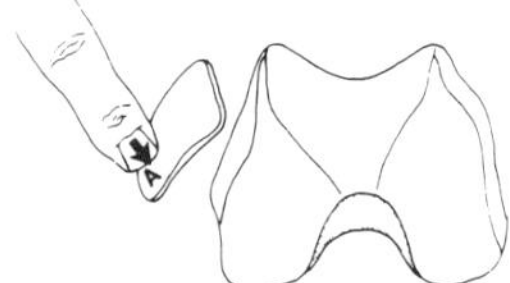
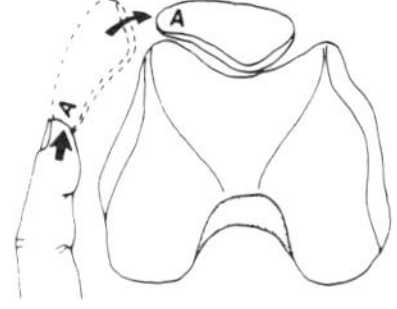

Fig 4–33.—A downward force applied to the lateral facet produces an external rotatory force on the patella. This unlocks the medial facet from the lateral condyle and facilitates a successful reduction. (Courtesy of Roger DJ, Williamson SC, Uhl RL: *Orthop Rev* 21:1333–1341, 1992.)

be considered in patients with an acutely dislocated patella that has the knee in nearly full extension and does not respond to conventional reduction maneuvers.

▶ Lateral dislocation of the patella is fairly common and can often be the result of congenital malformations in the tibiofemoral region. In normal cases, the reduction is fairly uncomplicated, if painful, for the patient. The authors present cases of apparent lateral dislocations that failed to easily reduce; further investigation demonstrated that, in addition to the dislocation, the patella had rotated 90 degrees internally. A standard reduction procedure in such cases would fail; the authors recommend that downward pressure be used when guiding the patella back into joint proximity. Internal rotation should be suspected when a patient has had an acute dislocation, when the knee is kept in full extension, and when the knee fails to respond to standard reduction procedures.—D.J. Lawrence, D.C.

High Tibial Osteotomy and Ligament Reconstruction in Varus Angulated, Anterior Cruciate Ligament-Deficient Knees: A Two- to Seven-Year Follow-Up Study

Noyes FR, Barber SD, Simon R (Cincinnati Sportsmedicine Ctr; Deaconess Hosp, Cincinnati, Ohio)

Am J Sports Med 21:2–12, 1993 4–71

Objective.—The short-term surgical results were reviewed in 41 patients having both anterior cruciate ligament (ACL) deficiency and varus alignment. All patients had a high tibial osteotomy. Fourteen also had a lateral iliotibial band extra-articular procedure because of symptoms of giving way. Sixteen patients underwent intra-articular ACL allograft reconstruction after osteotomy. The mean postoperative follow-up interval was 58 months.

Initial State.—All but 1 of the patients sustained ACL rupture 2 years or longer before osteotomy, the mean interval being almost 10 years. Thirty patients had sports-related injuries. In all cases, the ACL was totally ruptured or absent at preoperative arthroscopic examination. Twenty-two patients had abnormal lateral joint opening on varus stress testing. Ninety-four previous operations had been carried out.

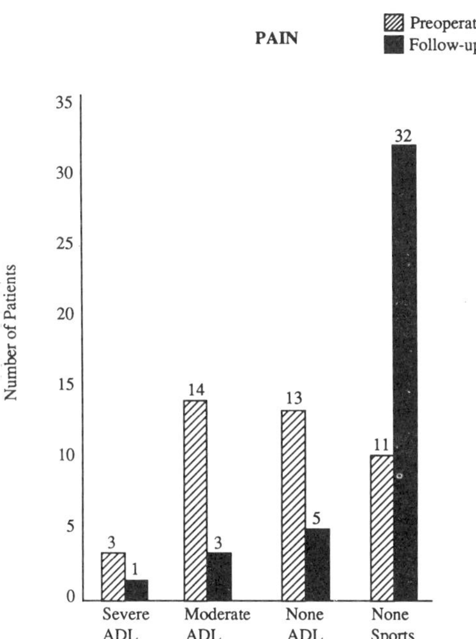

Fig 4–34.—The distribution of patient responses (n = 41) to the pain scale is shown preoperatively and at follow-up. The improvement was statistically significant (P < .05). (Courtesy of Noyes FR, Barber SD, Simon R: *Am J Sports Med* 21:2–12, 1993.)

Results.—Pain, swelling, and giving way all improved to a significant degree after surgery. Only 11 patients had been able to engage in light sports activity without pain before surgery, whereas 32 had no pain on light sports activity postoperatively (Fig 4–34). Symptoms of subchondral bone exposure usually had significant symptomatic improvement. All but 12% of patients would have had the operation again (Fig 4–35). Postoperative displacement in the anteroposterior plane was least in patients having allograft reconstruction of the ACL.

Discussion.—Osteotomy is indicated to eliminate symptoms in patients who have significant medial tibiofemoral arthrosis and symptoms during daily activities. Less severely affected patients who wish to return to strenuous activity may require ligament reconstruction.

▶ Why include a paper that deals solely with the result of surgery? There are several reasons: (1) some chiropractic patients will have been treated surgically before their chiropractic visit; (2) some will ultimately need to be referred for surgical consult; and (3) we need to be familiar with standard medical procedures and the reasons why they are used, as well as their rates of success. The high tibial osteotomy is used in situations where there is anterior cruciate deficiency coupled with varus angulation; the procedure helps to redistribute loads on the knee onto its lateral aspect and thus decrease

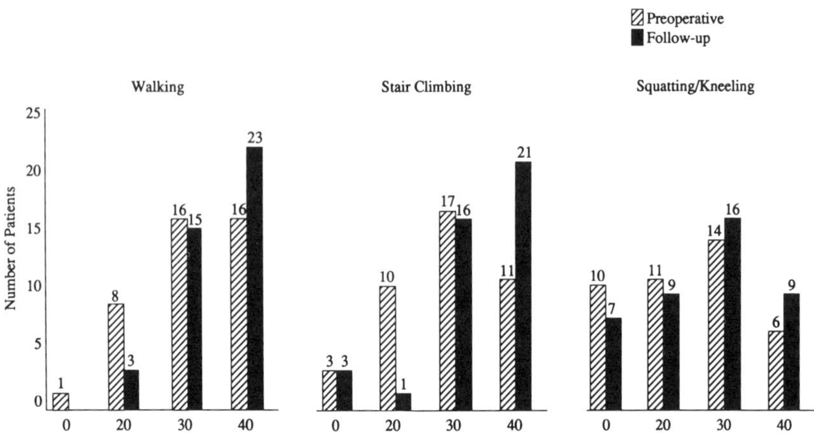

Fig 4–35.—The distribution of patient responses ($n = 41$) to the 3 functions of daily living are shown preoperatively and at follow-up. The population showed statistically significant improvement in stair climbing ($P < .05$). (Courtesy of Noyes FR, Barber SD, Simon R: *Am J Sports Med* 21:2–12, 1993.)

mechanical abnormality. Although the operation is well accepted, its success rate has not been adequately established. Fortunately, a relatively small percentage of anterior cruciate ligament–deficient knees are recommended for this surgery; there also several known complications for the procedure, including reoccurrence of varus angulation, development of patella baja, and arthritic formation.—D.J. Lawrence, D.C.

The PCL Line: An Indirect Sign of Anterior Cruciate Ligament Injury

Schweitzer ME, Cervilla V, Kursunoglu-Brahme S, Resnick D (VA Med Ctr; Univ of California, San Diego)

Clin Imaging 16:43–48, 1992 4–72

Objective.—Although several studies have demonstrated that MRI is highly accurate for anterior cruciate ligament (ACL) injury, others have failed to reproduce these results. When the ACL is injured, the tibia can shift forward, causing a change in the orientation of the posterior cruciate ligament (PCL) on MRI. A more vertical orientation of the distal PCL was studied as a useful secondary MRI sign of ACL injury.

Methods.—The MRI findings of 31 patients with suspected ACL injuries and 50 normal controls were examined. Using the image in which the distal PCL was best observed, a line was drawn along the posterior margin of the linear distal portion of the PCL and was extended proximally to show the ligament's relation to the femur. A positive line did not intersect the medullary cavitiy of the femur, whereas a negative line intersected the medullary cavity within 5 cm of its distal aspect.

Results.—Twenty-two of the 31 patients with suspected ACL injury were later confirmed as having a tear; a positive PCL line correctly predicted injury in 19 of the 22. The 3 patients with false negative PCL lines were noted on review to have hyperextension of the knee. The PCL line was negative in 47 of 50 controls. The sensitivity of the PCL line was 86%; specificity, 94%; positive predictive value, 86%; and negative predictive value, 94%.

Conclusion.—When MRI examination is inconclusive about the presence of an ACL tear, the PCL line is useful aid in diagnosis. When MRI is done with the knee in slight flexion, the relaxation of fascicles interferes with visualization. When ACL function is lost, it will change the position of the tibia at the limits of normal motion. Some patients will have a false negative PCL line if MRI is done with the knee in hyperextension.

▶ The standard MRI appearance of a torn ACL is discontinuity with a focal mass nearby that has increased signal on T2-weighted images. Like many other imaging studies, there is a modest probability that the MRI may fail to demonstrate these findings, thus leading to misdiagnosis. In this study, a new method was demonstrated that involved drawing a line along the posterior margin of the PCL and extending it proximally. If that line intersects the medullary cavity of the femur, it is a negative PCL sign. This procedure can help augment the accurate diagnosis of ACL tear where clinical impressions may be confusing. It does, however, need to undergo further established and refined before coming into common use.—D.J. Lawrence, D.C.

The Predictive Value of Radiographs in the Evaluation of Unilateral and Bilateral Anterior Cruciate Ligament Injuries

Schickendantz MS, Weiker GG (Cleveland Clinic Found, Ohio)

Am J Sports Med 21:110–113, 1993 4–73

Purpose.—Despite extensive literature about anterior cruciate ligament (ACL) injuries, there is little information on the uncommon bilateral ACL injury. The relatively few studies of the intercondylar notch have suggested that its shape or size may play an important role in the development of complete tears of the ACL, although this concept is controversial.

Methods.—Two hundred fifty patients undergoing surgical reconstruction of the ACL were reviewed to identify the prevalence of bilateral injury, the variables increasing the likelihood of bilateral ACL injury, and the role of radiographs and intercondylar notch measurements in the assessment of ACL injuries. The prevalence of bilateral injuries was assessed, and these patients were compared to patients with unilateral ACL injuries. In addition, standardized measurements of intercondylar notch height and width, and medial and lateral femoral condyle height and width on routine notch view radiographs were compared in 31

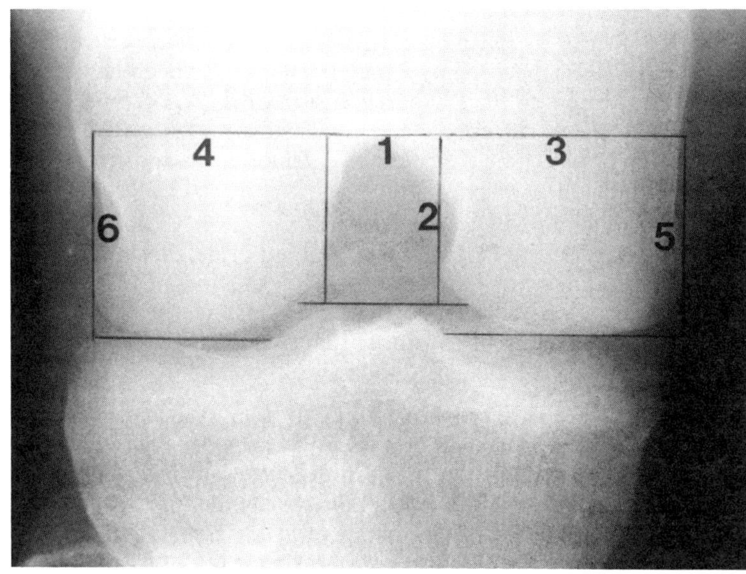

Fig 4–36.—Notchview radiograph demonstrating standardized measurements. *1,* notch width; *2,* notch height; *3,* medial condylar width; *4,* lateral condylar width; *5,* medial condylar height; *6,* lateral condylar height. (Courtesy of Schickendantz MS, Weiker GG: *Am J Sports Med* 21:110–113, 1993.)

knees of patients with bilateral ACL injuries, 30 knees of patients with unilateral injury, and 30 knees of patients with no injury (Fig 4–36).

Findings.—Twenty-four of the 250 patients had bilateral complete ACL tears, for a prevalence of nearly 10%. Twenty of the bilateral group had previous reconstruction of 1 ACL before rupture of the other. In 12 cases, the injury occurred during the same activity that had caused the initial opposite injury. An average of 29 months elapsed between reconstruction and rupture of the opposite ligament. The bilateral and unilateral groups showed no significant differences in other clinical or demographic characteristics. The radiographic analysis showed no significant differences among the 3 groups in any of 8 ratios calculated from the measurements described.

Conclusion.—Other than a previous complete rupture of the opposite ACL, sustained during the same or different activity, no significant clinical or demographic differences were identified between patients with bilateral vs. unilateral ACL injuries. In contrast to previous reports, radiographic measurements of the intercondylar notch are not reliable or reproducible predictors of ACL injury, and they are not needed for patient counseling.

▶ Ruptures of the ACL are career-threatening injuries to athletes. If predictors of this injury are found to exist, it would have a profound impact on training programs and rehabilitation plans. One of the methods advocated involves measuring the parameters of intercondylar notch and femoral condyle sizes. A strength of this study is that the author has populations of patients with one ligament damaged or 2 ligaments damaged, and also a set of normals for comparison. In this study, these measurements were not found reliable, and the authors therefore do not recommend their use. This seems a prudent recommendation. Chiropractors treating athletes may want to use other procedures in determining future prognoses for patients who have had cruciate ligament damage.—D.J. Lawrence, D.C.

Evaluation of Soft Foot Orthotics in the Treatment of Patellofemoral Pain Syndrome

Eng JJ, Pierrynowski MR (Univ of Waterloo, Ont, Canada; McMaster Univ, Hamilton, Ont, Canada)

Phys Ther 73:62–70, 1993 4–74

Background.—Patellofemoral pain syndrome (PFPS) is the main cause of chronic knee pain among adolescents. Its cause is unknown, but it is thought to result from abnormalities of the patellofemoral mechanics, causing uneven distribution of shear and compressive forces on the patellofemoral joint during normal activities. The effectiveness of foot orthotics in the treatment of PFPS has received limited attention.

Methods.—This randomized study compared the effects of soft foot orthotics plus an exercise program vs. exercise alone in the treatment of PFPS. The subjects were 20 adolescent girls (mean age, 15 years) with diagnosed bilateral PFPS and excessive forefoot varus or calcaneal valgus. All patients took part in a program of quadriceps femoris and ham-

TABLE 1.—Characteristics of Subjects ($n = 20$)

	Control Group* (n=10)		Treatment Group† (n=10)	
Variable	**$\bar{X}$**	**SD**	**$\bar{X}$**	**SD**
Age (y)	15.1	1.4	14.4	1.1
Height (cm)	160.5	9.6	159.4	4.0
Mass (kg)	53.2	10.0	50.2	8.0
Q-angle (°)	16.0	3.9	14.9	1.7
Forefoot varus (°)	12.6	2.8	12.4	3.7
Calcaneal valgus (°)	4.3	2.9	6.6	4.7
Knee pain (m)	9.7	9.9	10.0	9.8
Activity (h/wk)	7.4	5.2	7.2	5.6

* Control group = exercise only.
† Treatment group = exercise and orthotics.
(Courtesy of Eng JJ, Pierrynowski MR: *Phys Ther* 73:62-70, 1993.)

TABLE 2.—Analysis of Variance Summary for the Pain Response

Source	*df*	SS	MS	*F*	*P*
Group	1	831.37	831.37	7.92	.012
Error	18	1889.40	104.97		
Week	3	263.97	87.99	25.72	.0001
Week × group	3	39.32	13.10	3.83	.015
Error	54	184.72	3.42		
Activity	5	277.29	55.46	4.82	.0006
Activity × group	5	83.70	16.40	1.45	.21
Error	90	1035.48	11.50		
Week × activity	15	17.34	1.16	1.13	.33
Week × group × activity	15	19.12	1.27	1.24	.24
Error	270	277.04	1.03		

(Courtesy of Eng JJ, Pierrynowski MR: *Phys Ther* 73:62–70, 1993.)

string muscle strengthening and stretching exercise; half were also fitted with bilateral foot orthotics. Pain during the 8-week study was assessed by a visual analogue scale.

Results.—Baseline pain scores and descriptive variables were not different between the 2 groups (Table 1). Although both groups noted a significant decrease in pain, the treatment group achieved greater pain reduction (Table 2). The difference became significant beginning at 4 weeks for running, climbing stairs, going down stairs, and squatting.

Conclusion.—Soft foot orthotics plus exercise appears to be an effective treatment for adolescents with PFPS, at least for a short term. The benefits of orthotic treatment may relate to the motion of the tibiofemoral joint and the distribution of forces between the medial and lateral femoral condyles or the contact pressure and pattern between the patella and femoral condyles. The soft foot orthosis, an inexpensive and simple treatment, should be tried for at least 4 weeks because significant reduction in pain was not documented before that time.

▶ Foot orthotics are a very common device used in chiropractic practice. Great debate exists concerning whether weight-bearing or non–weight-bearing orthotics are best for common pedal and knee problems, but there is a paucity of research available to answer the question. As a result, use of these orthotics is largely based on clinical experience. Because patellofemoral pain syndrome is highly associated with pronation of the foot, use of an orthotic seems to make sense. In this study, although both groups benefited from therapy, the group using a soft orthotic responded more forcefully; they had better results. One potential problem in interpreting this study is that it was only extended for 8 weeks; therefore, the long-term benefits cannot be assessed. It may be that further down the line, the results between the groups may equalize.—D.J. Lawrence, D.C.

The Popliteal Artery Entrapment Syndrome in Children

Cummings RJ, Webb HW, Lovell WW, Kay G (Nemours Children's Clinic, Jacksonville, Fla)

J Pediatr Orthop 12:539–541, 1992 4–75

Introduction.—Although the clinician considers vascular insufficiency as a possible cause of leg pain in adults, it may not be considered in children. Forty-one cases of poplitel artery entrapment syndrome in young people were reviewed.

Patients.—Males predominated by a ratio of 3 to 1, and most patients were 16 to 17 years of age. The right leg was involved in 21 cases, the left leg in 12, and both legs in 7. The symptoms had been present for an average of 1 year before the diagnosis was made. Symptom onset could be acute or insidious. The pain was often typical of claudication but with bizarre features, such as pain when casual walking but not when running.

Discussion.—Popliteal artery entrapment syndrome in children usually results from either an anomalous course of the artery around a muscle or an anomalously located muscle. The condition is managed surgically, with release of the constricting muscle or fibrous band and, possibly, thrombectomy or bypass grafting. Popliteal artery entrapment syndrome is easily diagnosed, but because it is uncommon in children, the examiner may overlook it.

▶ If there is one point that this article hammers home, it is that vascular insufficiency can occur in the child, although we are not accustomed to thinking of this type of condition in the young. Therefore, in children complaining of leg pain and those who have no traumatic insult, the possibility of popliteal artery entrapment must be considered.—D.J. Lawrence, D.C.

Results of Conservative Treatment for Recalcitrant Anterior Knee Pain in Active Young Adults

Edeen J, Dainer RD, Barrack RL, Alexander AH (Naval Hosp, Oakland, Calif; Trivallery Orthopaedic and Sports Med Group, Pleasanton, Calif; Tulane Med School, New Orleans, La)

Orthop Rev 21:593–599, 1992 4–76

Objective.—The efficacy of a standard rehabilitation protocol was studied in 139 active young adults with resistant pain in the anterior knee. The patients, all military personnel, had a mean age of 25.5 years

TABLE 1.—Mechanism of Injury

Mechanism	Number of Cases
Fall	22
Direct trauma	17
Twisting injury	6
Running	4
Skiing	3
Valgus injury	2
Unspecified	3
Dashboard injury	2
Horse riding	2
Basketball	1
Obstacle course	1
Lacrosse	1
Climbing ladder	1
Softball	1
Volleyball	1
Jumping	1
Loading cargo	1

(Courtesy of Edeen J, Dainer RD, Barrack RL, et al: *Orthop Rev* 21:593–599, 1992.)

and included 16 women. Sixty-eight patients had a definite history of trauma.

Treatment.—The average duration of supervised physical therapy was 5.3 months. The patients warmed up on an exercise bicycle and performed multiple-angle quadriceps isometrics, 4-directional straight leg

TABLE 2.—Demographic Data

Patient	Success	Failure	P Value
Age (years)	27.4	24.5	< 0.01
Rank	E5	E4	< 0.05
Duration of service (months)	98	51	< 0.001
Duration of rehabilitation (months)	2.97	7.47	< 0.001
Supervised physical therapy sessions	14	16	> 0.05 (NS)
Duration of symptoms (months)	25.11	24.98	> 0.05 (NS)
Gender (M/F)	42/5	81/11	> 0.05 (NS)
Branch of military (USN/USMC/USCG)	40/7/0	71/19/2	> 0.05 (NS)
Station (ship/shore)	18/29	29/52	> 0.05 (NS)
Pain type (traumatic/insidious)	23/24	45/47	> 0.05 (NS)
Symptom type (bilateral/unilateral)	21/26	48/44	> 0.05 (NS)
Symptom onset (EPTE/DNEPTE)	4/43	23/69	> 0.05 (NS)

Abbreviations: USN, United States Navy; *USMC,* United States Marine Corps; *USCG,* United States Coast Guard; *EPTE,* existed prior to enlistment; *DNEPTE,* did not exist prior to enlistment; *NS,* not significant.

(Courtesy of Edeen J, Dainer RD, Barrack RL, et al: *Orthop Rev* 21:593–599, 1992.)

raises, and isotonic terminal extension quadriceps exercises. A short-arc range-of-motion isokinetic program began several weeks after symptoms started improving, and patients gradually entered a walk/jog program.

Results.—Thirty-four percent of the patients returned to full duty and were able to run 1.5 miles in a prescribed time limit. These patients were somewhat older, on average, than those who failed to improve. Failure was more frequent when there was a history of previous anterior knee pain. Injury was more frequent in those who were not rehabilitated. The

TABLE 3.—Results of Physical Examination

	Success		Failure	
Examination	% Normal	% Abnormal	% Normal	% Abnormal
Gait	70	30	69	31
Extension	94	6	97	3
Flexion	94	6	91	9
	% Present	% Absent	% Present	% Absent
Apprehension	19	81	33	67
Compression	71	29	83	17
Inhibition	80	20	84	16
Effusion	6	94	6	94
Crepitus	81	19	65	35
J-sign	8	92	18	88
Atrophy	30	70	37	63

(Courtesy of Edeen J, Dainer RD, Barrack RL, et al: *Orthop Rev* 21:593–599, 1992.)

mechanisms of injury are listed in Table 1. The outcome did not relate significantly to gender or unilateral vs. bilateral knee involvement (Table 2), or to the physical findings (Table 3). Three of 5 successfully rehabilitated patients had abnormal bone scan findings.

Discussion.—The duration of rehabilitative efforts (Table 4) is an important factor in the ultimate outcome. Rehabilitation of patients with recalcitrant anterior knee pain continues to be a difficult challenge.

▶ Patellofemoral pain is a complex problem with many possible theories concerning its cause: excessive lateral pressure causing pain through a tight lateral retinaculum, synovial fringe entrapment, osteoarthritic cartilage damage, and patellar malalignment. Because the cause cannot be so easily determined, surgical intervention seems senseless. Therefore, the question regards which conservative therapy will best treat the anterior pain. The physicians in this study used a program of quadriceps isometrics, straight leg raises, and so on. Although they had good results with this program, there is

TABLE 4.—Physical Therapy Regimens

Regimen	Description	Example
sometric	The muscle is exercised with the joint set at a given angle.	Quadriceps setting exercises
Isotonic	The muscle is exercised with a constant resistance through a range of motion.	Knee extensions with free weights
Concentric	The muscle is contracted causing a decrease in length of the muscle.	Hamstring curls with free weights
Eccentric	The muscle is contracted allowing an increase in the length of the muscle.	The descent phase of a squat
Isokinetic	The muscle is exercised with the speed of joint motion held constant	Knee extention on Cybex machine
Closed kinetic chain	The muscles are exercised with the foot and ankle in a fixed and loaded position.	Squats or lunges
Open kinetic chain	The muscles are exercised with the foot and ankle free and unloaded.	Leg extensions with free weights

(Courtesy of Edeen J, Dainer RD, Barrack RL, et al: *Orthop Rev* 21:593–599, 1992.)

no control group against which it can be compared. In future studies, it would be nice to test other procedures (e.g., manipulation or physical therapy), as well as have a control group, so that the very best conservative program can be developed.—D.J. Lawrence, D.C.

Occupational and Sports Injury

In Search of the Pathogenesis of Refractory Cervicobrachial Pain Syndrome: A Deconstruction of the RSI Phenomenon

Cohen ML, Arroyo JF, Champion GD, Browne CD (St Vincent's Hosp, Darlinghurst, Australia)

Med J Aust 156:432–436, 1992 4–77

Introduction.—Studies from both the medical and nonmedical literature dealing with refractory cervicobrachial pain (or repetitive strain injury)—mostly since 1980—were evaluated. The medical, psychiatric, and sociologic perspectives were examined, and the validity of their conclusions were judged to formulate a hypothesis of the origin of disordered nociception.

Hypothesis.—Refractory cervicobrachial pain is viewed as a reflex neuropathic state dependent on an ongoing afferent barrage from pain and mechanical receptors in the spinal zygapophyseal joints or related structures, or in muscles, tendons, and joint capsule tissues in the upper limb. The dorsal root ganglion, dorsal root, or peripheral nerve also may be affected. Sustained afferent activity in pain fibers supplying somatic structures may be a primary factor. An afferent barrage can result from constrained work postures and movements. Paresthesias may be projected into extended receptor fields. Hyperalgesia can reflect an amplified sensory input at the dorsal horn level.

Implications.—This hypothesis explains why measures blocking sympathetic efferents are only partly successful in relieving symptoms. Treatment directed toward central nociceptive mechanisms may be more effective than those based on activation of peripheral pain receptors. The hypothesis predicts that manipulating spinal zygapophyseal joints or proximal neural tissue may worsen pain.

▶ This theoretical discussion suggests that refractive cervicobrachial pain extends to a facilitation of the dorsal root ganglion. If this hypothesis is valid, blocking of the sympathetic efferents may be ineffective, and manipulation of the zygapophyseal joints may worsen the condition. This is an important concern to the chiropractor.—R.B. Phillips, D.C., Ph.D.

Factors Important in the Genesis and Prevention of Occupational Back Pain and Disability

Andersson GBJ (Rush-Presbyterian-St Luke's Med Ctr, Chicago)
J Manipulative Physiol Ther 1:43–46, 1992 4–78

Introduction.—Back injuries occurring at work typically are a result of overexertion, and only rarely are they caused by direct trauma. Fatigue

TABLE 1.—Occupational Factors Associated With an Increased Risk of Low Back Pain

Heavy Physical Work
Static Work Postures
Frequent Bending and Twisting
Lifting, Pushing and Pulling
Repetitive Work
Vibrations
Psychological and Psychosocial

(Courtesy of Andersson GBJ: *J Manipulative Physiol Ther* 1:43-46, 1992.)

TABLE 2.—Individual Factors Often Discussed as Potential Risk Factors in Low Back Pain

Factor	Importance
Age	Certain
Sex	Probable (age-dependent)
Posture	Low (severe only)
Anthropometry	Low (extremes only)
Muscle strength	Low (work-related)
Physical fitness	Low (work-related)
Spine mobility	Low
Smoking	Probable

(Courtesy of Andersson GBJ: *J Manipulative Physiol Ther* 1:43–46, 1992.)

injury may become evident only when complete failure takes place, and the final event may occur outside the workplace. Sustained static loading of tissues can cause injury through interfering with muscle blood flow.

Occupational Factors.—The most frequently implicated occupational factors associated with an elevated risk of low back pain are listed in Table 1. Much evidence implicates heavy work as an important factor in back pain, sciatica, and disk herniation. Static work postures include long-term sitting and driving. Psychological and psychosocial work factors have received increasing attention. Both monotony and poor satisfaction with work may be risk factors for back pain.

Individual Factors.—Low back pain often begins early in life. Among adults, it is most prevalent at ages 35–55 years. Women appear to be more vulnerable (Table 2). Postural deformities are not a major factor in low back pain and sciatica, and no strong association with body size or build is evident. Poor abdominal and back muscle strength is a frequent finding in those with chronic back pain. Smoking correlates closely with back pain, possibly because of the mechanical strain of coughing and also a reduction in oxygen tension in disk tissue.

Prevention.—Optimization of posture and regulation of permissible loads can help lower the risk of back pain at work. It is important to match the worker with the job, and also to teach workers how to prevent work-related symptoms.

▶ To prevent low back pain, one must recognize its cause. This article provides an accurate and concise review. The factors that increase the risk of low back pain are divided into occupational and individual groups. The author points toward the importance of prevention through the elimination of risk factors, a rational approach.—R.B. Phillips, D.C., Ph.D.

Trunk Muscle Strength and Back Muscle Endurance in Construction Workers With and Without Low Back Disorders

Holmström E, Moritz U, Andersson M (Bygghälsan, Malmö, Sweden; Univ of Lund, Sweden)

Scand J Rehabil Med 24:3–10, 1992 4–79

Background.—Investigators have come to different conclusions about the relationship of trunk muscle strength to low back pain, but several studies have found a relationship between isometric back muscle endurance and low back pain. Whether men without a low back disorder who are exposed to heavy work have better trunk muscle strength and back muscle endurance than men with the same work exposure who have a definite or probable low back disorder was investigated, as was the relationship between back muscle strength and endurance.

Method.—In an epidemiologic survey, 1,773 construction workers answered a questionnaire about musculoskeletal symptoms and their work environment. A control group of men (group A) with no history of lifetime low back trouble was compared with a group of men with a probable low back disorder (group B) and a group of men with a definite low back disorder (group C). These 3 groups underwent a personal interview and physical examination.

Findings.—The intraindividual maximum trunk extension/flexion ratio was 1.29 in group A, men with no history of low back disorder, compared to 1.19 in group C, men with clinically positive back disorder. The isometric trunk extensor endurance was also significantly lower in group C than in both group A and B. The groups did not differ in mean values for maximum isometric trunk extension and flexion strength.

Conclusion.—In a comparison of construction workers with no low back disorder, suspected disorder, and positive disorder, there was an association between isometric muscle strength and low back disorders.

▶ This study attempts to confirm a relationship between muscle strength and the absence of low back pain. Isometric trunk extensor endurance and extension/flexion ratios were found to be significantly higher in the non–low back pain group. This is also clinically significant, because all subjects were drawn from a heavy labor construction industry. Two assumptions are at issue: the use of muscle strength as a predictor of low back pain, and the potential of increasing strength as a method to prevent low back pain. The relationship of muscle strength to back pain is close but not unique, with other variables intervening in the relationship.—R.B. Phillips, D.C., Ph.D.

Low-Back Pain in Commercial Travelers

Pietri F, Leclerc A, Boitel L, Chastang J-F, Morcet J-F, Blondet M (INSERM U 88; Centre d' Information des Services Medicaux d' Entreprises et Interentre-

prises, Paris)
Scand J Work Environ Health 18:52–58, 1992 4–80

Background.—The incidence of low back pain has been studied in both the general population and the work environment to determine the role of individual, social, and occupational factors in the occurrence of this disorder. In the work environment, the activities most consistently associated with low back pain are lifting heavy loads and motor vehicle driving. This study focuses on low back pain in relation to life-style and the work environment in a group of commercial travelers in France.

Method.—The cross-sectional phase of the study (T_0) included interviews with 1,719 commercial travelers in several French towns during the employees' annual medical examination. Interview questions related to current life-style and occupational factors associated with low back pain during the previous 12 months. A subsample of 1,118 individuals was reinterviewed 12 months later (T_1) to study the association between the incidence of low back pain during the year of follow-up and the risk factors at T_0.

Findings.—The 1-year prevalence of low back pain was 25.1% to 28.2% for the men and 34.9% to 37.5% for the women. There was a borderline significant increase in the 1-year prevalence of low back pain with age and an association of gender with low back pain with a higher risk among women. The risk among current and ex-smokers was significantly elevated compared with nonsmokers, and there was a strong association of low back pain with psychosomatic factors. The occupational factors associated with low back pain at T_0 were the time spent driving per week, the comfort of the car seat, carrying loads, and standing. At T1, driving 10 hours per week or more, seat comfort, and psychosomatic factors were associated with the first occurrence of low back pain.

▶ This study linked low back pain with occupations fitting the job descriptions of commercial travelers; manufacture's agents; technical sales advisors; and insurance, real estate, and securities sales people. The presence of back pain was shown to be related to the time spent driving, the comfort of the car seat, carrying loads during work, long periods of standing, smoking, and psychosomatic factors. With so many variables contributing to the presence of low back pain, it is impossible to specify the weight of each variable. The generic classification of commercial traveler is broad, although clinical practice will seem consistent with the findings of this study.—R.B. Phillips, D.C., Ph.D.

Pre-Employment Musculoskeletal Assessment: The Imperative for Outcome Studies

Ebrall PS (Australian Centre for Chiropractic Research, Melbourne)

Chiroprac J Aust 22:9–14, 1992 4–81

Background.—Work-related mechanical low-back pain is a common, costly occupational problem. Chiropractic management is currently shown as being most cost effective. It is commonly thought that a preemployment muscoloskeletal evaluation can effectively predict which individuals are more prone to low back injury. The preemployment assessment of physical health was discussed.

Discussion.—The validity of preemployment chiropractic assessment has not been satisfactorily determined. A number of musculoskeletal conditions correlated for low back pain have been identified in the literature, but their predictive value for work-related low back injury remains questionable. The Metrecom is a computer-assisted goniometer that appears to have some potential for use in assessment, but there has been little published supportive data. The imperative for a prospective, longitudinal study of a cohort of new employees has been demonstrated. Each subject would be documented by a nominated screening procedure, and the subgroup that eventually has work-related low back pain would be identified. The common musculoskeletal findings of this subgroup can then be determined. Evidence of any predictive value for a suspected correlate would be the outcome to look for. The Australian Centre for Chiropractic Research has proposed to do such a study.

Conclusion.—The validity of preemployment chiropractic musculoskeletal evaluation has not been established. Although numerous correlates have been reported in the literature, their value as predictors of low back injury among workers remains questionable.

▶ Although the author strongly advocates the importance of preemployment assessment for identification of at-risk employees, he points out the absence of acceptable methods of evaluation. Although many tests have been shown to correlate with the presence of back pain, few have been shown to be good predictors of work-related onset of back pain. This paper proposes the use of computer-assisted goniometry as an approach to preemployment evaluation. The author needs to consider the issues of reliability and validity as they relates to this type of instrumentation.—R.B. Phillips, D.C., Ph.D.

Osteoarthritis of the Hip: An Occupational Disease in Farmers

Croft P, Coggon D, Cruddas M, Cooper C (Univ of Manchester, England; Southampton Gen Hosp, England; Bristol Royal Infirmary, England)

BMJ 304:1269–1272, 1992 4–82

TABLE 1.—Risk of Osteoarthritis According to Duration of Farming

	No. of subjects assessed	No. of cases	Odds ratio (95% confidence interval)* Adjusted for age alone	Adjusted for all variables †
Controls	83	2	1.0	1.0
1-9 Years' farming	52	6	5.8 (1.1 to 31.5)	4.5 (0.8 to 26.3)
≥ 10 Years' farming	115	22	10.1 (2.2 to 45.9)	9.3 (1.9 to 44.5)

* Adjusted for age in 2-year intervals.
† Adjusted for height (3 strata), weight (3 strata), and presence of Heberden's nodes (absent, possible, or definite).
(Courtesy of Croft P, Coggon D, Cruddas M, et al: *BMJ* 304:1269–1272, 1992.)

Background.—Farming appears to be associated with high rates of surgery for hip osteoarthritis. However, farmers may seek treatment more often than other occupational groups because they are more handicapped by hip osteoarthritis when it occurs, not because it occurs at a higher incidence. Establishing whether hip osteoarthritis is a true occupational hazard is important so that preventive measures can be initiated. A population-based survey comparing the prevalence of hip osteoarthritis in farmers and other groups was reported.

TABLE 2.—Occupational Activities Reported by Farmers With and Without Hip Osteoarthritis

Activity	No. (%) of farmers with hip osteoarthritis (n = 28)	No. (%) of farmers without hip osteoarthritis (n = 139)
Hand milking	23 (82)	109 (78)
Machine milking	18 (64)	84 (60)
Lifting churns	23 (82)	110 (79)
Using horses	22 (79)	102 (73)
Driving tractors	20 (71)	96 (69)
Regularly driving a tractor for at least 3 months/year	17 (61)	76 (55)
Regularly driving a tractor for at least 4 hours/day	10 (36)	42 (30)
Machine threshing	19 (68)	82 (59)
Combining	7 (25)	22 (16)
Lifting or moving weights of 25 kg or more by hand	27 (96)	125 (90)

(Courtesy of Croft P, Coggon D, Cruddas M, et al: *BMJ* 304:1269–1272, 1992.)

Methods.—One hundred sixty-seven male farmers, aged 60–76 years, and 83 control subjects with primarily sedenatry jobs were studied in 5 rural general practices. Subjects without previous hip replacement had radiography of the hip. The main outcome measures were hip replacement for osteoarthritis or radiographic signs of the condition.

Findings.—The prevalence of hip osteoarthritis was found to be higher in the farmers than in the control subjects. The prevalence was particularly higher in men who had farmed for more than 10 years, who had an odds ratio of 9.3. The excess risk could not be attributed to any 1 type of farming. Heavy lifting seems to be the most likely explanation (Tables 1 and 2).

Conclusion.—These and previous findings strongly suggest that hip osteoarthritis is an occupational hazard of farming. The exact nature of this hazard is unclear. Possible explanations include heavy lifting, exposure to whole body vibration from agricultural machinery, and stress on the hip from walking over rough ground.

▶ This study confirmed a higher incidence of hip osteoarthritis in farmers who had farmed for more than 10 years compared with controls in 5 other sedentary occupations. There are several risk factors described in the farming experience that would contribute to degenerative joint disease. Caution is recommended in using these findings to influence public policy. There is a need to more clearly define the farming experience and to draw comparisons with other occupations of a similar nature. Movement and function are beneficial for joint maintenance as long as they do not become abusive. More research is needed in this area.—R.B. Phillips, D.C., Ph.D.

Personal and Job Characteristics of Musculoskeletal Injuries in an Industrial Population

Tsai SP, Gilstrap EL, Cowles SR, Waddell LC Jr, Ross CE (Shell Oil Co, Houston)

J Occup Med 34:606–612, 1992 4–83

Background.—Work-related musculoskeletal injuries have been studied extensively, especially among patients with low back pain. However, little is known about non-work-related musculoskeletal injuries among workers. Personal and job characteristics of such injuries in an industrial population were investigated.

Methods.—The subjects were 10,350 full-time regular employees at Shell Oil Company's manufacturing facilities between 1987 and 1989. Two hundred seventy-five workers with low back injuries, 456 with non-low back musculoskeletal injuries, and 8,295 workers without musculoskeletal injuries in this period were compared. Morbidity data were collected from a prospective health surveillance system.

Findings.—The estimated relative risks for low back injuries were significantly higher among smokers and overweight individuals. The risks were also higher in smokers and overweight individuals for non-low back musculoskeletal injuries. Workers whose jobs were potentially more physically demanding had an increased relative risk for both low back and non-low back musculoskeletal injuries.

Conclusion.—It may be possible to decrease the impact of musculoskeletal injury by implementing an integrated injury prevention program. Such programs would include the traditional elements of assessment and modification of job factors, employee education and training, and overall increased attention to ergonomics as well as medical counseling and support for personal fitness programs, workplace smoking cessation programs, and weight-reduction programs.

▶ This study addresses the personal characteristics of individual sufferers of back pain to determine their significance. Smoking and overweight contributed to high relative risks for low back pain and other non–low back musculoskeletal injuries. More physically demanding jobs also created higher risks. The authors suggest the need for preventative programs in the workplace to reduce risk. Such a suggestion is consistent with the wellness concept found in the chiropractic paradigm.—R.B. Phillips, D.C., Ph.D.

Low Back and Neck/Shoulder Pain in Construction Workers: Occupational Workload and Psychosocial Risk Factors: Part 1. Relationship to Low Back Pain

Holmström EB, Lindell J, Moritz U (Bygghälsan, Malmö, Sweden; Research Found for Occupational Safety and Health in the Swedish Construction Industry, Danderyd; Univ of Lund, Sweden)

Spine 17:663–671, 1992 4–84

Background.—The physical work load has often been reported as a risk factor for low back pain (LBP). Studies have noted a high frequency of musculoskeletal complaints in construction workers, but the relationship of these complaints to ergonomic and psychosocial factors has not been established. The prevalence of LBP in construction workers was assessed and its relationship to physical and psychosocial factors was analyzed.

Methods.—A questionnaire that addressed individual and employee-related factors, locomotor disorders, physical work load, and psychosocial factors was sent to a random sample of 2,500 active construction workers. After exclusion of ineligible subjects and nonrespondents, 75% of this population was included in the study sample. Eight materials handling indices and 10 psychosocial indices, based on findings from factor analysis, were used to assess work load.

Results.—There was a 54% 1-year prevalence of LBP and a 7% incidence of severe LBP. The relationship with heavy manual materials handling varied with age such that it could be interpreted as a healthy worker effect. There was a dose-response relationship between severe low back pain and both stooping and kneeling. The stress index and the psychosomatic and psychic indices were the psychosocial factors most prominently associated with LBP and severe LBP. When workers reporting high stress were compared to workers reporting low stress, the age-standardized prevalence rate ratio of LBP was 1.6 and that for severe low back pain was 3.1.

Conclusion.—This analysis of LBP in construction workers suggests that age is the most obvious risk factor for severe LBP. However, when all other factors are equal, stooping and kneeling are significantly associated with severe LBP. Older workers should be given less strenuous working tasks. Low back pain does not appear to be affected by experienced social support.

▶ The relationship of back pain, occupational work load, and psychosocial risk factors is important to understand if progress is to be made in this area. This study found age to be the most evident risk factor. Back pain becomes more likely with advancing age. Controlling for age, the actions of kneeling and stooping become significant risk factors. Stress levels also become important contributing factors to severe low back pain. Once again, we see a display of multiple factors contributing to a very broad category of back pain. The potential of multiple etiologies makes the art of predicting risk factors and relationships most difficult.—R.B. Phillips, D.C., Ph.D.

Predicting Return to Work for Lower Back Pain Patients Receiving Worker's Compensation

Lancourt J, Kettelhut M (North Dallas Orthopedics and Rehabilitation; Humana Advanced Surgical Inst, Dallas)

Spine 17:629–640, 1992 4–85

Objective.—The problem of low back pain (LBP) is exacerbated by high cost claims. A more comprehensive model of treatment that considers the nonorganic signs and psychological factors is needed. The development of predictive indices for estimating the probability that patients with lower back injuries would return to work was reported.

Methods.—The subjects were 161 consecutive patients with LBP who were receiving worker's compensation. Demographic, personal, physical, and diagnostic data were collected for each patient.

Findings.—Work- , personal- , and family-related problems were more common in patents who did not return to work. In terms of the physical organic findings, the only significant difference was muscle atrophy, with patients who did not return to work having a statistically higher incidence. Outcome was significantly related to time off work. For those off work less than 6 months, important predictors were a high Oswestry score, a history of leg pain, family relocation, short time on the job, verbal magnification of pain, moderate to severe pain on superficial palpation, and positive reaction to a sham sciatic tension test. For those off work more than 6 months, the significant factors were previous injuries and stability of family living arrangements. Three significant factors were developed from a larger group of 92 factors. These measures more accurately predicted return to work than the total set of factors did.

Conclusion.—This study confirms the importance of personal, job, family, and stress-related factors in predicting return to work of worker's compensation patients with LBP. A short set of indicators for predicting which patients will and will not return to work is presented. Although the model is limited and preliminary, it provides a basis for further research and validation with other groups of patients with back injury or chronic back pain.

► Although some attempts have been made to pre-screen potential patients who would be at risk for back pain in a particular work environment, this study is attempting to predict the return to work. Once a patient has missed work as a result of back pain, which factors will limit the possibility of returning to work? Some of the factors found to be important contributors to limiting return to work include previous compensation, time off work, family living arrangements, job status, stress levels, and nonorganic signs of back pain.—R.B. Phillips, D.C., Ph.D.

A Prospective Evaluation of Preemployment Screening Methods for Acute Industrial Back Pain

Bigos SJ, Battié MC, Fisher LD, Hansson TH, Spengler DM, Nachemson AL (Univ of Washington, Seattle; Sahlgren Hosp, Göteborg, Sweden; Vanderbilt Univ, Nashville)

Spine 17:922–926, 1992 4–86

Introduction.—Preemployment screening has long been used in an attempt to decrease back injury claims. Methods of screening have moved from radiographic factors to clinical examination. The use of preemployment screening information was evaluated for its ability to predict individuals at risk for acute back injury.

Methods.—The prospective, longitudinal study included 3,020 hourly workers at an aircraft factory. All subjects had a physical examination of anthropometry, posture, and flexibility, as well as a clinical back evaluation including reflexes, straight-leg raising, and circumferential leg measurements. Demographic and psychosocial information was available for 54% of workers. The workers were followed up for as long as to 4.25 years.

Findings.—Back problems were reported by 279 subjects, including 9.9% of those who did not provide demographic and psychosocial data and 8.7% of those who did, a nonsignificant difference. Univariate analysis found that younger age, higher education, smoking, several past medical history variables, and various physical examination findings were significant predictors of acute back pain. However, on multivariate analysis, the predictive power of these variables for men was explained by a greater history of treatment for pain over the past 2 years and history of seeing a chiropractor for any reason.

Conclusion.—In preemployment screening, physical factors do not add any significant predictive value over simple historical information about previous pain treatment. Preemployment screening appears ineffective because of problems with statistical evaluation of the data, the poor predictive ability of those factors associated with back problems, and the fact that back problems do not fit into the injury model very well.

▶ This report is one of many generated by the large prospective Boeing study on back pain. The authors suggest that physical factors do not add any significant information over that gained by obtaining a thorough history, including previous pain treatments. This paper provides an excellent discussion regarding why preemployment screening has not been successful in identifying potential risks for injury. The discussion reviews the issues related to statistical limitations, the low predictive capabilities of the factors being considered, failure of back pain to fit the injury model and psychosocial issues chiefly related to compensation.—R.B. Phillips, D.C., Ph.D.

Electromyographic Fatigue in Neck/Shoulder Muscles and Endurance in Women With Repetitive Work

Hansson G-Å, Strömberg U, Larsson B, Ohlsson K, Balogh I, Moritz U (Univ Hosp, Lund, Sweden)

Ergonomics 35:1341–1352, 1992 4–87

Objective.—Workplace automation may result in repetitive motion that places a static muscle load on the neck and shoulders. Patients with occupational cervicobrachial pain complain of aching, stiff muscles, often with palpable tender spots. The cause of the problem is unknown. Also unknown is whether the static load affects the long-term function of the muscle or whether subjects with neck and shoulder muscle disorders differ from unaffected patients in terms of muscle function.

Methods.—Electromyography (EMG) was used to evaluate possible differences in muscle fatigue during isometric endurance testing with a static workload in women with and without neck and shoulder disorders. The EMG recordings were made from the trapezius and deltoid muscles using surface electrodes. The following 3 groups of women were studied during a static endurance test at approximately 20% of maximal voluntary contraction: 22 industrial workers who performed repetitive, short-cycled work tasks, half with and half without neck and shoulder disorders; and a reference group of 11 women who did not perform such work. Isotonic regression was used to assess the amount of fatigue, assuming that the root mean square (RMS) curve increases and the mean power frequency (MPF) curve decreases with time.

Results.—An increase in RMS values was the most notable sign of fatigue for the trapezius muscles; for the deltoid muscles, it was a decrease in MPF values. The symptomatic women had a significantly shorter endurance time than either of the other 2 groups. The EMG fatigue measures were not significantly different among the 3 groups, and endurance time appeared unrelated to EMG parameters.

Conclusion.—Women with shoulder or neck disorders exposed to repetitive, short-cycled work show a shorter endurance time and more pronounced EMG signs of fatigue than do asymptomatic women doing similar work or women who do not do such work. The EMG findings suggest that neck and shoulder disorders are not associated with divergent mechanisms of muscle fatigue. The shorter endurance time may result from the sensory output of pain or chemical receptors in the muscle or both.

▶ The occurrence of occupational neck and shoulder problems is increasing. Some have attributed this rise to the increase in automation, where workers undergo day-long episodes of repetitive motions, increasing the loads on the neck and shoulder muscles. Under repetitive motion, the muscles of these areas become fatigued; however, there is little difference in the fatigue created by repetitive work and fatigue resulting from other causes. It may behoove us to recommend that those patients with cervical or shoulder problems who must undergo repetitive motion be allowed to shift responsibility over the course of the day to decrease the possibility of the involved muscles becoming fatigued.—D.J. Lawrence, D.C.

Intercollegiate Ice Hockey Injuries: A Case for Uniform Definitions and Reports

Pelletier RL, Montelpare WJ, Stark RM (Univ of Ottawa, Ont, Canada; Ottawa Civic Hosp; Brock Univ, St Catharines, Ont, Canada)

Am J Sports Med 21:78–81, 1993 4–88

Purpose.—Although injuries are common in ice hockey, the risks are unclear, partly because of lack of agreement on definition of terms and consistent reporting strategies. One researcher reported a rate of 1 injury per game in college hockey, but this estimate failed to account for the number of persons at risk. A standardized reporting method and defined terminology were used to describe Canadian intercollegiate ice hockey injuries during a 6-year period.

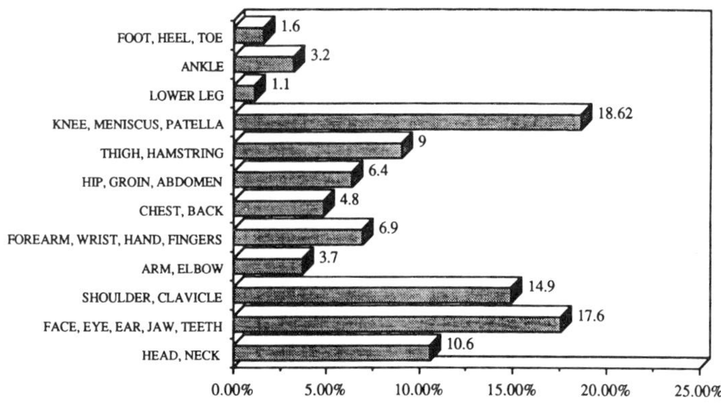

Fig 4–37.—Percent of reported injuries classified by body part. (Courtesy of Pelletier RL, Montelpare WJ, Stark RM: *Am J Sports Med* 21:78–81, 1993.)

Methods.—The data were drawn from the Canadian Athletic Injuries/Illness Reporting system for the years 1979 through 1985. This system observes uniform reporting procedures and clear definitions of a reportable injury or illness, participant, and participation.

Results.—The incidence of injuries was estimated at 20 per 1,000 player-games. The knee was injured most commonly, accounting for 19% of injuries, followed by the facial area, shoulder or clavicle, and head and neck (Fig 4–37). Forwards accounted for two thirds of the injuries. Forty-five percent of injuries resulted from body contact for which no penalty was called, 28% from accidental collisions, and 24% from fighting and illegal play. More than half of the injuries were sprains and

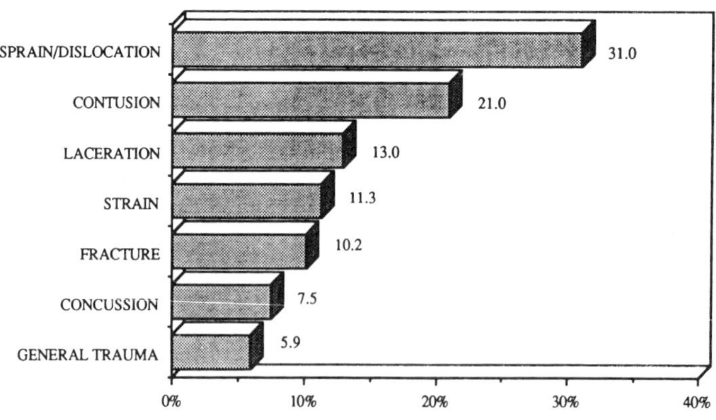

Fig 4–38.—Percent of injuries reported classified by type of injury. (Courtesy of Pelletier RL, Montelpare WJ, Stark RM: *Am J Sports Med* 21:78–81, 1993.)

contusions. Compared with previous studies, the rate of hockey injuries appeared to have decreased during the past 15 years (Fig 4–38).

Conclusion.—The prevalence of injuries in collegiate ice hockey appears to be declining, probably because of the use of helmets and visors. These safeguards have been especially effective in reducing the incidence of puck- and stick-induced injuries to the face. Standardized reporting strategies and uniform definitions should be used in future epidemiologic research on sports injuries.

▶ On average, there is 1 hockey injury per game played. For those involved in sports chiropractic practice, it might be well to "play the odds" and know what the frequencies of these injuries are. Sprains and dislocations are most frequent, especially affecting the knee; contusions to the face area are also quite common. It might be well to design exercise and strengthening programs, especially at the junior level or lower, to prevent these injuries. In the case of facial injuries, newer designs in protective gear have decreased the loss of teeth and other damage.—D.J. Lawrence, D.C.

Frequency and Perception of Spinal Manipulation in College Athletics

Jacobson BH, Gemmell HA (Oklahoma State Univ, Stillwater)

Chiroprac Sports Med 6:16–20, 1992 4–89

Objective.—Because a very large but unknown number of athletes receive spinal manipulation, a survey of 105 college athletes was undertaken to determine how frequent spinal manipulation is and why it is carried out. The group included 75 men and 30 women, most of whom played football or women's basketball. Manipulation was defined as any physical adjustment using the hands or whole body tension, thrust, or stretch.

Item 1.—Have You Had Your Back Adjusted (Popped)?

Sport	Yes Answers (%)
Football (FB)	94
Basketball (BB)	63
Wrestling (WR)	100
Track (TR)	72
Softball (SB)	78
Total	81.4

(Courtesy of Jacobson BH, Gemmell HA: *Chiroprac Sports Med* 6:16–20, 1992.)

Findings.—Four of 5 athletes, and nearly all of those engaging in contact sports, had received spinal manipulation at some time (table). More than half had had their backs adjusted at least once a month, most often for perceived stiffness. Teammates performed manipulation in about one third of the cases, and athletic trainers performed manipulation in about 30%. Nearly 90% of the subjects stated that their back felt better after manipulation. Direct thrust was most frequently used. Two thirds of the respondents acknowledged that the procedure carries some risk.

Conclusion.—Athletes very often undergo possibly unnecessary spinal manipulation, which frequently is done by unqualified individuals. More educational efforts are needed.

▶ This article highlights the unwarranted use of spinal manipulation by athletes. Investigation on a larger scale would provide further insights into the prevalence of this phenomena.—A.H. Adams, D.C.

The Nature of Dance Injuries

Kerr G, Krasnow D, Mainwaring L (Univ of Toronto; York Univ, North York, Ont)

Med Probl Perform Art 7:25–29, 1992 4–90

Background.—Although dancers and athletes have much in common, there are unique differences that may affect the nature of the injury process in dance. The number, severity, and anatomic location of dance injuries and the hypothesized relationship between postural alignment and such injuries were investigated.

TABLE 1.—Number of Injuries Incurred Over 8 Months ($n = 39$)

No. of Injuries	*No. of Dancers*	*Percentage*
0	1	2.5
1	12	31.0
2	10	26.0
3	8	20.0
4	5	13.0
5	2	5.0
6	1	2.5
Totals	39	100.0

(Courtesy of Kerr G, Krasnow D, Mainwaring L: *Med Probl Perform Art* 7:25–29, 1992.)

TABLE 2.—Anatomical Location of Reported Injuries

Anatomical Location	*No. of Injuries*	*Percentage*
Back	24	26.0
Knee	16	17.4
Foot	11	11.9
Shoulder	8	8.7
Ankle	7	7.6
Shin splints	4	4.3
Achilles tendon	4	4.3
Quadriceps	3	3.3
Hamstring	3	3.3
Calf muscle	3	3.3
Neck	3	3.3
Groin	2	2.2
Hip	2	2.2
Elbow	1	1.1
Thumb	1	1.1
Totals	92	100.0

(Courtesy of Kerr G, Krasnow D, Mainwaring L: *Med Probl Perform Art* 7:25–29, 1992.)

Methods.—Thirty-nine female university students majoring in dance were studied during an 8-month period, ranging from preseason to peak season. Injury records were maintained; posture was assessed 4 times.

Findings.—The injury rate was 97%. Only 1 dancer sustained no injuries. The rest had a mean of 2.4 injuries during the study. Most injuries occurred to the lower back, followed in prevalence by knee and foot injuries. Most interfered with training for 3 weeks. In 6 dancers, injuries interfered for 4 months or more. The injury rate increased significantly when the season began and remained at this level throughout the study. Postural alignment worsened at each evaluation (Tables 1, 2, and 3).

Conclusion.—These findings do not provide support for the proposed negative relationship between injuries and postural alignment. The seriousness of the injury problem among dancers is significant. Further research is needed to study the interrelationships between training and performance demands, injuries, and postural alignment.

▶ The nature and extent of musculoskeletal injuries in dancers deserves more attention from the chiropractic profession. It would be interesting to see studies that address the effectiveness of chiropractic care in the management and prevention of dance related injuries.—A.H. Adams, D.C.

TABLE 3.—Duration of Time That the Injury Interfered With Regular Training or Performance Over an 8-Month Period

Duration of Time	*No. of Injuries*	*Percentage of Injuries*
< 7 days	12	13.0
7–13 days	17	18.5
14–20 days	23	25.0
21–27 days	14	15.2
28–34 days	5	5.4
35–41 days	4	4.3
42–48 days	3	3.3
49–55 days	3	3.3
56–62 days	2	2.2
63–69 days	3	3.3
> 70 days (10 weeks)	6	6.5
Totals	92	100.0

(Courtesy of Kerr G, Krasnow D, Mainwaring L: *Med Probl Perform Art* 7:25–29, 1992.)

Measurement of Reactive Vasodilation During Cold Gel Pack Application to Nontraumatized Ankles

Taber C, Contryman K, Fahrenbruch J, LaCount K, Cornwall MW (Northern Arizona Univ, Flagstaff)

Phys Ther 72:294–299, 1992 4–91

Background.—Research on local vascular response during cryotherapy has yielded conflicting results. Cold packs were applied to nontraumatized ankles to determine whether blood volume decreased.

Methods.—Thirteen individuals, aged 18–30 years, volunteered for the study. An impedance plethysmograph and venous occlusion was used to assess the changes in local blood volume at the ankle for 20 minutes. Measurements were obtained in 3 conditions: rest, room-temperature gel pack application, and cold gel pack application.

Findings.—Local blood volume in the cold gel pack condition was significantly reduced compared with the resting condition. This decrease was attributed to pressure from the weight of the cold gel pack combined with the pack's temperature. The maximum reduction in blood volume occurred at 13.5 minutes after the cold gel pack was applied. No reactive vasodilation was seen.

Conclusion.—A cold gel pack applied to the untraumatized ankle for 20 minutes at 10°F to 20°F significantly decreases the local increase in blood volume during venous occlusion. This reduction was sustained.

This effect appears to result from the combination of pressure from the weight of the cold pack and the cold stimulus. Another important finding of this study was the absence of reactive vasodilation.

► The influence of cryotherapy on local vascular response has been an area of contention among sport injury specialists. Two important findings were prouced by this study. First, application of a cold gel pack to the ankle for 20 minutes at a temperature of 10°F to 20°F produced an immediate and sustained reduction in local blood volume increase during venous occlusion. Second, reactive vasodilation was not observed during the cold gel pack application. These findings suggest the value of cold gel pack application for control of local circulation immediately after soft tissue trauma. Further studies in subjects with acute local soft tissue trauma are required to validate these findings.—A.H. Adams, D.C.

Subject Characteristics and Low Back Pain in Young Athletes and Nonathletes

Kujala UM, Salminen JJ, Taimela S, Oksanen A, Jaakkola L (Helsinki Research Inst for Sports and Exercise Medicine; Turku Univ Hosp, Finland)
Med Sci Sports Exerc 24:627–632, 1992 4–92

Background.—The effects of athletic training type, intensity, and frequency on the incidence of low back pain (LBP) during growth are not well understood. Also unknown are the intrinsic factors predisposing to LBP during growth and whether children with LBP during growth develop chronic LBP in adulthood. The relationships among LBP, athletic training, and different subject characteristics were studied in 2 male and 3 female cohorts of young athletes and nonathletes.

Methods.—Factors associated with LBP were elicited from 138 adolescents using a questionnaire and physical measurements. One hundred were athletes. Ages ranged from 10.3 to 13.3 years.

Findings.—No significant differences were found in the occurrence of LBP between athletes and nonathletes. Among athletes, training duration in the preceding 12 months was higher in those with LBP in the past

Hip Flexor Tightness (Degrees) in Study Subjects With and Without Lifetime LBP History

	No Back Pain		Back Pain	
	Mean	SD	Mean	SD
Boys	166	5	163	7
Girls	175	7	171	4

(Courtesy of Kujala UM, Salminen JJ, Taimela S, et al: *Med Sci Sports Exerc* 24:627–632, 1992.)

12 months, compared with asymptomatic subjects. Similar differences were also observed between those with positive lifetime histories of LBP and asymptomatic adolescents. There were various differences in measures of anthropometry, flexibility, and strength between athletes and nonathletes and boys and girls. A multivariate analysis showed that the cumulative incidence of lifetime history of LBP was related to tightness of hip flexor muscles only. Low back pain in the past 12 months was associated only with the amount of training in the past 12 months (table).

Conclusion.—High training duration appears to predispose young athletes to LBP. In athletes, the associations between subject characteristics such as mobility and LBP may differ compared with those in nonathletes.

▶ This study reports that athletic participation alone is not a causative factor for low back pain in adolescents. However, the association between the amount of training and the occurrence of low back pain suggests that extreme training during the growth period in pre-adolescents may be harmful. Clinicians working with children and adolescents who participate in organized athletic activities should pay particular attention to the training regimens of athletes seen with low back pain.—A.H. Adams, D.C.

Avulsion Fracture of the Anterior Superior Iliac Spine in a Collegiate Distance Runner

Draper DO, Dustman AJ (Brigham Young Univ, Provo, Utah; Illinois Wesleyan Univ, Bloomington)

Arch Phys Med Rehabil 73:881–882, 1992 4–93

Mechanisms.—Apophysitis, or inflammation of the epiphyseal growth plate, occurs when traction is applied by the attaching tendon; it may culminate in avulsion fracture. The most common pelvic sites of avulsion fracture are the ischial tuberosity where the hamstrings attach; the rectus femoris attachment to the anterior inferior iliac spine; and the sartorius attachment to the anterior superior iliac spine.

Case Report.—A distance runner, 20, felt a snap in his left hip while turning left during an interval workout, and he fell to the ground. Point tenderness and swelling were noted over the left anterior superior iliac spine. Radiographs revealed an avulsion fracture of this structure that was classified as a Salter-Harris type II epiphyseal injury. The patient was allowed non-weight-bearing exercises a week later; a week after that, he was free of pain and had good strength. He effectively competed in a cross-country race less than 3 weeks after the injury.

Discussion.—Overuse injuries of the hip and pelvic region make up less than 10% of running injuries. A conservative approach to avulsion fractures of the anterior superior iliac spine allows union at a nearly normal level without functional problems for athletes.

▶ Avulsion fractures in the pelvis are typically seen in athletes involved in contact sports such as football. In all injuries to the hip, the avulsion fracture of the anterior superior iliac spine accounts for, at best, 1.5%; its presence in a distance runner is exceedingly rare. The mechanism for the fracture in this case involved the runner making a sharp turn around a tree, which apparently created sufficient force to tear the fragment. Surgery is not usually considered for these fractures. Treatment consisted of rest and a decrease from weight-bearing for a period of 3–4 weeks; the fragment typically unites with little problem. Sports chiropractors should be aware of this injury, particularly those who see a high percentage of runners.—D.J. Lawrence, D.C.

Effect of Vitamin and Trace-Element Supplementation on Immune Responses and Infection in Elderly Subjects

Chandra RK (Mem Univ of Newfoundland)

Lancet 340:1124–1127, 1992 4–94

Background.—Impaired immune responses and increased infection-related morbidity accompany aging. The effect of physiologic amounts of vitamins and trace elements on immunocompetence and occurrence of infection-related illness was investigated.

Methods.—Ninety-six healthy elderly individuals living independently were randomly assigned to receive nutrient supplementation or placebo. Nutrient status and immunologic variables were evaluated at baseline and at 12 months. The frequency of illness from infection was determined.

Findings.—Subjects receiving the supplement had higher numbers of certain T-cell subsets and natural killer cells, improved proliferation response to mitogen, and increased interleukin-2 production. They also had higher antibody response and natural killer cell activity. Subjects given the supplement were less likely to have illness caused by infections than subjects given placebos.

Conclusion.—These findings support the hypothesis that nutritional status is an important determinant of immunocompetence in old age and that optimal micronutrient intake is needed for enhanced immune responses in elderly persons. The intervention described resulted in a striking decrease in illness.

▶ Elderly subjects receiving vitamin and trace element supplementation were found to be less ill than patients who did not receive those compounds. The authors recommend that an optimum intake of micronutrients can help to increase immunocompetence in old age. This should be done cautiously, in recognition that megadoses of certain vitamins can be toxic; before the initiation of a program of micronutrient supplementation, the nutritional status of the patient should be carefully assessed.—D.J. Lawrence, D.C.

Low-Back Injuries in a Heavy Industry I: Worker and Workplace Factors

Clemmer DI, Mohr DL, Mercer DJ (Tulane Univ, New Orleans, La; Univ of North Florida, Jacksonville)

Spine 16:824–830, 1991 4–95

Background.—An ongoing study of injuries among petroleum drilling workers suggests that an increasing percentage of the injuries involve the low back (LB). As the rate of other injuries has declined, the rate of LB injuries has remained stable, and the incidence of LB injuries involving lost time has increased. The costs and circumstances of LB injuries, both those resulting from body motion and those resulting from impact, were examined and compared with non-LB injuries.

Methods.—The analysis included data for a 6-year period on worker injuries occurring on a large fleet of mobile off-shore drilling units in the Gulf of Mexico. The data were reported in standardized fashion, including employment and job at the time of injury; site and severity of injury; time, type of energy involved, and nature of the injury; the worker's activity just before the event; and possible contributing factors. After excluding 150 LB injuries in which other body sites were involved, the final analysis included 543 "pure" LB injuries and a comparison group of 4,222 non-LB injuries.

Findings.—Sixteen percent of LB injuries resulted in lost time, compared to 9% of non-LB injuries. The LB injuries resulting from impact accounted for more than one third of the 88 lost-time LB injuries. The average cost per claim was 3 times higher with LB vs. non-LB injuries. The workers who performed the heaviest physical labor had the highest risk of LB injury and accounted for the greatest number of injuries. The LB strain injuries occurred in workers older than the workers with LB impact injuries or non-LB injuries, but this difference was only significant for workers performing the heaviest physical labor. Floorhands and derrickhands were nearly 3 times more likely, and roustabouts 2 times more likely to have a lost-time LB strain injury than those in other jobs, after adjustment for age and length of service.

Conclusion.—Low-back injuries among oil rig workers result mainly from falls, although LB strain injuries are most common in workers doing the heaviest physical labor. Specific recommendations for prevention are presented, including prevention or reduction of hazards, prevention or modification of the release rate of hazards, separation of the hazard from the host, modification of the harmful characteristics of the hazard, increasing host resistance to the hazard, limiting damage done, and rehabilitating injured workers.

▶ It appears that the incidence of LB pain in industrial settings is increasing at the same time that other injuries are decreasing. One of the goals of this study was to try to identify the workplace factors that are associated with LB pain. In doing so, there were few surprises; those doing heavier labor had more injury, and those who were older also had more injury when compared among oil rig workers. The import here is that a task analysis may need to be done in most industrial settings to gain an understanding of the risks that may cause LB pain. When these risks are identified, then a prevention program can be specifically designed to help reduce or minimize the dangers associated with those activities. The authors provide a thorough set of recommendations for the prevention of LB injury in a heavy industrial setting; the reader would do well to keep these in mind in establishing industry-related prevention programs.—D.J. Lawrence, D.C.

5 Professional Issues

Health Services

Unconventional Medicine in the United States: Prevalence, Costs, and Patterns of Use

Eisenberg DM, Kessler RC, Foster C, Norlock FE, Calkins DR, Delbanco TL (Harvard Medical School, Boston; University of Michigan, Ann Arbor; Chicago College for Osteopathic Medicine)

N Engl J Med 328:246–252, 1993 5–1

Purpose.—The prevalence, costs, and patterns of use of unconventional therapies in the United States were determined by a national telephone survey.

Methods.—A total of 1,539 randomly selected adults from a national sample were asked about their medical conditions and the use of 16 commonly used interventions neither taught widely in United States medical schools nor generally available in United States hospitals during the past 12 months.

Results.—One in 3 respondents had used unconventional therapy in the past year. One third of these respondents had made an average of 19 visits to a provider of unconventional therapy. The rates of use varied widely across all sociodemographic groups, being most common among non-black individuals aged 25–49 years with relatively more education and higher incomes. Unconventional therapies were generally used as adjuncts to conventional therapy and for chronic, non–life-threatening conditions, such as back problems, anxiety, headaches, chronic pain, and cancer or tumors. Among those who used unconventional therapy for serious medical conditions, 83% also saw a medical doctor for the same condition, but 72% did not inform their medical doctor that they did so. Extrapolation to the United States population suggested that the estimated number of visits to providers of unconventional therapy exceeded the number of visits to all primary care medical doctors nationwide in 1990. In addition, the amount spent out of pocket on unconventional therapy was comparable to that spent for all hospitalizations in the United States.

Implications.—The use of unconventional therapy is far more common than previously reported. Medical doctors should ask about their patients' use of unconventional therapy whenever they obtain a history, and information about unconventional therapy and the clinical social sciences should be included in the medical curriculum.

▶ Here we have a paper with what appears to be a most positive finding: the use of "unconventional therapies," including chiropractic therapy, is higher than had previously been reported. From this finding, the authors have managed to put forth a most negative interpretation of their data: (1) users of unconventional therapy don't discuss their use of these therapies with their medical doctors because of a lack of communication resulting from the doctors' belief that patients don't routinely use these therapies; and (2) this poses a danger to patients and is not in their best interest because these therapies are potentially dangerous. What, then, is Dr. Eisenberg and colleagues' answer? To have the medical doctor ask about the patient's use of unconventional therapy (a term I loathe, because who decided what constitutes the conventional therapy?) and to have medical colleges add courses about these therapies in their curriculum. It never occurs to the authors to attempt to create interdisciplinary interactions. Rather than let the individual with the best training become involved in the therapy (for example, a chiropractor for back pain), Dr. Eisenberg would prefer to have medicine co-opt the treatment, although certainly not at the level of training that a chiropractor receives. Although I can't fault the research in this paper, the conclusions represent a seeming arrogance with which I am uncomfortable.

If we extrapolate these data, nearly one third of Americans saw an alternative health-care practitioner during the past year, representing nearly 14 billion dollars in expenditures. It is patently obvious that these practitioners offer health care that is beneficial to the patient. This article seems to miss this point in its call for medicine to gain more knowledge of these forms of health care. Simply because they don't fit the reigning paradigm does not mean they are ineffective. In the case of the chiropractic profession, it is abundantly clear that the care we offer is effective for a wide variety of health-care situations, and that research is demonstrating just how effective it can be.

Finally, Dr. Eisenberg notes that the majority of patients who saw alternative health-care practitioners did not inform their medical doctor. To him, that is a problem. All I can say is, "Why should they?"—D.J. Lawrence, D.C.

Utilisation of Chiropractic Services by Members of One Private Health Fund in Victoria, 1990

Ebrall PS (RMIT Univ, Melbourne, Victoria, Australia)

Chiroprac J Aust 22:122–128, 1992 5–2

Background.—In Australia, where cooperative health-care plans have long been in place, reimbursement of expenses for chiropractic treatment is limited to a set amount per visit (mean, $16); a set amount once per year for an initial consultation (mean, $19); and a set limit per year (up to $600 per family). In the United States, one community-based study of the use of chiropractic services found a substantial tail to the right, with 2% of the total person-years examined accounting for 10% of the total number of visits.

Methods.—A study of 252,193 payments for chiropractic services made during 1 year by a major private health fund in Victoria, Australia, sought to determine whether a similar positive skew existed and whether its characteristics might be valid indicators of the use of chiropractic services. A utilization index of services per eligible member was calculated by dividing the number of services reimbursed by the fund by the number of eligible members.

Results.—Similar to the United States study, a considerable tail to the right was identified, with just 2% of practice locations generating 15% of all initial services. In addition, 2% of practice locations generated 15% of subsequent visits. The typical practice location accepted 7 to 10 initial consultations and generated 168 to 243 subsequent services during the study. Certain regions could be identified as having more than marginally atypical utilization.

Conclusion.—A positive skew in chiropractic use in 1 private health fund in Victoria, Australia was documented. Indicators of atypical use identify regions in which there are more practice locations than expected by chance. If such high utilization levels are accepted as a normal variant, the economic implications to insurers are vital. If they reflect a practice aberration, they may be containable by insurers.

▶ Studies that examine chiropractic utilization patterns are important in the new and developing health-care environment. These studies result, in part, from escalating costs and the needs of third-party payers to keep costs within manageable levels. However, these studies are difficult to manage and few of them exist. Studies in the United States show a distinct skew to the right, where few practice locations account for great percentages of utilization. This study, done in Australia, demonstrated similar findings. Health-care policy planning will need to be mindful of these patterns.—D.J. Lawrence, D.C.

Acute Low Back Pain and Economics of Therapy: The Iterative Loop Approach

Lawrence VA, Tugwell P, Gafni A, Kosuwon W, Spitzer WO (Univ of Texas, San Antonio; McMaster Univ, Hamilton, Ont, Canada; McGill Univ, Montreal)

J Clin Epidemiol 45:301–311, 1992 5–3

Introduction.—Acute and subacute nonspecific low back pain consumes considerable resources in medical care, absence from work, and workers' compensation. Furthermore, the effectiveness of therapies for the treatment of nonspecific low back pain has not been proven. The measurement iterative loop, a model for the critical appraisal of the

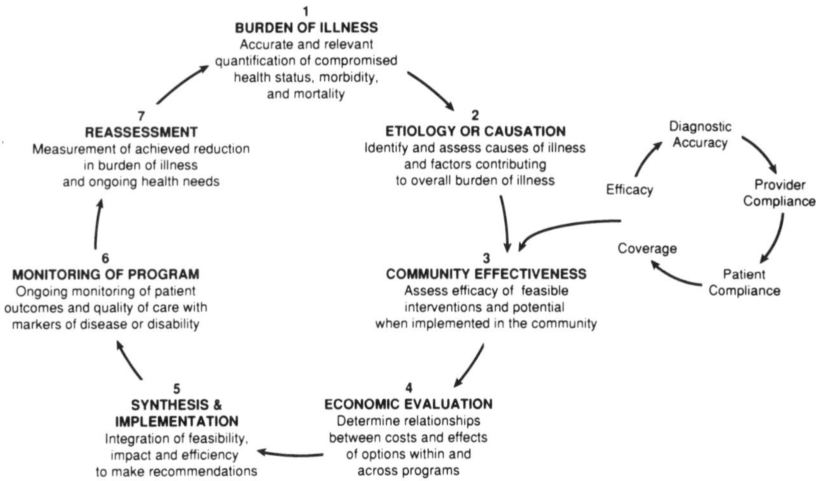

Fig 5–1.—The measurement iterative loop: a framework for the critical appraisal of need, benefits, and costs of health interventions. (Courtesy of Lawrence VA, Tugwell P, Gafni A, et al: *J Clin Epidemiol* 45:301–311, 1992.)

need, benefits, and costs of health interventions (Fig 5–1), was used to examine nonspecific low back pain.

Measurements.—Although there is evidence that acute and subacute nonspecific low back pain causes substantial burden of illness, precise estimates of compromised health status and morbidity are not available. Difficulty in obtaining specific diagnoses contributes to the lack of accurate information.

Therapy.—Although many therapies for the treatment of nonspecific low back pain have been proposed, the usual prescription includes bedrest, nonsteroidal anti-inflammatory analgesics, back school, physical therapy, and possibly muscle relaxants. A review of randomized controlled clinical trials of various treatment modalities showed some evidence of benefit for bedrest, back school, and physical therapy, but insufficient evidence of benefit for other therapeutic modalities, including spinal manipulation. The management of low back pain, as recommended by the Quebec Task Force on Spinal Disorders (QTFSD), combines a short period of bedrest with physical therapy and back school.

Cost-Benefit.—Analysis of the cost-benefit of bed rest, back school, physiotherapy, and QTFSD management reveals that bedrest at home plus analgesics and possibly muscle relaxants is the most economically efficient therapy (table).

Conclusion.—The measurement iterative loop reveals that the burden of illness associated with acute nonspecific low back pain is substantial but inaccurately measured to date. Bedrest appears to be economically superior to all other treatment modalities, followed closely by the management as recommended by the QTFSD.

Summary of Modified Cost-Benefit Analysis (CBA)

	CBA assuming equal community effectiveness for all four therapies					
	Direct * medical cost	Days lost from work	Indirect cost of lost earnings	Total cost	Cost averted with bedrest	Threshold values for recurrence rates compared to bedrest: reduced rate of recurrence needed to equal bedrest in cost
Physiotherapy	$1084	26.5 [12]	$2533	$3617	$3065	6.6
Back School	1313	20.5 [12]	1960	3273	2721	5.9
QTFSD†	1340	8.4 [66]	803	2143	1591	3.8
Bedrest	256	3.1 [33]	296	552	—	—

* Figures in 1985 Canadian dollars. Conversion factor to 1985 United States dollars is .7. Assumes equal use of analgesics and muscle relaxants among the 4 therapies.

† First step management recommended by the QTFSD.

(Courtesy of Lawrence VA, Tugwell P, Gafni A, et al: *J Clin Epidemiol* 45:301–311, 1992.)

▶ The iterative loop approach provides a useful model for the evaluation of various management strategies for low back pain. Economic evaluation becomes especially important when several treatment approaches are shown to be effective. The authors' review of treatment interventions suggests an inadequate evaluation of the evidence on spinal manipulation. Recent scientific overviews have documented the effectiveness of spinal manipulation in patients with certain types of acute and subacute low back pain.—A.H. Adams, D.C.

Patient Satisfaction With Chiropractic Care

Sawyer CE, Kassak K (Northwestern College of Chiropractic, Bloomington, Minn)

J Manipulative Physiol Ther 16:25–32, 1992 5–4

Introduction.—Studies of patient satisfaction determine how the patient feels about the process and result of care. The patient's viewpoint cannot be replaced by direct observation; it gives the provider useful information for predicting patient behavior. Patients' attitudes about the process and outcome of chiropractic care were surveyed to identify characteristics predicting patient satisfaction.

TABLE 1.—Satisfaction Survey Content and Organization

Scale/subscale	Item no.	Question
General satisfaction	1	I am satisfied with the care I received.
	9	The care I received was just about perfect.
	18	I would recommend this doctor to a friend or relative.
	20	The care I received could have been better. *
	24	I expected better results from the treatment I received.*
	26	Improvements in my condition took longer than I expected. *
Access to the doctor		
Convenience of location	2	My doctor's office was easy to get to.
	32	It takes me a long time to get to my doctor's office.*
Appointments	7	I had to wait a long time before I could see this doctor for my first visit*
	14	I was able to schedule appointments that were convenient for me.
	30	In an emergency, it was hard for me to get in to see my doctor quickly.*
	23	My doctor's office hours were convenient for me.
Finance	5	The cost of treatment has caused a financial burden for me.*
	10	My doctor's fees were reasonable.
	15	My insurance provided adequate coverage for the cost of my care.
	27	My doctor's payment policies posed no problems for me.

Methods.—A patient satisfaction questionnaire was mailed to 541 new and returning chiropractic patients who received care during a 1-year period. The survey consisted of 32 attitude statements with a 5-point Likert scale (Table 1) and a personal information questionnaire. Clinical information was provided by the chiropractor. The response rate was 70%.

Findings.—Women were somewhat more satisfied with their care than men; gender was the only characteristic affecting general satisfaction. Twenty-eight percent of patients said that improvement of their condition took longer than expected, but almost all said they would recommend the practitioner. Access to the practitioner was the area with which patients were most satisfied. Patients were least satisfied with the

Doctor conduct		
Competence	3	My doctor was not as thorough as he/she should have been. *
	8	My doctor was interested in all my health problems.
	11	Some of the examination procedures my doctor used were unnecessary*
	29	I feel I had to see my doctor more than I should have. *
	31	My doctor was very careful to check everything when examining me.
Communication	4	All of my questions were answered by my doctor.
	17	My doctor didn't give me suggestions on what I could do to help my problem. *
	19	My doctor gave me advice on how to prevent health problems from occurring.
Humaneness	6	My doctor did his/her best to keep me from worrying about my problem.
	12	My doctor treated me with respect and concern.
	16	My doctor made me feel foolish.*
	22	I think that my doctor should have spent more time with me. *
	28	My doctor acted as though I was important.
	33	My doctor avoided unnecessary patient expenses.
Facilities	21	My doctor's staff was helpful and courteous.
	13	I think my doctor's office has everything needed to provide good chiropractic care.

* Negatively worded questions for which scoring direction was reversed (*1* = strongly disagree).
(Courtesy of Sawyer CE, Kassak K: *J Manipulative Physiol Ther* 16:25–32, 1992.)

TABLE 2.—Patient Satisfaction Scores

Scale/subscale	Mean *	SD	Chronbach's alpha
General satisfaction	1.89	0.63	0.86
Access	1.69	0.48	0.62
Convenience of location	1.74	0.71	0.63
Appointments	1.66	0.54	0.59
Finance	2.24	0.70	0.60
Doctor conduct	1.76	0.46	0.88
Competence	1.89	0.56	0.67
Communication	1.73	0.58	0.55
Humaneness	1.71	0.47	0.74
Facilities	1.60	0.54	0.52
Total satisfaction	1.89	0.46	0.92

* A mean of 1 for questionnaire scales and subscales would indicate strong agreement with survey items (or strong disagreement with negatively worded items) and, consequently, a high level of satisfaction.

(Courtesy of Sawyer CE, Kassak K: *J Manipulative Physiol Ther* 16:25–32, 1992.)

financial aspects of treatment, particularly those with lower incomes or no insurance (Table 2). The most important predictor of patient satisfaction was treatment outcome, with the 12% of patients who reported minimal or no improvement also reporting a slightly greater degree of dissatisfaction.

Conclusion.—A high level of patient satisfaction with chiropractors and the care rendered was found. Women expressed slightly more satisfaction than men, but satisfaction was otherwise unaffected by characteristics such as education, income, employment status, or previous chiropractic care. Further research on the relationship between rendering chiropractic care and patient satisfaction is needed.

▶ This study adds to the literature regarding chiropractic patients' satisfaction with the health care they receive. An expected finding in this study was that treatment outcome was predictive of patient satisfaction, i.e., the more positively a patient perceived his or her response to therapy, the more positive was his or her satisfaction level. We must keep in mind that not all patients will have positive treatment results, despite the best efforts of the chiropractor; therefore we need to be sensitive to the patient's perception of our care.—D.J. Lawrence, D.C.

CPT/EM Codes in the 1990s

Murkowski KS

ICA Review 49:49–53, 1993 5–5

Introduction.—The Current Procedural Terminology (CPT) coding system was derived from the California Relative Value System, which was first published in 1956; it includes more than 7,000 codes and descriptions for reporting the services and procedures performed by physicians and other health-care providers. Its objective is to provide a uniform language describing medical, general, surgical, and diagnostic services, and to allow nationwide communication among physicians, patients, and third-party carriers. The CPT also is used for administrative management purposes.

Use of CPT E/M.—Health-care providers are still attempting to interpret the 1992 CPT Evaluation/Management (E/M) Service Code numbers. These Codes provide a new way of classifying how physicians work with patients. The basic format includes a code number; the place and/or type of service; the content of the service; the nature of the presenting problems, usually with a given level; and the time expected for services. Practicing physicians have been surveyed to determine the amount of time and work associated with typical E/M services.

A 6-Step Guide.—After meeting with office staff to itemize all procedures used in the office, copies of the current CPT manual are distributed, and a super bill is created to record all charges. A master reference 92 CPT Code list should be available for services used most often in the office. Check with the state association and/or the Peer Review Committee to solicit opinions. Looking to the future, it may be desirable to establish a "case fee basis" with written guidelines.

Overview.—Doctors of chiropractic must consider establishing a profile in 1993 by listing all procedures done in their offices. Many third-party reimbursing agencies are implementing payment on the new E/M Codes and rejecting claims not based on them.

▶ As most of us are now aware, the new CPT codings are far more complicated than the simple codes used before 1992. Dr. Murkowski discusses the options available to chiropractors under the new coding system. I believe that this might have been made stronger by the use of several sample calculations using established patient records; however, the general basis for the new system is well elaborated.—D.J. Lawrence, D.C.

A Study of Patients and Patient Complaints at Chiropractic Teaching Clinics

Walsh MJ (Phillip Inst of Technology, Bundoora, Victoria, Australia)

Chiroprac J Aust 22:61–64, 1992 5–6

Objective.—Although teaching clinics are commonly used data sources for research purposes, it is unknown whether the findings can be generalized to the at-large population of chiropractic patients. The characteristics of patients attending 3 Australian teaching chiropractic clinics were compared, and the patient characteristics of North American teaching clinics were compared with the Australian results. Also, a data base for comparing patients at teaching and private clinics was provided.

CHIEF PRESENTING COMPLAINTS (%)

Complaint	Abbotsford (n=166)	Bulleen (n=75)	Summerhill (n=69)	Total (n=310)
Low Back	34.9	25.3	33.3	33.2
Cervical	15.7	34.7	21.2	23.6
Thoracic	19.8	17.3	18.2	16.5
Shoulder	7.8	6.7	3.0	6.4
Elbow	3.0	1.3	0.0	1.9
Wrist	1.2	0.0	1.6	1.0
Hip	1.2	0.0	0.0	0.6
Knee	3.6	4.0	0.0	2.9
Ankle	1.8	1.3	6.2	2.6
Headache	6.0	5.3	16.7	8.1
Other visceral	4.8	4.0	0.0	3.2

$\chi^2 = 20.2$; $df = 14$; $P > .05$ (the categories elbow, wrist, hip, knee, and ankle have been grouped together for this calculation).

(Courtesy of Walsh MJ: *Chiroprac J Aust* 22:61-64, 1992.)

Methods and Findings.—The analysis included 310 patients seen by interns during a 1-year period at 3 clinics associated with 1 Australian school of chiropractic and osteopathy. There were slightly more females than males, and the median patient age was 34 years. One of the clinics had a significantly greater proportion of patients in the under-20-years group. Most patients were in nonmanual occupations, followed by light manual, unemployed, and heavy manual. Spinal problems accounted for about three fourths of the chief complaints at all 3 clinics, with one third consisting of low back pain (table). Nearly half of the complaints were of unknown cause, with trauma accounting for most of the rest. Most of the complaints had been present for at least 2 months before presentation, and 91% represented only the first or second episode of the complaint.

Conclusion.—Few differences were found among patients at 3 teaching chiropractic clinics in terms of sociodemographic characteristics and types and characteristics of complaints. Thus, studies could be performed using pooled data from the 3 clinics. The data are similar to those reported in US and Canadian clinics; the data will be compared with data from private clinics. There was a high incidence of cause unknown for the chief complaint, probably more attributable to the insidious nature of the complaint than to lack of memory.

▶ There are 2 basic reasons for examining the incidence of patient complaints at chiropractic teaching clinics. One is that the profession needs to assure itself that its students are being exposed to a wide range of problems so that they gain some expertise before graduation; the other involves the development of a data source for clinical research. Past studies have been fairly uniform in their findings, and this one is no exception. The majority of patients seek chiropractic care for musculoskeletal complaints, primarily for spinal problems and then for extremity conditions. Visceral problems account for a relatively small percentage of visits. We need to examine the reasons for this if the chiropractic profession is to seek primary-care status nationwide; there must be greater exposure to organic problems, even if the end result is a referral to a medical practitioner.—D.J. Lawrence, D.C.

Proposal for Establishing Structure and Process in the Development of Implicit Chiropractic Standards of Care and Practice Guidelines

Hansen DT, Adams AH, Meeker WC, Phillips RB (Los Angeles College of Chiropractic, Whittier, Calif; Palmer College of Chiropractic-West, Sunnyvale, Calif)

J Manipulative Physiol Ther 15:430–438, 1992 5–7

Introduction.—In an area of increasing accountability in health-care practice, the chiropractic profession must create its own implicit standards and guidelines for care. Failing this, outside public and private sector purchasing groups will do so. The need for standards of care in chiropractic were examined, and a proposal for developing such standards was offered.

Discussion.—A number of state chiropractic associations have already been pressured into unsophisticated attempts at creating guidelines, which lack input from the national chiropractic associations or their representatives. The literature clearly defines the process of creating guidelines by various consensus methods, and gives information on measuring outcome once the guidelines have been developed. Now the United States Congress has directed the Agency for Health Care Policy and Research, a new federal agency, to oversee the development of standards and monitor the outcome of quality improvement programs.

Proposal.—The chiropractic profession should now define its own role in health-care delivery and create implicit standards and practice guidelines. A panel of experts, commissioned to represent the academic and clinical chiropractic profession, should manage the standard development effort. The protocol for selecting the panel and the appropriate method for development of standards remain to be decided. Having defined the structure and process of standard development, the chiropractic profession can bring it to federal and state agencies, private-sector health-care purchasers, patient advocacy groups, and others. The profession will be legitimized by providing a mechanism for internal consensus and by the establishment of a research agenda to evaluate chiropractic procedures.

Summary.—A structure is proposed by which to create implicit standards of care and practice guidelines for the chiropractic profession. A preliminary definition of the structure and process, with a "seed" policy statement and decision flow chart for guideline development, are included in the proposal. By legitimizing the chiropractic profession, this effort will probably expedite research funding by federal agencies.

▶ The controversy surrounding the development of standards of care within the chiropractic profession seems destined to increase, at least over the short term. Part of that controversy arises from a lack of understanding concerning the processes used to set the standards. Because there is a wide range of ethical practice protocols within the chiropractic profession, how can a set of standards be determined? These authors show the methods by which the profession can begin the process of handling the massive volumes of information necessary to meet the requirements of the groups seeking to impose standards upon us, yet they allow us to be proactive in determining just what those standards should comprise.

The 2 consensus methods widely used in the chiropractic profession are the nominal group and the Delphi methods. In the nominal group procedure, a panel is asked to independently list answers to specific questions. Each panelist presents a single answer (the most important one first) in round-robin fashion, until the lists are exhausted. These answers are recorded, discussed and, finally, ranked by each panelist. At the end, the group discusses the views presented. Delphi methodology involves a poll of experts with questionnaires, and it is done in rounds as each set of answers is gathered. It is competed when there is convergence of opinion.

These procedures allow for a consensus to develop, which can then be used by organizations to set standards. The attributes of chiropractic standards are provided by the authors in an appendix to this paper.—D.J. Lawrence, D.C.

The Descriptive Profile of Low Back Pain Patients of Field Practicing Chiropractors Contrasted With Those Treated in the Clinics of West Coast Chiropractic Colleges

Phillips RB, Mootz RD, Nyiendo J, Cooperstein R, Konsler J, Mennon M (Los Angeles College of Chiropractic, Whittier, Calif; Palmer College of Chiropractic-West, Sunnyvale, Calif; Western States Chiropractic College, Portland, Ore; Pasadena College of Chiropractic, Calif; Cleveland Chiropractic College, Los Angeles)

J Manipulative Physiol Ther 15:512–517, 1992 5–8

Background.—Patients seeking chiropractic care for back pain may do so from a licensed chiropractor or from an outpatient teaching clinic at a chiropractic college. No studies have compared the practice of chiropractors in these 2 practice settings. The differences and similarities were assessed in a survey analysis of new patients at private practices vs. teaching clinics.

Methods.—New patients were randomly selected from 10 chiropractic offices located near 6 west coast chiropractic colleges during a 10-year period. The self-report study was limited to patients with low back pain.

The data were compared to the findings of a previous study of consecutive new patients in a similar time frame from chiropractic teaching college clinics (CTCCs).

Results.—The analysis included data on 392 patients, 141 of whom had low back pain as their main complaint. This represented a 65% response rate, compared to 99.5% for the CTCC study. The 2 patient groups were similar in terms of gender distribution, job description, and education. However, 61% of those in the CTCC group made less than $20,000/year vs. 37% of the private practice group. Twenty-nine percent of the CTCC group lost no work time, vs. 43% of the private practice group. Severity and functional disability were also greater in the private practice group.

Conclusion.—Chiropractic teaching college clinics and private practice patient populations are comparable in terms of sociodemographic characteristics. There is clinical variation, however, including a higher percentage of patients with chronic and mild low back pain in the CTCC setting. These differences should be accounted for in extrapolating research findings from the teaching clinic setting to the chiropractic profession in general.

▶ Because the chiropractic profession has traditionally found it difficult to obtain federal research money, we have had to turn to other sources for funding. The difficulty of running clinical trials is compounded by the difficulty in recruiting patients for those studies. No clinical trial is worth the money and trouble if its results are not in some manner applicable to the real world. Because the likeliest location for clinical trials resides within the chiropractic colleges, the most likely source of subjects for studies is from the population of patients who visit CTCCs. However, are these individuals a reasonable representation of the "real world"? This study discusses the demographics of patients who visited 6 west coast college clinics; it found that they are similar to patients who visit private chiropractic clinics. The population of patients from CTCCs are, therefore, worthy of inclusion in large-scale clinical trials.—D.J. Lawrence, D.C.

Strategies for Improving and Expanding the Application of Health Status Measures in Clinical Settings: A Researcher-Developer Viewpoint

Deyo RA, Carter WB (Seattle Veterans Affairs Med Ctr)

Med Care 30:176MS–186MS, 1992 5–9

Purpose.—Health status measures can be used for a wide range of purposes in clinical practice, including screening for functional problems, monitoring disease progression or therapeutic response, improving communications between clinician and patient, assessing quality of care, and comparing outcomes between patient groups. Such applications have been hindered, however, by conceptual, practical, and attitudinal barriers. The ways in which health status measures affect the process and outcomes of care were described, and strategies to enhance and expand their application were presented.

Education.—An important step in broadening the application of health status instruments is training health-care providers in the various measures, their validity, and the available instruments. Scores may be made more meaningful by comparing newer functional measures with the older scales that clinicians are familiar with. There should be better data for selection of instruments, and their responsiveness to clinical changes should be improved.

Strategies.—In direct patient care, the goal of the health status measure determines its selection, the types of patients it will be used for, and the frequency with which it is used. To fit into the office routine, the instruments must be brief, easily interpretable, and without the need for complicated training. Clinicians should be provided with information on management and community resources to consider in addition to functional status scores. Third-party payers must be convinced that the health status measures are providing useful information. Quality assurance applications must include adjustment of average scores for groups of patients for disease severity, comorbidity, demographic characteristics, socioeconomic status, and baseline health status. Often, the most severely ill or vulnerable patients in the clinical population may be least able to provide valid information on health status. As these patients are likely to alter the average scores for the overall population, the methods to ensure complete ascertainment must be considered.

Conclusion.—Health status measurement can be useful in routine care settings for a variety of purposes. Education of health-care practitioners is a vital step in the dissemination of such measures. Special considerations to remember when using health status measures in the management of individual patients were outlined.

▶ Dr. Deyo is one of the true innovators and leading researchers in epidemiologic low back pain research. In this study, he discusses some of the impediments to the use of health status measures in clinical research. He considers 3 main groups of barriers: attitudinal, methodologic, and practical. Training chiropractors in the use of these instruments (e.g., the Roland-Morris Disability Scale) would help to overcome at least 2 of these barriers, leaving only practical considerations as the main impediment. There are many health status tools that chiropractors can use; many don't, leaving the measurement of outcomes more suspect than necessary. This must change, given the drive toward accountability that all health-care professions are experiencing.—D.J. Lawrence, D.C.

Benefits and Obstacles of Health Status Assessment in Ambulatory Settings: The Clinician's Point of View

Wasson J, Keller A, Rubenstein L, Hays R, Nelson E, Johnson D, Dartmouth

Primary Care COOP Project (Dartmouth-Hitchcock Med Ctr, Hanover, NH; Univ of California, Los Angeles; RAND Corp, Santa Monica, Calif; Hosp Corp of America, Nashville, Tenn)
Med Care 30:42MS–49MS, 1992 5–10

Background.—Standard medical care has traditionally emphasized diagnosis and treatment of conditions, overlooking global function and quality of life. Health status, or functional, assessment would appropriately be performed in the clinic setting, but time constraints and the lack of reimbursement pose problems. Ways in which the clinician can identify and manage functional problems during brief, outpatient visits were studied.

Discussion.—The clinic must address 4 important issues before adopting health status assessment: why function is measured; how it is fit into a brief patient encounter; what is done with the assessment information; and when functional status measurements are done. The reason for health status assessments is now generally understood; clinicians now need answers to the other questions. There are many problems associated with integrating measurement into clinical practice, which are not always recognized. The clinician must pay careful attention to the office ecosystem and overcome barriers through improved communication with other clinicians, staff, and patients. Individual tasks must be jointly assigned to incorporate assessment procedures with no adverse effect on patient flow. Integration will be easier if the instrument is simple and easy to use. However, the clinician must choose among competing priorities for unreimbursed time and may be obligated to document action once poor function is detected.

The results of health status screening must be transformed into a functional diagnosis, which is based on an understanding of the measure's sensitivity, specificity, and predictive value. Establishing the specific functional diagnosis may require additional measurements, known as assessment linkage. Having identified the cause of the dysfunction, the clinician must determine the need for special services, known as resource linkage.

Summary.—A clinician's perspective on the integration of health status assessment into the busy ambulatory care setting was examined. Steps are provided by which to overcome the obstacles to performing such assessments as a routine part of clinical care.

▶ This article provides a contrast to the paper by Deyo and Carter (Abstract 5–9). By clarifying a clinical perspective on the use of health status assessment, the authors remind us of the good they can do. Their point is that it is extremely difficult to integrate measurement procedures into practice operations; by keeping mindful of the reasons the measures are used, the patient and the doctor ultimately benefit.—D.J. Lawrence, D.C.

Family Physicians, Chiropractors, and Back Pain

Curtis P, Bove G (Univ of North Carolina, Chapel Hill)

J Fam Pract 35:551–555, 1992 5–11

Background.—Back pain is the second leading reason that patients report for visiting physicians. Chiropractors account for about twice the number of visits for back pain as physicians. Patient satisfaction reported in a health maintenance organization population indicated significantly greater satisfaction with chiropractic care than with family physician care, primarily because patients perceived that family physicians were not able to provide as clear or rational an explanation of the problem to the patient and that they did not individualize management as well as chiropractors. Although the American Medical Association's ethical prohibition against referral to a chiropractor has been overturned, many physicians are reluctant to make specific referrals. Guidelines published by the RAND Corporation in 1991 assessed the appropriateness of spinal manipulation for low back pain. The guidelines may be useful for primary-care physicians and the health insurance industry in deciding which patients may benefit from referral to a chiropractor or an osteopath.

Method.—The expert-panel approach relied on literature review and complex consensus development to develop guidelines on the indications and time frames to be expected for manipulative treatment and recovery. Guidelines on identifying a competent chiropractor were also developed (Table 1).

Recommendations.—A favorable previous response to manipulation is a good sign that chiropractic treatment may be helpful again. Absent or

TABLE 1.—Guidelines for Identifying a Competent Chiropractor

- Treats mainly musculoskeletal disorders with manual manipulative techniques
- Does not do routine radiographs on every patient
- Does not extend duration of treatment unnecessarily (see Table 2)
- Writes a response to a referral and outlines evaluation and therapy
- Does not charge "front end" lump sum for whole treatment program
- Graduated from a school accredited by the Council on Chiropractic Education
- Is willing to have physician visit the office to observe treatment
- Good feedback from patients on care given

(Courtesy of Curtis P, Bove G: *J Fam Pract* 35:551–555, 1992.)

TABLE 2.—Clinical Profiles Appropriate for Manipulation

Problem	Duration of Treatment*
Acute low back pain (<3wk) Previous good response to manipulation Normal or abnormal radiographs Radicular pain None or minor neurologic signs	3 to 5 treatments, maximum of 10 before reevaluation
Subacute low back pain (3-12 wk) Previous good response to manipulation Normal or abnormal radiographs No neurologic signs	Unclear
Chronic low back pain (>3 mo) Previous good response to manipulation Normal radiographs/imaging No neurologic signs	3 treatments/wk for up to 8 wk before reevaluation

* Estimates, not consensus.
(From Curtis P, Bove G: *J Fam Pract* 35:551–555, 1992. Adapted from Shekelle PG, Adams AH, Chassin MR, et al: *The Appropriateness of Spinal Manipulation for Low-Back Pain. Indications and Ratings by a Multidisciplinary Panel.* Santa Monica, Calif, RAND Corp, 1991.)

minor neurologic signs and normal radiographic findings in the presence of acute, subacute, or chronic low back pain are clinical profiles appropriate for manipulation (Table 2).

Conclusion.—Guidelines developed with an expert panel approach and reported by the Rand Corporation identify the clinical profiles of patients who are appropriate candidates for manipulation by a chiropractor. A previous good response to manipulation is one of the strongest indicators of future success with manipulation.

▶ The authors, one of whom is a chiropractor, provide a set of guidelines for medical professionals to use in referring their patients to a chiropractor. The practice of manipulative therapy is explained in detail, and a list of contraindications and indications for its use is provided. Some of the contraindications may seem controversial or even specious. One contraindication for manipulation is arthritis; another contraindication is neurologic disease (for which specific neurologic diseases are the authors making this recommendation?). A stronger case for chiropractic might have been made here, based upon the available evidence, only some of which the authors cite. Still, the recommendations for selecting a chiropractor to work with are prudent, and the overall tone of the paper is quite positive.—D.J. Lawrence, D.C.

Chiropractic Adjustment in the Management of Visceral Conditions: A Critical Appraisal

Jamison JR, McEwen AP, Thomas SJ (Phillip Inst of Technology, Victoria, Australia)

J Manipulative Physiol Ther 15:171–180, 1992 5–12

Introduction.—The rationale for spinal intervention in managing visceral conditions is based on empiricism. The current study was performed to determine whether Australian chiropractors consider spinal adjustment an intervention option for patients with visceral conditions and to determine the preferred level of adjustment for patients with migraine, asthma, hypertension, or dysmenorrhea.

Methods.—All 1,311 chiropractors registered in Australia were surveyed. Their opinions on the usefulness of spinal adjustment in treating patients with visceral conditions were elicited. Practitioners were asked to comment on the appropriate level of adjustment in managing different conditions based on their personal clinical experience.

Results.—Twenty-two percent of the chiropractors responded to the survey. More than half favored a role for spinal adjustment in such patients. The perceived usefulness of spinal adjustment and the preferred level of adjustment varied according to the condition being managed. Respondents who were able to identify vertebral levels that they associated with the greatest success were most likely to do so in the treatment of migraine and were least likely in hypertension. Most respondents said they adjust the atlas, axis, or upper cervical vertebrae in patients with migraine. Most reported adjusting lower cervical and/or upper thoracic vertebrae in patients with asthma or hypertension. In women with dysmenorrhea, the lumbar and lumbosacral region were prime therapeutic targets.

Conclusion.—Even though this intervention is regarded as an obstacle to the recommendation of public funding for chiropractic services in Australia, Australian chiropractors continue to use spinal adjustment in the management of visceral conditions. Further study of the validity of the chiropractic management of visceral conditions is needed.

▶ There is great controversy and debate in Australia regarding chiropractic involvement in treating and diagnosing organic disease. The Australian Medical Association has gone on record as being opposed to chiropractic involvement with such disorders, and the profession itself is split regarding the issue. Dr. Jamison surveyed all chiropractors in Australia regarding their opinion on this subject. In particular, she was interested in the use of manipulation for managing visceral disease. Although she received only a 22% response, there did seem to be some consistency among respondents regarding the levels to adjust for certain diseases (e.g., upper cervical region for migraine, and the lower cervical or upper thoracic region for asthma). Although there has been a great deal of conflicting data regarding manipulation and visceral disease over the years, the majority of papers published (and we must acknowledge the osteopathic profession in particular here) are positive in their findings. Dr. Jamison notes 4 points worth discussion: (1) clearly delineate diagnostic criteria; (2) discriminate between objective clinical outcomes and subjective responses; (3) take the natural history of the process into account; and (4) compare therapeutic interventions. The third point in particular is often missed by chiropractors. Often, cases are written that describe a manipulative intervention in a disease process and indeed the patient gets better. However, is this the result of the intervention. If the natural history is that patients generally get better within 5 days and it took the patient 5 days to respond, then did the therapy do anything at all?

The Australian chiropractors face an uphill fight to gain public funding for managing visceral conditions with manipulation. Only more and better research will allow them coverage; public health agencies do not generally offer coverage to speculative procedures.—D.J. Lawrence, D.C.

Factors Influencing the Adoption and Maintenance of Canadian, Facility-Based Worksite Health Promotion Programs

Wolfe R, Slack T, Rose-Hearn T (Univ of Alberta, Edmonton, Canada)

Am J Health Promot 7:189–198, 1993 5–13

Purpose.—Worksite health promotion programs have increased significantly in recent years. These programs offer a variety of valuable services—smoking cessation, stress management, weight control, exercise and fitness, health risk appraisal, blood pressure screening, nutrition education, prevention of back problems, and prevention of accidents. They are associated with such benefits as decreased absenteeism, health-care costs, and turnover. However, because of discrepant motivations and objectives between executives and health professionals, the continued growth and long-term viability of these programs may be in jeopardy. The rationale of senior management for adopting and maintaining worksite health promotion programs was surveyed and compared with the objectives of the health professionals managing the programs.

Methods.—Using a multiple case-study design, 9 major Canadian organizations with facility-based health promotion programs were included. Data were collected by semistructured interviews, questionnaires, and internal reports. The respondents were senior managers involved in adopting the program, senior managers responsible for program budgets, and senior health promotion professionals.

Findings.—The motivation for adopting the health promotion program was related more to tangential issues—moving to a new building or gaining access to unused space—than with concerns about the health of employees or the performance of the organization. The program was most commonly adopted because of its potential recruiting benefits. The rationale for maintaining the program generally concerned process issues, such as participation rates and quality of activity offerings, more

Program Objectives According to Organizational Managers and Program Managers

	Sample	Management	Professionals
Human Relations	19.35 *	18.63	20.00
	(5.18)	(6.21)	(4.40)
Improve morale			
Improve cohesion			
Decrease conflict			
Positively affect human relations			
Rational Goal	17.56	17.33	17.78
	(6.21)	(6.21)	(6.57)
Increase profit			
Achieve company goals			
Contribute to efficiency			
Contribute to productivity			
Open Systems	16.29	15.38	17.11
	(6.25)	(8.02)	(4.51)
Contribute to competitiveness			
Increase flexibility			
Help meet challenges			
Improve external image			
Internal Processes	15.83 †	16.33	15.33
	(4.79)	(5.36)	(4.42)
Improve workforce stability			
Improve workforce continuity			
Increase interaction			
Improve communication			

Note: Response options ranged from 1 (low importance) to 7 (high importance); the scales, therefore, could range from 4 (1 × 4) to 28 (4 × 7).
* Significantly greater than † at the .05 level.
(Courtesy of Wolfe R, Slack T, Rose-Hearn T: *Am J Health Promot* 7:189–198, 1993.)

than health or organizational outcomes. Both the health professionals and senior managers stated that the human relations and morale aspects of the program were more important than saving money, although the health professionals considered the cost savings more important than did the senior managers (table).

Conclusion.—In the adoption and maintenance of worksite health promotion programs, health professionals should develop program objectives in common with those of senior management. These programs reflect the realization by business leaders that the traditional corporate view must include a focus on the human element. Expanding on an organizational innovation model, a comprehensive worksite health promotion program adoption model is presented (Fig 5–2).

▶ The implementation of a work-based health promotion program is based, in part, on the goals of senior management. Often times, the selection of a program may be based on cost-containment issues rather than health-related ones. In this study, 2 groups of individuals involved in setting up health promotion programs were studied to investigate these attitudinal issues. The health professionals involved in these programs more often considered cost

2) Organization Policy
— aggressive recruiting policy
1) Appropriate Context
— competitive labor market
— increased global competition
— program institutionalization
3) Preinnovation Condition
— program champion
4) Innovation Adoption
— program adoption
Innovation Process Initiator
— availability of corporate space

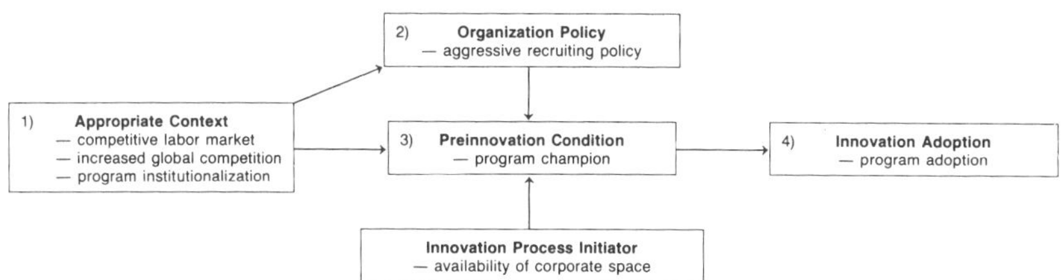

Fig 5–2.—Worksite Health Promotion Program Adoption Model. (Courtesy of Wolfe R, Slack T, Rose-Hearn T: *Am J Health Promot* 7:189–198, 1993.)

issues; senior management looked more at human relations and morale issues. Future programs may need to examine their outcome measures when these programs are initiated. This study may also be limited by its small sample size, and it should be extrapolated into different industrial and occupational settings.—D.J. Lawrence, D.C.

Arthritis: The Cumulative Impact of a Common Chronic Condition
Yelin E (Univ of California, San Francisco)
Arthritis Rheum 35:489–497, 1992 5–14

Objective.—The number of individuals with arthritis among working-age and elderly individuals who meet the criteria for disability defined by the recently enacted Americans with Disabilities Act (ADA) was estimated.

Methods.—The prevalence of arthritis-related disability among working-age adults, aged 18–64 years, was determined using the data from the 1970–1987 National Health Interview Survey (NIS), an annual survey of the noninstitutionalized population of the continental United States. In the NIS, arthritis is defined by self-report of symptoms and diagnoses. The prevalence of arthritis-related disability among adults aged 70 years and older was determined using data from the Longitudinal Study on Aging survey.

Results.—Among 71.429 million working-age men, 3.734 million reported having arthritis, of whom 2.208 million reported limitation in physical activity. Among 75.689 million working-age women, 5.649 million reported having arthritis, of whom 3.390 million reported activity limitation. Labor force participation rates were about 20% lower among men and about 25% lower among women with arthritis than they were among those without arthritis. Of 15.613 million community-dwelling elderly individuals aged 70 years and older, 55% reported having arthritis. More than 75% reported limitation in physical activities and more than one-third reported limitations in an activity of daily living (ADL), with 6% reporting limitations in 5 or more ADLs. Furthermore, disability rates among persons with arthritis appears to be on the rise, and the health status among the elderly with arthritis appears to be deteriorating.

Conclusion.—Persons with arthritis experience a disproportionate amount of disability relative to those with other chronic disorders.

▶ Arthritis is undoubtedly one of the most common conditions to be seen in a chiropractic office. It can cause serious limitations in the normal activities of daily living, and it has major impact on the labor force in general. The incidence of the condition may be increasing because of the increased life expectancy.—D.J. Lawrence, D.C.

Chiropractic Principles

The Embryology of Chiropractic Thought

Keating JC Jr (Palmer College of Chiropractic-West, Sunnyvale, Calif)
Eur J Chiroprac 39:75–89, 1991 5–15

Background.—The basic theory and method of chiropractic, thought to have been fixed by its founder in 1985, appears to have undergone a good deal of evolution during the subsequent decade. Some of the earliest documents of D.D. Palmer were examined and illustrated at least 3 stages of conceptual development in Palmer's professional career.

"Vital Magnetic" Healing (1886–1896).—Palmer had been led to the practice of magnetic healing in the 1880s. By 1897, he spoke of chiropractic as both an extension of his magnetic practice and as a quantum improvement over other forms of magnetic healing. The magnetic Palmer sought to identify diseased or dysfunctional organs by touch and to deliver a healing life force from his hands. Within a few years, however, the "magnetic manipulator" had become a "chiropractic manipulator."

First Stage Chiropractic/"Magnetic Manipulation" (1897–1902).—Like Old Dad Chiro, who compared the human body to a machine, Palmer likened the human body to a valuable watch that required all of its parts to be in their proper place for optimal functioning. Palmer also expressed devotion to the bone-setting tradition, healing by manipulative methods and stressing the relationship between the spine and disease. Another area of interest was osteopathy, but it is not known whether Palmer studied under osteopathic practitioners. The Palmer School of Magnetic Cure, founded in 1986, taught various trade secrets, including the theory of "hot spots" along the spine. His technique of nerve-tracing, an integral component of his overall theory of tone, inflammation, and disease, appears to have been based upon Old Dad Chiro's vibratory nerve theory.

The Second Theory of Chiropractic (1903–1933).—Palmer went on to distinguish his methods from those of osteopathy and to abandon whole body manipulation in favor of joint-only adjusting. Other practitioners and writers of the time, such as Solon Massey Langworthy (Palmer's former pupil) and A.T. Still, may have also played a role in narrowing the chiropractic rationale. "Adjusting" began to take the place of "manipulating" in Palmer's language.

Conclusion.—A review of Palmer's early writings raises questions about his views and practice and suggests that chiropratic theories have never been fixed. Chiropratic practitioners can choose their guiding principles from among the various areas explored by Palmer and other early writers.

▶ This article clearly supports the premise that chiropractic thought and philosophical development has been a developing process. Even the "founder," D.D. Palmer, evolved the chiropractic concept in his own mind. Such a position may threaten the foundation of dogmatisim that persists within the chiropractic profession. As scientific investigation and intellectual thinking continue to evolve (as demonstrated by Keating's article), chiropractic will continue in its professional development.—R.B. Phillips, D.C., Ph.D.

Integrate Osteopathic Principles and Practices in Postgraduate Medical Education—*Now*

Kasovac M, Jones JM III (College of Osteopathic Medicine of the Pacific, Pomona, Calif)

J Am Osteopath Assoc 93:118,123–125, 1993 5–16

Background.—Is the practicing doctor of osteopathy (DO) truly an osteopathic physician who teaches and uses hands-on osteopathic diagnostic and manipulative techniques, or merely a "generic physician"? Calling for a "renaissance" in the teaching of osteopathic principles and

Workshops Offered at the College of Osteopathic Medicine of the Pacific

- Osteopathic structural screening as part of the history and physical examination
- Osteopathic approaches to care of hospital patients
- Structural approaches to intensive care unit patients, with a cardiopulmonary emphasis
- Balancing the four diaphragms
- Treatment of the postabdominal surgery patient
- Cervical/lumbar techniques in the bedridden patient
- Headache: Considerations in diagnosis and manipulative treatment
- Techniques for treating labor and postpartum in the obstetric patient
- Techniques for the pediatric hospital patient
- Repetitive motion injury: Etiologic and therapeutic considerations

(Courtesy of Kasovac M, Jones JM III: *J Am Osteopath Assoc* 93:118, 123–125, 1993.)

manipulative techniques, a postdoctoral seminar series that integrates osteopathic principles and practice is described.

Discussion.—Osteopathic training has changed considerably in recent years, with students serving clerkships in osteopathic, allopathic, or mixed-staff hospitals. Osteopathic principles are easily integrated into the educational process, but questions remain as to how these techniques will be integrated into the clerkships and osteopathic medical internships and residency programs. The integration of osteopathic manipulation into all postgraduate medical education programs is recommended. The workshops offered at a college of osteopathic medicine cover specific clinical situations and the application of osteopathic manipulative techniques (table). Making graduates feel competent using these techniques allows them to serve as role models for current students. Interns and residents must be taught to do an osteopathic medical examination on every patient, just as they would a cardiac or neurologic evaluation. The osteopathic examination must be time efficient as well as appropriate. Active participation by directors of medical education, residency program directors, teaching faculty, and others is needed. Using guidelines for osteopathic care, clinical research protocols can be developed to confirm the efficacy and cost effectiveness of osteopathic manipulative therapy.

Conclusion.—Every DO must be involved in the "osteopathic medical renaissance." A fresh start to the second century of osteopathy, with a renewed commitment to osteopathic heritage and to delivering the health care services expected by the public, is needed.

► Osteopaths have seen the practice of manipulation fall by the wayside in their quest for general medical acceptance. The authors implore their colleagues to not lose these osteopathic principles embodied by their manipulative arts, echoing a common battle cry within the chiropractic profession. How far can the profession go before it is subsumed by medicine? Perhaps the major difference between the chiropractic profession and osteopathy is that chiropractors have never given up their manipulative procedures; virtually all chiropractors use manipulation as their main therapeutic intervention. In the case of osteopathy, the number of manipulation adherents is small (perhaps only 5%) and seems to be decreasing. Osteopathy may have gained general acceptance only by loss of identity. The case for chiropractic is more complex. The profession has, in a sense, remade itself by increasing its amount of quality research, but it has not been at the expense of manipulation. There are those, such as Dr. Barge, who view these increases as an indication of potential loss of identity, but the profession remains the strongest alternative to medical practice in history; it will not be so easily lost.—D.J. Lawrence, D.C.

The Reflex Effects of Spinal Somatic Nerve Stimulation on Visceral Function

Sato A (Tokyo Metropolitan Inst of Gerontology, Japan)

J Manipulative Physiol Ther 15:57–61, 1992 5–17

Introduction.—Somatovisceral reflex responses at various sites have been examined in anesthetized animals to eliminate emotional factors. Various forms of somatic sensory stimulation can produce different autonomic reflex responses.

Cardiovascular Responses.—Most anesthetized cats and rats have a reflex increase in heart rate after such stimuli as pinching or brushing anywhere on the body surface. Substances that excite small muscle afferents, such as KCl or bradykinin, can alter the heart rate when injected into a muscle artery of the hindlimb. Activation of knee joint afferents can alter the heart rate, blood pressure, and efferent cardiac sympathetic nerve activity. Stimulation of the spine may lower blood pressure and reduce muscle blood flow.

Gastrointestinal Responses.—Pinching of the abdominal skin usually inhibits gastric motility, while pinching the hindpaw may enhance gastric motility in the anesthetized rat. No such facilitatory response is seen in the cat.

Bladder Responses.—Mechanical stimulation of the perineal skin produces a transient rise in intravesical pressure. Noxious stimulation of the perineal, abdominal, or chest skin leads to reflex inhibition of micturition contractions. These contractions also are inhibited when thin afferent fibers in hindlimb muscle nerves are stimulated.

Adrenal Medullary Responses.—Noxious pinching of the lower chest or hindpaw leads to reflex increases in adrenal sympathetic efferent nerve activity and catecholamine secretion in the rat and cat. Movement of the knee joint beyond the normal range increases both adrenal nerve activity and catecholamine secretion. Mechanical stimulation of vertebral joints in the rat decreases and then increases adrenal nerve activity.

▶ This work supports many of the contentions of spondylotherapy or metric system adjusting. The use of somatoautonomic reflexes has a long and honored history within the chiropractic profession, as well as the osteopathic profession, going back at least as far as the 1920s. The work of Sato has been instrumental in placing the clinical practice of spondylotherapy on an electrophysiologic basis; he has helped to understand mechanisms. His work revolves around stimulating the afferent nerve with nociceptive and nonnociceptive stimuli and then measuring visceral organ responses. For example, using cat models, he found that any type of stimuli (usually mechanical, thermal, or chemical), either nociceptive or not, caused acceleration of cardiac responses; in the gastrointestinal tract, there were differing responses depending on what part of the body was stimulated (for example, pinching the abdomen inhibits gastric motility, whereas pinching the face stimulates it). This work has wide implications for chiropractic intervention in a host of organic conditions, and it lays the framework for understanding somatoautonomic reflexes in the clinical setting.—D.J. Lawrence, D.C.

Education

Case Study Research Designs: Their Place in Chiropractic

Waalen JK (Canadian Mem Chiropractic College, Toronto)

J Can Chiroprac Assoc 36:29–32, 1992 5–18

Background.—The research method of the case study arises from a desire to understand the complex processes and broad issues and may involve nonclinical aspects of practice. Information on the case study as a research strategy, including appropriate topics, elements that make up a good design, and ways to formulate ideas before undertaking case study research, was discussed.

The Case Study.—Doing a case study involves a distinct research approach. Case studies are often confused with case reports, case series, cases used in rounds, and cases without control groups or baseline measures. The case study approach provides a way to explore broad chiropractic issues, policies, or practices in real settings. This research design is appropriate in clinical and nonclinical settings. Careful planning is needed when doing a case study, including a literature review to define the scope of the research question, a specification of the unit of analysis, a method to link the question to its measurements, and a graphic portrayal of the criteria used to evaluate the results. Case studies require good conceptual skills, not elaborate equipment; extensive thinking time but not sophisticated statistical analysis; and a well-designed protocol but not control groups or randomization. Most of all, case study research in chiropractic requires curiosity about the profession: case studies can highlight the "culture" of chiropractic, rather than focusing on treatment modalities and their outcomes.

Conclusion.—Case study research is often misunderstood. Yet hundreds of compelling, informative case studies exist. Reading a few of them will provide insight into the flexibility of this type of research. With case study approaches, the researcher can investigate contemporary aspects of the chiropractic profession in the context in which they occur. By contrast, experimental research focuses on conditions and their treatment.

▶ A case study is useful to illustrate a chiropractic procedure or report on an interesting condition and its clinical outcome in a patient. This is particularly true for cases that are unique or have an unexpected association, an important variation, or unexpected event. Well-designed case reports can provide information from which observational and experimental research studies may be developed. Also, case studies provide essential information for chiropractic education. The use of small-group active-learning techniques, such as problem-based learning, require "real world" cases.—A.H. Adams, D.C.

Research

The Evolution and Importance of Spinal and Chiropractic Research

Haldeman S (Univ of California, Irvine)

J Manipulative Physiol Ther 15:31–35, 1992 5–19

The Past.—Spinal pain is as old as recorded medical history and, throughout the history of medicine, the spine and nervous system have occupied a central position in anatomical, physiologic, and pathologic research. Chiropractic has evolved quite rapidly during its history of less than 100 years. Chiropractic theory began primarily as a vitalistic viewpoint at a time when the medical scientific community was rejecting vitalism. The chiropractic profession then went through a period of speculative theorizing based on perceived neurologic or pathologic observations. A chiropractic emphasis on subluxation conflicted with a medical focus on disk herniation.

The Future.—More scientific approaches to problems of mutual chiropractic and medical concern are emerging. The coming years probably will see increased interest in social research into the clinical efficacy of treatments, the prevention of back pain, and patient satisfaction.

Large, expensive, controlled clinical trials will likely be carried out. Neurophysiologic studies will help define the role of neural reflexes, neuronal plasticity, and central control mechanisms in pain and other spinal disorders. Research also will concern itself with issues of genetics, aging, immune function, and vascular factors. In addition, the chiropractic profession is not exempt from concern over rising costs, and cost effectiveness should be studied.

▶ Research is vital for further development of the chiropractic profession. The profession's distinctive body of scientific knowledge will influence its role in the health-care system. This article lays out a research agenda for chiropractic.—A.H. Adams, D.C.

Homeopathic Treatment of Plantar Warts

Labrecque M, Audet D, Latulippe LG, Drouin J (Université Laval, Sainte-Foy, PQ)

Can Med Assoc J 146:1749–1753, 1992 5–20

Background.—Homeopathic treatments are popular, but there is a lack of published studies providing evidence of the efficacy of such drugs. The efficacy of a homeopathic treatment of plantar warts was investigated.

Outcome of Treatment at 6, 12, and 18 Weeks by Treatment Group

Outcome	Treatment group; no. (and %) of patients: Homeopathic	Placebo	Difference between groups (and 95% CI),%
Healed			
6 wk	4 (4.8)	4 (4.6)	0.2 (-6.2 to 6.5)
	(n = 84)	(n = 87)	
12 wk	11 (13.4)	11 (13.1)	0.3 (-10.0 to 10.6)
	(n = 82)	(n = 84)	
18 wk	16 (20.0)	20 (24.4)	-4.4 (-17.2 to 8.4)
	(n = 80)	(n = 82)	
Self-assessed	22 (27.5)	27 (32.9)	-5.4 (-19.5 to 8.7)
improvement at 18 wk	(n = 80)	(n = 82)	
Side effects	2 (2.4)	4 (4.6)	-2.2 (-7.7 to 3.3)
	(n = 84)	(n = 87)	

Abbreviation: CI, confidence interval.
(Courtesy of Labrecque M, Audet D, Latulippe LG, et al: *Can Med Assoc J* 146:1749–1753, 1992.)

Methods.—Patients were recruited by various methods for this randomized, double-blind, placebo-controlled trial. Of 853 patients screened, 174 met the eligibility criteria and agreed to participate. The patients were required to be between 6 and 59 years of age and have 1 or more plantar warts untreated in the preceding 3 months. One hundred sixty-two patients (93%) completed the study. Homeopathic treatment, administered for 6 weeks, consisted of thuya 30 "centésimal hahnemannien" (CH), antimonium crudum 7 CH, and nitricum acidum 7 CH. Placebo pellets and treatment pellets were identical in taste and appearance. The patients were followed up for 18 weeks.

Outcomes.—Healing was defined as the disappearance of all warts. At 6 weeks, 4.8% in the homeopathic group and 4.6% in the placebo group were healed. At 12 weeks, 13.4% and 13.1%, respectively, were healed. At 18 weeks, healing had occurred in 20% of those taking homeopathic treatment and in 24.4% of those taking placebo (table).

Conclusion.—In this series, homeopathic treatment was no more effective than placebo in the treatment of plantar warts. The rate of healing with the homeopathic treatment was much lower than previously reported rates.

▶ There are very few published studies examining the efficacy of homeopathic remedies for the treatment of specific conditions. As an "alternative health-care" field, it has not had access to the funding agencies that medicine has; in this respect, it is similar to the chiropractic profession. However, there are far more numerous reports of chiropractic research than homeopathic ones. The decision was made to study homeopathic treatment of plantar warts, because protocols for such treatment did exist. The results of this study showed that the homeopathic therapy was no more effective than placebo. Although this is not a blanket condemnation of homeopathy, it does demonstrate that homeopathy, like the chiropractic profession, is studying its therapeutic interventions. Will homeopathic practitioners now discard the useless procedure? Or, like some chiropractors, will they continue to use an outmoded and ineffective therapy despite the lack of science to support it?—D.J. Lawrence, D.C.

Role for the Cervical Sympathetic Trunk in Regulating Anaphylactic and Endotoxic Shock

Waddell SC, Davison JS, Befus AD, Mathison RD (Univ of Calgary, Alta)

J Manipulative Physiol Ther 15:10–15, 1992 5–21

Background.—There is increasing interest in the possibility of an intimate relationship between neurologic and immunologic functions. Manipulative therapy has been linked with autonomic regulation of blood flow and, because hyperemia is a normal part of the response in inflated tissues, biomechanical manipulations could contribute to the management of inflammatory disorders.

Objective and Methods.—Modulation of systemic inflammatory responses by sympathetic nerves in the thoracic spinal cord was studied in rats sensitized to the nematode *Nippostrongylus brasiliensis.* Pulmonary inflammation resulted from anaphylaxis in these animals. Anaphylaxis was induced a week after bilateral decentralization (through removing a segment of the nerve joining the middle and superior cervical ganglia) or bilateral ganglionectomy. Other animals received endotoxin intravenously.

Observations.—Both decentralization and ablation of the superior cervical ganglia reduced pulmonary inflammation after induction of anaphylaxis. Hypotensive responses to intravenous endotoxin were lessened in sensitized rats, and the surgical procedures prevented endotoxic shock in unsensitized animals.

Conclusion.—The spinal cord may have an important role in regulating immune function, particularly the processes of anaphylaxis and endotoxemia. Neurologic and immune functions also are interrelated at the level of the sympathetic ganglia.

▶ Neuroimmunology is one of the more exciting areas of research for chiropractic, because it has implications regarding our effect on general immune competence and quality of life. This study indicates that the sympathetic nervous system may play an important role in body responses to anaphylaxis and endotoxemia. The role of the nervous system in immune system function remains very poorly understood long after Hans Selye's seminal work.—D.J. Lawrence, D.C.

Appendix: Chiropractic-Related Health Science Information

NEHMAT G. SAAB, M.A., M.L.S.
Director, Library Services, Los Angeles College of Chiropractic, Los Angeles, California

SHOREH SALJOOGHI, M.L.S.
Assistant Librarian, Los Angeles College of Chiropractic, Los Angeles, California

The purpose of this article is to present a description of sources for chiropractic-related health science information research and to guide the interested searcher in obbtaining the needed references. Similar to information from any health-care field, this information can be retrieved from textbooks, monographs, periodicals, indexes, and computerized on-line databases.

Books and Periodicals

To obtain a global coverage of monographs and textbooks, consulting the publication "Selected List of Books and Journals" by Adams et al. is recommended. The subjects suggested in the list are sciences considered basic to chiropractic, such as anatomy, biochemistry, biomechanics, kinesiology, neuroscience, pathology, physiology, chiropractic principles, diagnosis, laboratory and physical, radiology, exercise physiology and athletics, geriatrics, the spine, osteopathy, physiologic therapeutics, psychology, public health, rehabilitation, rheumatology, and chiropractic technique.

The subjects are listed to acquaint the reader with the topics with which the chiropractic profession and related health sciences are concerned. A list of scientific and peer-reviewed periodicals appears at the end section of the list. The subjects covered are primarily chiropractic, research, manipulation, technique, nutrition, education, orthopedics, and sports medicine. Also relevant are the periodicals and books from the current "Brandon Hill Selected List of Books and Journals for the Small Medical Library".

Indexes and Databases

An index is a publication that presents the information necessary to locate an original item or reference according to its author or subject area. Indexing is usually done by scanning information (e.g., periodical articles) and then referring to the gathered information by its author and/or subject. This process usually makes it easy for the searcher to find the needed information on a particular subject by examining the relevant indexes. Indexes usually are assigned subjects or assigned keywords, known as a thesaurus, under which articles are classified and cumulated regularly and periodically. Very often, the information from the indexes is not current. There is at least a 6-month lag between the indexing date and the date the index is actually published, unless the index is updated on a monthly regular basis, such as the *Index Medicus*. Another reason to use the automated database is the possibility of combining 2 or more subjects and finding information by using bolean logic, whereas in indexes, only the subjects listed one by one can be looked up as references. For current information, the use of a database is recommended and, if not available, the use of current awareness tool.

Information obtained from indexes or databases is referred to as bibliographic reference information, and each reference designates the author of the article, the title, the source, the date, and the pages of the references in the publication in which they were published.

Indexes of Use to Chiropractic Literature

Chiropractic Research Abstract Collection (CRAC)

The first volume was published by the Canadian Memorial Chiropractic College in 1984 and, at that time, the word Archives was used in the title rather than Abstract. The second and third volumes followed in 1985 and 1986, respectively, and in 1990 Williams & Wilkins published the fourth volume. The subjects covered in the index are chiropractic, osteopathic, and other related health-care subjects. The information indexed is obtained from chiropractic monographs, journals, and other health-related publications.

The index covers the following parts:

1). A thesaurus of subject headings for the index that are chiropractic, and the National Library of Medicine (NLM) medical subject headings are referred to as MeSH

2). A list of journals indexed in addition to those indexed by the NLM's *Index Medicus*

3). A list of monographs and other publications indexed

4). The abstracts are arranged in numerical order and are referred to from the author and subject indexes

5). An author index with names in alphabetical order and the abstract number next to each reference

6). A subject index in alphabetical order with the abstract number next to each reference

Index to Chiropractic Literature (ICL)

This annual index was first published in 1980 as a joint effort of the member librarians in the Chiropractic Library Consortium (CLIBCON). Up to this date, volumes have been published, with a cumulative volume covering the years 1985–1989. This last volume is also available on floppy disk, and it is a useful tool for quickly referencing information on chiropractic and other related subjects.

The index covers the following parts:

1). A list of terms used, which are mainly from a chiropractic thesaurus developed and updated by CLIBCON

2). A subject index

3). An alphabetical author index

The references cited in each volume are indexed from periodicals published during the current publication date.

Cumulative Index to Nursing and Allied Health Literature (CINAHL, or the RED BOOKS)

The first volume of the *Cumulative Index to Nursing and Literature* appeared in 1956, and it was limited to indexing 12 nursing journals only. In 1977, the editors widened the scope of the index and changed its name to the *Cumulative Index to Nursing and Allied Health Literature* (referred to as CINAHL). This is a bimonthly publication for 10 months of the year, and it indexes 300 English language journals and scans more than 2,600 biomedical journals from *Index Medicus* for related material. The subjects the index covers are nursing, occupational therapy, physical therapy, and rehabilitation, as well as other health-related subjects.

The index covers the following parts:

1). A subject section, which is mainly the thesaurus coined by CINAHL

2). An author section arranged alphabetically

3). A list of the journals and serials indexed

The *Cumulative Index to Nursing and Allied Health Literature* became available on-line in 1983, and article abstracts became available as of 1986. The database is accessible through NLM, DIALOG, AND BRS. The compact disc version is available from different vendors and comes with regular up-dates.

Index Medicus

Index Medicus, published by the National Library of Medicine in Bethesda, Maryland, is considered the mother index of all indexes. The first volume was published in 1879. Since then, the index has undergone several changes, and in 1960 it became a regular monthly index with an *Annual Cumulative Index Medicus.* The index covers biomedical information such as medicine, nursing, occupational therapy, physical therapy, biology, nutrition, etc.

The monthly index is made up of the following three parts

1). A bibliography of medical reviews that contains the review articles for that month

2). A subject section

3). An alphabetical author section

The National Library of Medicine indexes almost 3,000 journals using the MeSH. The thesaurus is updated on an annual basis and is published seperately. There is a smaller, concise form of *Index Medicus* that is a monthly publication and was first published by the NLM in 1970. There are 118 core journals in different biomedical fields indexed in this version, which is known as the *Abridged Index Medicus. Index Medicus* is available on-line from 1966 to the present, and it is known as MED-

LINE. It is also available through DIALOG, BRS, and compact disc from different vendors.

Excerpta Medica

This index was first published in 1946 by Excerpta Medica of Elsevier Science Publishing, Amsterdam, The Netherlands. There are 52 sections to the index. Of interest to the chiropractic profession is the section on rehabilitation and physical medicine, which publishes 8 issues each year.

Each issue has the following parts:

1). A table of contents defining the subjects under which the articles are indexed

2). An abstract section in which the citations are listed by abstract number

3). A subject index with abstract numbers next to each reference

4). An author index with an abstract number next to each reference

Nutrition Abstracts and Reviews

This publication was first created in 1931, when the need for a nutrition review was needed. It was published by the joint efforts of the Imperial Agricultural Bureaux Council, The Medical Research Council, and the Reid Library. It is now prepared on a monthly basis by the C-A-B International Bureau of Nutrition, and it indexes literature by scanning articles from journals on nutrition published worldwide and articles from nonjournals, such as books, reports, and conferences. This index covers 2 series. Series A is Human Experimental, and series B is Livestock, Feeds, and Feeding.

The index covers the following sections:

1). A table of contents

2). Abstracts numbered consecutively

3). An author index that includes the abstract number with each reference

4). A subject index with an abstract number for each reference

Nutrition Abstracts and Reviews is accessible on-line through DIALOG from 1972 to the present, and through BRS from 1973 to the present.

Chiropractic Literature Analysis and Retrieval System (CHIROLARS)

This chiropractic database was very recently developed and compiled by Ronald Rupert, Action Potential. Rupert, who is a chiropractor and was interested in indexing the information for his personal use, found that what he amassed was so vast that he decided to automate the compiled information and make it accessible to those who would be interested. The database underwent several improvements and was finally made available on-line as of March 1991. The coverage includes chiropractic and related health sciences, and it contains references from more than 700 chiropractic and biomedical publications; as of March 1993, there were citations from more than 16,000 published articles. This makes CHIROLARS the largest and only computerized index of chiropractic literature. The subjects included are chiropractic, etiology, diagnosis, exam, prevention and treatment of neuromuscular disorders, anatomy, physiology, and biomechanics. This continuously expanding database is kept current by regular monthly updates. The citations are complete with number, author, title, subject, source, and abstract. Users may retrieve information by using the controlled thesaurus for subject or subjects or by using the author's name.

To subscribe to the database or to request articles, contact Ronald Rupert, P.O. Box 50837, Denton, TX 76206; Telephone: (817) 898-0234

How to Locate Information

Information has become part of our lives, and there is no professional health-care provider not involved with its management. Computer literacy is essential and a powerful means of information management. Our purpose is to provide helpful suggestions for locating a needed document, whether it is a monograph, a periodical article, or an audiovisual. Thousands of books and articles on biomedicine are published every month, and it is becoming harder and harder for health professionals to locate needed literature relevant to their field of interest. To make searching for the literature easier and user friendly, the National Library of Medicine modified the MEDLARS system in 1986 and developed a software for searching known as GRATEFUL MED. GRATEFUL MED is available for the IBM personal computer or any compatible personal computers (version 6.0 was released in April 1991). Retrieving information from the indexes and databases mentioned above is also possible. The professional health-care provider can either perform and tailor his/her own searches from any of the databases, or he/she can request the help of a librarian. The citations obtained from most indexes or from an on-line database usually provide an abstract and the source of the information. Full texts could be obtained by contacting a library of your choice, which would then be considered your provider library. Contacting one library only would be sufficient to put you in touch with a network of biomedical libraries, the number of which may exceed 3,000. The problem of locating documents has been solved thanks to the National Library of Medicine's development of a system for requesting information and directing it to the appropriate source.

How Does the Network System Work?

The National Library of Medicine has assigned Regional Medical Libraries to organize a networking system between the biomedical libraries. The purpose of this system is to provide high-quality information services to the nations' health professionals. There are 7 regional medical libraries in the United States:

1). Greater Northeastern Regional Medical Library Program
The New York Academy of Medicine

2 East 103rd St
New York, New York 10029
Phone: (212) 876-8763
On-line Center for Regions 1 and 2 states served: Connecticut, Delaware, Maine, Massachusetts, New Hampshire, New Jersey, New York, Pennsylvania, Rhode Island, Vermont, and Puerto Rico
FAX: (212) 722-7650

2). Southeastern/Atlantic Regional Medical Library Service
University of Maryland
Health Sciences Library
111 South Greene Street
Baltimore, Maryland 21201
Phone: (301) 328-2855
(800) 638-6093
FAX: (301) 328-8403
States served: Alabama, Florida, Georgia, Maryland, Mississippi, North Carolina, South Carolina, Tennessee, Virginia, West Virginia, The District of Columbia, and the Virgin Islands

3). Greater Midwest Regional Medical Library Network
University of Illinois at Chicago
Library of the Health Sciences
P.O. Box 7509
Chicago, Illinois 60680
Phone: (312) 996-2464
FAX: (312) 942-1951
(312) 733-6440
TELEX: 206243
States served: Iowa, Illinois, Indiana, Kentucky, Michigan, Minnesota, North Dakota, Ohio, South Dakota, and Wisconsin

4). Midcontinental Regional Medical Library Program
University of Nebraska
Medical Center Library
42nd and Dewey Avenue
Omaha, Nebraska 68105-1065
Phone: (402) 559-4326
(800) MED-RML4
FAX: (402) 559-5498
States served: Colorado, Kansas, Missouri, Nebraska, Utah, and Wyoming
On-line Center for Regions 3, 4, and 5

5). South Central Reginal Medical Library Program
The University of Texas
Southwestern Medical Center at Dallas
5323 Harry Hines Boulevard
Dallas, Texas 75235-9049
Phone: (214) 688-2085

FAX: (214) 688-3277
States served: Arkansas, Louisiana, New Mexico, Oklahoma, and Texas

6). Pacific Northwest Regional Health Sciences Library Service
Health Sciences Library and Information Center
University of Washington
Seattle, Washington 98195
Phone: (206) 543-8262
FAX: (206) 543-8066
States served: Alaska, Idaho, Montana, Oregon, and Washington

7). Pacific Southeast Regional Medical Library Service
Louise Darling Biomedical Library
University of California
10833 Le Conte Avenue
Los Angeles, California 90024-1798
Phone: (213) 825-1200
FAX: (213) 206-8675
ONTYME: PSRMLS
States served: Arizona, California, Hawaii, Nevada, and United States Territories in the Pacific Basin
On-line Center for Regions 6 and 7

The Regional Medical Libraries were assigned to organize the networks in each of their own regions. Enrollment for membership in the RML was open to any information center or organization with a collection of health sciences materials (e.g., books, journals, or audiovisuals), from which information services are provided to health professionals. There are (at least) between 400 to 500 member libraries in each region, and the total is almost 3,000 libraries. Libraries in each region are linked together so they provide documents to one another when requested. Each member enrolled in the network is certified by the Director of the National Library of Medicine as a "Valued Member of National Network of Libraries of Medicine Dedicated to Providing High Quality Information Services to Health Professionals and Entitled to the Full Benefits of Network Membership."

The goals of the Regional Medical Libraries' network, as expressed by the National Library of Medicine, are to improve access and delivery of information to health professionals and to enhance sharing of resources between the network libraries' health professionals. One aspect of sharing information is the interlibrary loan services provided by an automated system known as DOCLINE. The system was designed to promote efficiency in document routing and delivery through a National Network of Libraries that include biomedicine and chiropractic libraries. It is a very simple and easy system to use, and it reduces the time required by the library staff to process interlibrary loans. Health professionals using the GRATEFUL MED version 5.0 are offered the option of using a document-ordering feature LOANSOME DOC, which can be linked to it. LOANSOME DOC provides a valuable link between the

GRATEFUL MED user and the library designated by the user as his or her provider of services. By means of the routing system, the request will still be fulfilled, even if the requested document is not available at the designated providing library. The routing takes place through a ladder of libraries. (See the diagram, which uses the LACC library as the designated provider.)

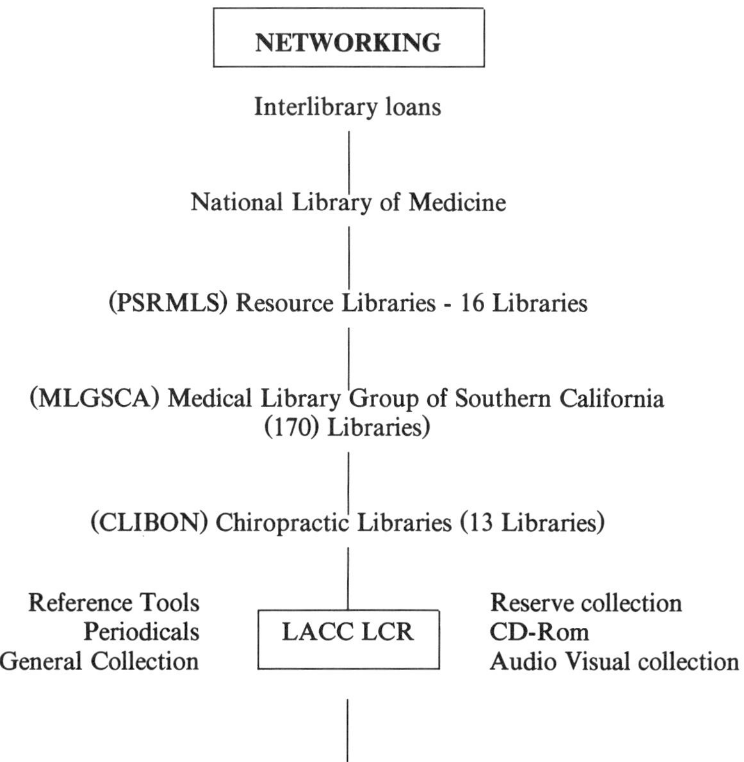

It is important to remember that the user's library serves as both the document delivery center and the contact point for information about obtaining documents.

Other services provided by the Network include answering or referring reference questions and performing computerized or manual bibliographic searches. We are witnesses to an age in which libraries have no boundaries, and the sharing and exchanging of resources is enhanced by automated linkage.

Within each region of the Regional Medical Libraries, information centers bonded together and formed Medical Library Groups (MLGs), such as the Medical Library Group of Southern California (MLGSCA). The MLGs also maintain the same goals, quality, and reciprocity of providing information services to health professionals. Specialized libraries, members in the Regional Medical Libraries network, also bonded together to form section membership of the National Library Medicine. Accordingly, CLIBCON was an acknowledged section of the National Library of Medicine in 1988.

Participating CLIBCON libraries include the following:

Canadian Memorial Chiropractic College (CMCC)
C.C. Clemmer Health Sciences Library
1900 Bayview Avenue
Toronto, Ontario
Canada M4G 3E6
Phone: (416) 482-2340, ext. 156
FAX: (416) 482-9745

Cleveland Chiropractic College (CCC)
Ruth M. Cleveland Library
6401 Rockhill Road
Kansas City, Missouri 64131
Phone: (816) 333-8230
FAX: (816) 361-0272

Cleveland Chiropractic College—Los Angeles (CLA)
Library
590 North Vermont
Los Angeles, California 90004-2196
Phone: (213) 660-6166, ext. 53
FAX: (213) 665-1931

Life Chiropractic College (LCC)
Nell K. Williams Learning Resource Center
1269 Barclay Circle
Marietta, Georgia 30062
Phone: (404) 424-0554, ext. 221/222
FAX: (404) 429-8359

Life Chiropractic College—West (LCCW)
Library
2005 Via Barrett
San Lorenzo, California 94580
Phone: (415) 276-9345
FAX: (415) 276-4893

Logan College of Chiropractic (LOCC)
Learning Resource Center
1851 Schoettler Road
P.O. Box 1065
Chesterfield, Missouri 63006-1065
Phone: (314) 227-2100, ext. 187
FAX: (314) 227-8503

Los Angeles College of Chiropractic (LACC)
Seabury-McCoy Library
16200 East Amber Valley Drive
P.O. Box 1166

Whittier, California 90609-1166
Phone: (310) 947-8755, ext. 566
FAX: (310) 947-5724

National College of Chiropractic (NCC)
Sordoni-Burich Library
200 East Roosevelt Road
Lombard, Illinois 60148
Phone: (708) 629-2000, ext. 101
FAX: (708) 629-9022

New York College of Chiropractic (NYCC)
Library
2360 State Route 89
P.O. Box 800
Seneca Falls, New York 13148-0800
Phone: (315) 568-3244
FAX: (315) 568-3015

Northwestern College of Chiropractic (NWCC)
Library
2501 West 84th Street
Bloomington, Minnesota 55431-1599
Phone: (612) 885-5417
FAX: (612) 885-5463

Palmer College of Chiropractic (PCC)
David D. Palmer Health Sciences Library
1000 Brady Street
Davenport, Iowa 52803
Phone: (319) 326-9894
FAX: (319) 326-9897

Palmer College of Chiropractic—West (PCCW)
Library
1095 Dunford Way
Sunnyvale, California 94087
Phone: (408) 983-4000
FAX: (408) 244-8975

Parker College of Chiropractic (PKCC)
Library
2500 Walnut Hill Lane
Dallas, Texas 75229
Phone: (214) 438-6932
FAX: (214) 357-3107

Texas Chiropractic College (TCC)
Mae Hilty Memorial Library
5912 Spencer Highway
Pasadena, Texas 77505
Phone: (713) 487-1170, ext. 246
FAX: (713) 487-4168

Western States Chiropractic College
W.A. Budden Library
2900 North East 132 Avenue
Portland, Oregon 97230
Phone: (503) 256-3180

Conclusion

Your local chiropractic library or any other Medical Library Group is the first point of contact for obtaining documents such as monographs, softwares, periodicals, articles, videotapes, etc. If you decide to do your own literature searches by connecting to the National Library of Medicine through GRATEFUL MED, you will be offered the option of requesting documents from a designated library through the services of LOANSOME DOC. The latter will establish an electronic link between the user and the providing library. GRATEFUL MED: Telephone, (800) 638-8480.

Bibliography

1. *Database Catalog 1992.* Palo Alto, Calif, DIALOG, 1993.
2. *Fact Sheet.* Bethesda, Md, National Library of Medicine, August 1992.
3. *Fact Sheet.* Bethesda, Md, National Library of Medicine, August 1991.
4. *Fact Sheet.* Bethesda, Md, National Library of Medicine, May 1989.
5. *Fact Sheet.* Bethesda, Md, National Library of Medicine, April 1989.
6. *Fact Sheet.* Bethesda, Md, National Library of Medicine, January 1989.
7. Feinglos SJ: *MEDLINE: A Basic Guide to Searching.* Chicago, Medical Library Association, Inc, 1985.
8. Gitelman R, Callaghan JC: CRAC: *Chiropractic Research Archives Collection.* Toronto, Canada, Canadian Memorial Chiropractic College, 1986.
9. *Index Medicus,* vol 33 (introduction), December 1992. Irvine K: *Index to Chiropractic Literature* (introduction). CLIBCON, 1991.
10. Mrozek JP, Schafer ME: CRAC: *Chiropractic Research Abstracts Collection* (introduction). Baltimore, Md, Williams & Wilkins, 1990.
11. Rupert RL: CHIROLARS: A computerized chiropractic literature database. *California Chiropractic Journal* 16:36–37, 1991.
12. *Status Report: CHIROLARS.* March 6, 1992.
13. Williams M, Baker LM, Marshall JG: *Information Search in Health Care.* Thorofare, NJ, Slack, Inc, 1992.
14. Woodbury M, Adler S: The literature of chiropractic: Journals, indexes and databases. *California Chiropractic Journal* 16:44–45, 1991.

Subject Index

A

B

C

D

E

F

G

J

K

L

M

N

Q

R

S

T

U

V

W

Author Index

A

B

C

D

E

F

Y

Z